Letters Home from Nigeria

1952 - 1962

Dr. D. S. H. Cannon

FRCGP, MRCS, DObst.

H/

First edition published by Hayloft 2012

Hayloft Publishing Ltd, South Stainmore,
Kirkby Stephen, Cumbria, CA17 4DJ

tel: 017683 41568 or 07971 352473
email: books@hayloft.eu
web: www.hayloft.eu

ISBN 1 904524 86 9

A CIP catalogue record for this book is available from the British Library.

Designed, printed and bound in the UK

Copies of this book can be purchased direct from the author at a price of £15
each including post and packing.

Dr. D. S. H. Cannon
Coldbeck Cottage
Ravenstonedale
Kirkby Stephen
Cumbria, CA17 4LW, UK

This book is dedicated to my colleagues at Ilesha.
We worked together, prayed together and played together,
creating bonds that cannot be broken.

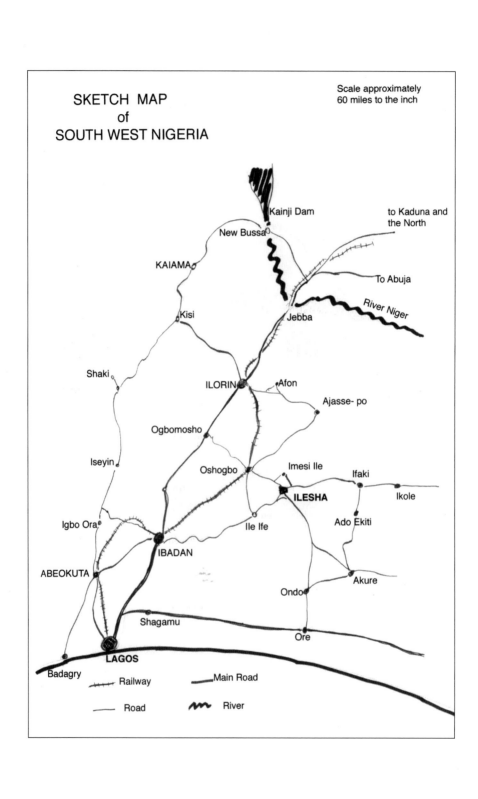

SKETCH MAP
of
SOUTH WEST NIGERIA

Scale approximately
60 miles to the inch

Kainji Dam

New Bussa

to Kaduna and
the North

KAIAMA

To Abuja

Kisi

Jebba

River Niger

Shaki

ILORIN

Afon

Ajasse- po

Ogbomosho

Iseyin

Oshogbo

Imesi Ile

Ifaki

Ikole

ILESHA

Igbo Ora

Ile Ife

Ado Ekiti

IBADAN

ABEOKUTA

Akure

Ondo

Shagamu

Ore

Badagry

LAGOS

Railway   Main Road

Road   River

CONTENTS

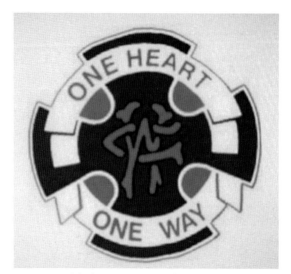

Methodist Wesley Guild logo.

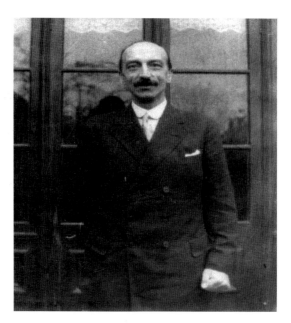

Dr. John R. C. Stephens

INTRODUCTION

David Cannon offered to serve as a Medical Missionary with the Methodist Church. The family had many connections with Methodism. His father was a Methodist Minister and his father's twin brother was a Methodist Missionary serving in the West Indes.

David qualified in 1950, aged 23, and after working at the London Hospital and the Bromley hospital, was appointed to the Wesley Guild Hospital in Nigeria, the work being supported by the Wesley Guild organisation of the Methodist Church.

Dr. J. R. C. Stephens was one of the first medically qualified doctors with the Missionary Society and he was posted to Nigeria in 1912. Initially he had a clinic in Igbo Ora but in 1913 moved to Ilesha and is reputed to have operated under a tree adjacent to the Methodist Church!

The First World War interrupted the work, which was restarted by Dr. E. U. MacWilliam in 1920, with the building of the first portion of the hospital.

Over the years the building has been added to as the need arose. When Dr. Andrew Pearson, who had been in China as a Medical Missionary for five years, and David, arrived in 1952, they realised the magnitude of the task they had been given. They were responsible for continuing the work of the hospital but also supervising the building of the new, larger hospital on the other side of the town.

These letters reveal the joys, sorrows and anxieties that were experienced.

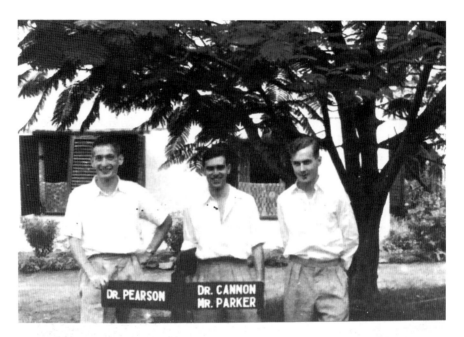

Andrew, David and Ken

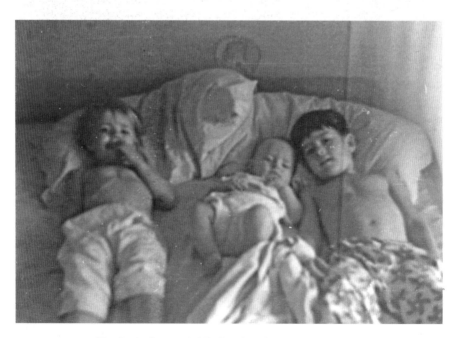

Elizabeth, Peter and Richard under a mosquito net

8

FIRST TOUR, May 1952 - February 1954

Elder Dempster Lines   On Board M.V. 'Apapa'
May 8th 1952

Dear Mother and Father
On board safely, no customs difficulties and had a good lunch whilst I am able. The food certainly promises to be good and my cabin companion congenial. Have not yet met Miss Compton,

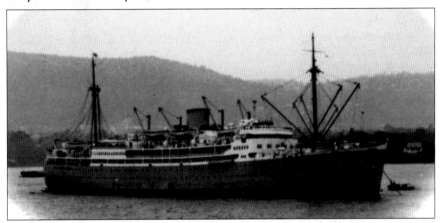

M.V. Apapa

My luggage from Allisons is not yet on board although my case is. (I have now asked purser and Allisons stuff comes on last). Will write and send it off from Las Palmas. Telegrams awaiting here from St. Andrews, the Hoopers and Ernest and Vivian - very nice.   Still very wet outside but pleasant here.
Much love   David

Sunday Morning, 11.5.52

The next available post goes by boat from the Canary Islands, at which we call next Tuesday - so I think that I ought to start writing the odd letter - how far I shall get I don't know because I have been frightfully ill, and in fact this is the first time I have felt anything like and even now it is as though I had had my T.A.B. injections both together in my abdomen. All went well until 4.00 am on Friday morning when we were somewhere off Wales when I began to be sick and it continued for 24 hours. I remained in pyjamas, unshaven wreck on my bunk the whole day.

Yesterday I dressed and shaved but had to keep lying down otherwise I felt awful. In the midst of my misery the Purser came in to ask me to take the service today - as there is no protestant male missionary on board except me! I protested, stating that I was a doctor, not a clergyman. The Purser, with a note or triumph, replied, 'I have looked on the next of kin and your Father is a vicar'! I said I would see how I feel tomorrow. Anyway this morning I felt better and I had breakfast in the dining room. I have just finished the service! About 60 present, Union Jack on the lectern, three hymns, prayers, readings, and an address. I have not spoken to anyone yet but they listened quite well.

My cabin mate is a nice enough chap - works in Barclays Bank, Lagos, and we knock along quite well together.

My camera etc. are in good condition - but as yet I have not been able to read the instructions with feeling ill - however that day will soon come. At the moment I am feeling quite fit despite what I call a pretty heavy swell but other people think it pretty flat.

Yesterday we travelled through the Bay - stormy most of the time with much pitching and tossing as well as rolling from side to side. The dining room steward said with some pride that there were only eleven people missing from breakfast today - the first day - Friday - only a handful turned up so I certainly was not the only one. The sun here is much warmer and the sea looks blue - and when I get my real sea legs and tummy I shall be on top.

Needless to say I was very pleased to take the service this morning and shall be interested to see if I am asked to do it next Sunday - if so I do not know what to talk about! Anyway there is a week to think about it.

The typewriter works well - I am writing this upstairs in one of the lounges, as the cabin is a bit close. The bunks are separate - we share a wardrobe - have a chest of drawers each, and a shower in a little offshoot,

Each one of us has been given a printed passenger list and list of entertainments, which I will bring home with me or send if the opportunity offers.

At mealtimes I share a table with Miss Humble and Miss Compton - the former played the piano for the service this morning - two very sort of missionary people.

On board I found a note from Michael, Auntie Sarah and Mary and two from the Mission House which was very nice, and telegrams from St Andrews, Ernest, and Mr Hird and one slips my mind, but I believe I mentioned them in my previous letter.

There are a number of children on board, and there is a special play pen and Nanny at the stern end where they can be left in safety.

The stewards are most helpful as are the officers which I have met so far. Well I will leave this now and go below I think and finish it sometime tomorrow if all is well.

Monday Afternoon and a pleasant day so far without unusual incident - warm but not too hot.

Still slightly queasy at times but otherwise well. I have located the leather trunk and pillows in baggage room - I expect the rest is in the hold.

Post is just about to go so I must close. Will write again soon.

Much love   David

Tuesday, May 13th, 3.15 pm

The Canary Islands are disappearing from view over the horizon, and I am sitting at ease on deck in a chair, having had an exhausting morning and the experience of being among people who did not understand what I said. It will be some time before I can post this letter and even then it will go by sea but there are no airmail letters available until we reach Africa.

Little of note has occurred, except a film show on deck last night, since I last wrote, but this morning we awoke to our morning cup of tea brought by the steward who said 'ten to seven sir' and the Canary Isles in two hours and sure enough we dropped anchor at 9.00 am or thereabouts. Most passengers went ashore and the four of us from our table went together.

On the quay I was offered a magnificent gold watch - worth £20-30 for £2 eventually, having started at £5 but I did not succumb to temptation. On the way back however we shall see!

Having reached the end of the quay - having been pestered to buy watches and pearls, Parker 51 pens (for five shillings), clothes etc. we caught a bus into town. The bus was full, and we sat on hard benches - quite an experience and 20 minute ride for 6d. seemed to be quite a goodly sum, because the conductor handed us out when we had reached our destination - the Cathedral. This is a plain affair for a Cathedral but quite pleasant. There was a festival in progress for St. Theresa, and all the people (Spanish) were dressed in their best and all women and children wore mantillas. Mass was being celebrated in the square with flags music etc. and all the officials in gorgeous robes. I got four photos of these people - and I hope they turn out OK.

The cathedral was full of schoolgirls so we could not see a lot of it but there are some very fine paintings in alcoves round it. Afterwards we strolled round the shops and prices much the same as in England.

The houses are stone built, light in colour and in Spanish fashion. The flowers are bright and the trees palms with the blue sky and blue sea - a very pretty picture.

Cars abound, British, American, Italian, French - all kinds, and the driving is on the right hand side of the road. To return to the boat we hired a taxi as the buses were full, having beaten the taxi man down from £1 to 10/- for the four of us we were in and away! Soon back on board again.

On my return I found an airmail from Michael written on May 6th - it was grand to see his writing and to hear that he has got an audition for the BBC - great stuff.

On board there was a man selling stamps on air letters, we could not find a post office in the town so I bought an envelope with 2/- worth of stamps on it and sent it to Michael so it may well arrive the first of my missives.

We have three full days at sea before we reach Freetown which is our next port of call. I am not sure if we shall be able to go ashore or not as our sister ship the Oriel is there at the same time and has precedence I believe. I will leave this now, and finish it in a day or two when we are nearer to African shores.

Friday 16th: Two days have gone since I started this letter, days of ease and sunshine, with little in the way of events to relieve the routine.

Wednesday evening was Carnival night when the majority of the passengers were in evening dress (the ladies are each night) and we were presented with balloons and paper hats. We were given a marvellous meal - seven courses of which turkey and plum pudding were two and followed by dancing on the afterdeck.

Yesterday the children had their sports - there must be about a dozen between two and five years and in the afternoon diving for pennies and the greasy pole. I have never seen the latter before and it was most amusing. I took one or two photos of it, which I hope will show it in action. This afternoon the finals of the deck quoits and deck tennis are being played so I must get a snap of them in action.

Last night we could see sixteen lighthouses off Cape Verde - my first glimpse of Africa! though I have not seen any land yet. Tomorrow we reach Freetown and we are intending to go ashore, but the Oriel of the same line as the Apapa is getting in first and may commandeer all the launches. There is insufficient depth of water at Freetown to go into dock so we anchor just outside. Anyway a post office official comes on board for us to buy stamps and to post our letters.

The food is excellent and has included duck, pheasant, and fresh salmon, though I think I enjoy breakfast as much as anything! We spend 50 minutes on breakfast an hour on lunch and one and a half hours over dinner! Fantastic really but there is not much else to do.

I am remarkably fit, eating and sleeping well and looking forward to the next week. I trust that all is well at home, the flowers and vegetables doing their bit. Looking forward to hearing from you,

Much love, David

Off the coast of Liberia
Sunday evening 18-5-52

It was good to receive your letter when we dropped anchor in Freetown yesterday. It had arrived on the fourteenth, which was very good. Little happened after I last wrote until I woke up yesterday morning, when the change in temperature was most noticeable - very hot and sticky. After shower and going up on deck Freetown lay on port beam, and very lovely it looked too with the hills covered with trees, rising steeply from the deep blue sea. The town lies in a sort of basin of hills on the shore and looked most attractive at a distance. We dropped anchor a little way from the shore because as yet there is no deep water quay. I bought some stamps on board and posted a letter that I hope you have got by this time.

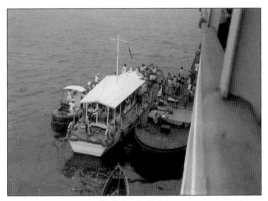

Going ashore

The three others on my table and myself went ashore in a launch and found the land very hot indeed. Miss Compton had stayed at Freetown at one time during the war, and so knew the way to the Mission House. Here we were made very welcome by the two missionaries stationed there, Miss Burness and Miss Mawson. They invited us to stay for lunch and I had some of the nicest fruit salad you can imagine, containing fresh pineapple, mango, guava, banana and so on. Water is however very scarce and in some parts of the town the fire wagon comes round doling out buckets full. There has been no water in the taps for six weeks now and they are all looking forward to the rain that is due to start in a few days time.

After lunch Miss Burness drove Miss Humble and myself up to Fourah Bay College, which has a marvellous position on one of the hills overlooking Freetown. The road up is the steepest road I have ever seen, with a precipice on one side and no fence. The car is a Standard 8. It got frightfully warm and smoke poured out of the engine and through the floor by my feet. We walked the last few hundred yards until we reached the house of the Rev. Ernest Sawyer who is one of the lecturers there. He is from Sierra Leone, and was at Durham University. Both he and his wife are very charming people. After seeing them we drove down to a Mrs. Stobart where we had tea. Miss Burness went to fetch the other two of our party down from the Wilberforce monument and got them safely down to the Mission House. Unfortunately the clutch on the car broke as she was coming back to collect us, and rushed back on foot to let us know. As it happened however, a friend of Mrs. Stobart's dropped in to use the phone and so was able to take us down to the quay just in time to catch the last launch back to the boat - a very near squeak! It was much cooler once we got back to the ship, which was a relief and we weighed anchor at six and stole quietly away. I shall never forget my first visit to Freetown. What impressed me most was the hospitality of those two ladies upon whom we dropped.

Yesterday was Sunday (I have written this in two sittings) and I woke feeling none too well, as there was a good storm blowing and I think that I must have eaten something in Freetown that did not agree with me entirely. However I took the service in the lounge and afterwards had a quiet day. Today however I am back to normal I am glad to say and eating well again. Tomorrow we reach the port of Takoradi, the port of the Gold Coast, now Ghana. Miss Compton leaves us, and then we sail for one more day to reach Lagos. I will post this in Takoradi if all is well.

It was grand to hear that Henry spoke at the fellowship on the eighth, perhaps he will write and tell me about it. It is interesting to hear of Michael's audition, if anything comes of it you must let me know and I will listen in. By the way the Mission House in London sends out the Methodist Recorder each week so there is no need for you to do it from home.

My typing is very bad I am afraid but it has to be done in the cabin with great difficulty and as it happens it is the one thing that if I do for long makes me feel dizzy. I am looking forward to using this machine which goes very well - on dry land. My space is gone so I must close, will write again soon.

Much love to you all, David

Wesley Guild Hospital
Ilesha, Nigeria
24.5.52

At last I have arrived in Ilesha in fact I have been here for just 24 hours.

We steamed into Lagos at 2.30pm on Wednesday and the entrance to the Lagos lagoon is a very lovely place, just as Hollywood technicolour would have us believe. Andrew was on the quay to meet us with Len Cooper who is the Methodist accountant in Lagos and in whose home Andrew and I stayed for two days. I had no trouble with the customs, paying nothing but I had to open one of the cases - the DSHC one. The kit car was there and with the help of the boys got the stuff loaded in and drove in style to the Coopers house which is more like a hotel there being many people staying there, twelve of them altogether. The Revd and Mrs. Angus are here in Ilesha on the Chairman's trek but I got the letter which you sent to me through him. I have just met Mr. Angus in fact and after a bath in a few minutes, am going with all the Europeans on the compound to a party at the Sousters in their and my honour. Lagos was very hot and sticky, with many white people and a great deal of poverty in some places. It is very strange being waited on by two boys who bring all the food round to you and nothing is left on the table, no vegetables that is. Sleeping under a mosquito net is a new experience but does not reduce the amount of air about.

Thursday Andrew and I spent shopping in Lagos getting drugs for the hospital and food and so on for the house. In one of the shops I was recognised by Norcross who was a contemporary of Michael's at Kingswood. He is in charge of one of the departments in one of the big stores.

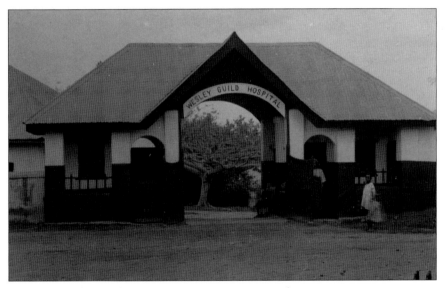

Entrance to compound

On Friday we set forth in the kit car with one of the hospital drivers driving. We called at the Girls High School Lagos and picked up Monica Humble's kit as she is being moved to the United Missionary College at Ibadan. We were finally on the road at 10am and made good progress on the tarred road, cruising with a ton of luggage and drugs at 45 mph! The tarred part of the road is not wide enough to allow two cars to pass without one going on the mud at the side. At one point there was a sign 'Dead Slow' at a point where the railway and road cross. We took this at 50 mph I thought that the end had come but the driver obviously knew the road and all was well. The road for most of the way runs through forest, with tall palms, types of mahogany trees lining the road, with occasional little villages by the roadside. We went through Abeokuta then Ibadan and then Ife. We arrived at Ilesha at 8.30pm and all the African staff were at the gate crying welcome to me as we drove in the compound arches of flowers, hibiscus were *made in my honour. It was most touching. I was met by Jean Pearson and Marion Souster, who are charming people. There are four children, Pheobe and Helen (S) and Michael and Roger (P). Jack was busy and came round later after dinner.*

The place is much more civilised than I had imagined it to be, cold water tap in the bathroom and so on but of course no drainage system. This morning I went to the hospital prayers where I was introduced to the nurses and then to the Sisters who seem very nice people. Jack then took me round the hospital that certainly needs rebuilding. The compound is quite big - nine acres altogether and contained lemon, orange, grapefruit, mango, pawpaw trees and coconut palms so you can see that most things are to hand. Meat is the biggest problem, and all the milk is dried - no fresh milk or fish. Food is good though, and plenty of it. I am living in the Pearsons' house as it is the larger of the two. They have a cook, a steward and a garden boy.

The most noticeable things are the ants, myriads of them flying and otherwise, and geckos (lizard like) of which there are hundreds. It is now dark and the light is on the verandah and a gecko about a foot long has been looking at me from the wall a few feet away. I have unpacked Allison's things and all has arrived safely, the clock and torch are very useful.

It is now Sunday and last night there was a party at the Sisters, with the Revd. and Mrs. Angus, the Sisters, and the rest of us. We had a turkey, which the Anguses had been given on their tour - it was very nice indeed.

This morning Andrew and I went up to the church for the service that was all in Yoruba, though the hymn tunes were the ones we know. I have just received your letter addressed here, which had been tucked away in the office and has just come to light. It was good to hear that you are all well, and enjoying some warmth. Here life is very full and when I get into the swing of it even fuller. However it is much as I expected.

Must close, much love, David.

29.5.52

I was very glad to receive your letter that arrived by lunchtime on Tuesday. It was good to hear of all your doings, especially that you are having a good time in Swanwick. I was disturbed that you have not had any letters from me, and consequently I will run over the places where they were posted although no doubt they may have started reaching you by this time. After the one on the boat the next were two from Las Palmas one by surface mail to you and one by air to Michael. The latter was really for the stamps as planes are very infrequent. I wrote both from Freetown and Takoradi by air to you, and then from Lagos to Stanley with some stamps. Finally a letter left here last Monday and should be nearly home by this time.

At present it is 85F in the shade a reasonable temperature for the middle of the afternoon. Paul, the cook, is just getting my tea, Andrew, Jean and the children being at Ikole - one of our dispensaries - they have been away since yesterday morning and are due back soon if the car hasn't broken down. The days seem quite long at the moment as everything is new, but most exciting. I am keeping very well in spite of the heat and the work, which I have started.

Last Sunday evening we all went to the service in the church that was taken in English by Miss Blake the Sister Tutor here. I wore my light suit, which was very cool nevertheless it was pretty hot, with the church packed, about 350 I believe.

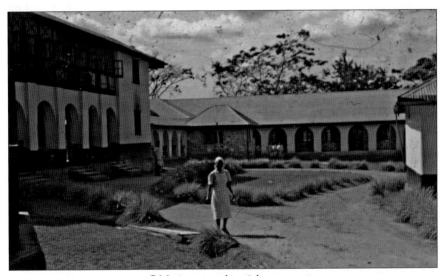

Old site wards with nurse

Monday I attended outpatients and watched Jack as he coped with all the problems. One of the things I find very strange is working through an interpreter all the time, and one cannot really get to feel what the patient is really worried about and what is their main complaint.

On Tuesday, I performed my first caesarean section and all went well although I ought to have been very much speedier in getting the baby out. However after a while the babe was fine and the mother is quite well too, so far. Needless to say I was very thrilled. In the evening Andrew, Jean and I were invited round to Miss Cutlers to dinner with the Mr. and Mrs. Angus and herself. The food was a bit unusual, and Mr. Angus was very tired, but despite these drawbacks it was a very nice change. One appreciates getting out of the compound to see fresh people, because there is not the fellowship or camaraderie with the Nigerian staff, which one might expect because of the very great difference in status or seniority between us. I have just had tea, bread and butter and Marmite, buns and a cup of tea, followed by a lesson in Yoruba given by another Mr. Ajayi from the boy's school in Ilesha. He is good and his fee is 3/6 an hour, which seems pretty steep, but comes from a Mission House grant of £10 per annum which is available for language teaching. Andrew has the same teacher on different days.

On Tuesday afternoon I went up to the new site and was very pleasantly surprised by the amount already built. Three of the blocks are completed and one or two others well on the way, but it will take some time to get it completed. One of our tasks is to arrange the work for the lorries and to pay the men who work on the lorries at the end of the day, so in fact it is the non-medical work which takes up much of the time and demands much patience.

Yesterday I did the female outpatients, getting on quite well. One of the odd things is collecting money for the medicines and examinations on the spot. Yesterday morning I collected five pounds from the outpatients I saw so you can see how the place is kept going. The turnover of the Hospital is £11,000 each year now and all this has to be balanced each week. What is needed much more than a third doctor is a hospital manager, but I understand that the Mission House is not sympathetic on this point. However Dr. Bolton asked me to write letting him know my first impressions, so I shall put it to him in a gentle manner. All the same the work is very worthwhile and enjoyable and I am sure this is the place for me so far as I can tell, in so short a time. There is so much to say that I don't know where to start but I will describe the compound first and then go on to this bungalow in my next epistle if all is well. Please ask me for any special topics you wish to hear about and I will endeavour to oblige.

The compound is nine acres in extent, and situated on a slight slope, the gate being at the top and the staff houses at the bottom. On either side of the gate are outpatients on the left and the welfare centre on the right. Through outpatients, across a piece of grass is the female ward with the children's ward above it. Continuing through that is the operating theatre, and then the maternity unit with the men's ward opposite. The next down the slope consists of offices and stores and engine house laundry and a small workshop. The third layer are the two doctors bungalows and the sisters house, the ground floor of which is the chapel in which we have prayers each morning, 50 nurses and the Sisters and Doctors plus wives and families at 7.00 am (note that Henry). Finally there are the nurses houses which I can see as I type this letter at my table on the verandah, My space has gone, looking forward to hearing how the garden and you all are! Much love, David

1.6.52

I am going to start this letter tonight although I do not think I shall get very far, as I am on duty at night this week, starting tonight and in a few minutes it will be time to do a night round and then go to the sing-song in the sisters' house at nine o'clock.

It was good to get your letter last Friday and to hear that at last some of my letters are beginning to get through. I was interested to hear that you had been comparing notes with Mrs. Pearson and that you both had a good time at Oxford - it must have been wonderful to see and hear the Bach Choir. Was Michael in his dinner suit? If so I expect he looked very smart. Henry too will be back from his visit by now, perhaps I shall hear tomorrow.

Thursday was the day I last wrote so I will pick up the thread on Friday. This is a very busy day with outpatients in the morning and a vast antenatal clinic in the afternoon, a most exhausting day. Yesterday was the coolest day we have had since I came and it was possible to work right through without having to rest during the afternoon. In the morning I assisted Andrew with his operating as I hadn't any from my ward and attempted a skin graft, which may or may not take. In the afternoon we all three went across the road to our settlement for the remaining sixteen leprosy patients. They are remarkably cheerful and practically self-supporting, but we are trying to close it before we move to the new site as their supervision there would be too much. Afterwards the other two with their children, went to a party given by the District Officer for the European children in the town. There are about eight of them I think.

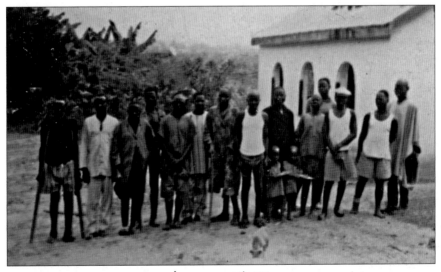

Leprosy patients

Have just returned from the hymn singing in the Sisters house. There has been a terrific storm so there weren't any folk from outside the compound and as a result the singing was not great in volume.

This morning we went to the service in the church that was taken by the superintendent minister Rev. Salako. After the morning service I was introduced to the congregation, about 400 of them and then the elders of the church welcomed me after which I had to reply with a few well chosen words. It was all done in front of the altar and through an interpreter. An interesting experience, but a bit harrowing, not knowing what was going to happen next! After it there was the Communion service, and from start to finish the whole lasted two hours and 20 minutes, and today is one of the hottest so far. This afternoon Andrew and I struggled with the accounts but unfortunately were six pounds out in a matter of £1500 so we had to leave it to Jack to sort out. It is going to be a real fag but I expect as we gain experience it will be easier.

It is now Monday evening and I have just finished lecturing to the nurses in midwifery, a very laborious process. They are unable to take notes and listen at the same time, so one has to have ones lecture notes typed out in full for them to copy. This morning I took the women's outpatients but there was nothing of great urgency. Afterwards I did a dilatation and curettage on one of the ward patients and I hope she will be better for my efforts.

I was going to describe this bungalow to you this week. It is raised up on metal piles about six feet from the ground and underneath is space which is filled with packing cases, and materials for the new hospital. The exterior walls, are of corrugated iron, and were made in sections in England and sent out many years ago, in fact the original prefab. The inside walls are made of plasterboard, which is quite suitable, except that it is not sound proof. There are three principal rooms, which cross the house as it were. The middle one is the living room with half a dozen chairs and poufs, small tables and so on.

On either side is a bedroom, one large which the Pearsons use, and a smaller one at my end, which is the spare one. Out of the big one opens a bathroom and a tiny room with two cots in for the children. Behind mine is the pantry and scullery. The kitchen as in all houses of Europeans out here is separate from the main building on account of the heat produced. They contain a range similar to those in England but run on wood of which there is plenty in the bush. Around all the rooms is a wide verandah on which I am now working and on which we have all our meals, There are shutters all round which we let down when the storms come though in fine weather the house is open all round it can be closed up if need be.

At some point Andrew and I have to go up to the photographers to have our photos taken for our driving licenses which out here are a thing like a passport, but when we shall get a moment I don't know. Just now we are busy getting our lectures in order. Once they are done they will be fixed for all time and won't have to be done again, but they do take some arranging.

Another thing, we have to write our own letters to Professors at Ibadan Hospital when we send specimens up for examination, which again takes time. The cold season is coming, and at night one is glad of the blankets on the bed. Space has once more, gone.

Much love, David

June 6th 1952

The days have slipped by since I last wrote and it is now Friday afternoon and there is just a short while before I have to lecture to the nurses. Your last letter arrived on Wednesday, and it was good to hear all your news. I had a letter from Michael written on the eve of the Keble Ball, which by this time will be old news and merely a memory. I do hope that all went according to plan and his dancing proved adequate. Father seems to have had a good time in Hull seeing all the old friends, and I expect Henry enjoyed his visit to Oxford. He certainly seems unsettled at the moment, it is really time he settled down and did something constructive.

Dr. Bolton wants some photographs for the September issue of Youth, of the new site of the hospital. Jack was quite impressed with my camera and so asked me to take some of it. This I did last Tuesday and yesterday I saw the negatives of the photos I took on the boat. They are first class, I am very thrilled with them, the camera is a very good one.

On Tuesday evening a patient was admitted saying he had tripped over a stick. In fact he had run it straight through his chest and at operation, which Andrew did under anaesthesia by me, he removed about three inches of wood from under his right lung. What is more he is still alive! There is a saying here that life is never dull and although I have only been out here a fortnight I can testify to its truth!

On Wednesday two prisoners were brought in. They had been handcuffed together and one had pulled the other underneath a lorry. Both of them were shaken up and one had a fractured neck of femur. Fortunately for us the government hospital at Ogbomosho said they wanted them so we were relieved of unwelcome customers. In the afternoon Louie Trott came down from Ikole where she is in charge of the small hospital and which a doctor visits once a month. She has a really forceful personality and is obviously an individualist. In the evening Andrew, Jean and I went round to Jacks where we played Rummy - which I won, having a most enjoyable evening.

Thursday was a public holiday because of the Queens Birthday making up for Whitsuntide that is not a holiday out here. In the morning I did a hernia operation, and afterwards incised an abscess. I then gave an anaesthetic for Andrew to do one or two things. In the afternoon I had a lesson from Mr. Ajayi and then walked up to the women's training centre, which is the nearest compound to ours, about ten minutes walk away. I was most impressed with the layout of the building and with the houses themselves. The Head, a Miss Saunders, has invited us to have a look round at the end of term in a few weeks time. In the evening I was called to see a new patient who, I thought, had an acute appendix as well as being pregnant. Andrew thought so too so at eight o'clock I opened her up and found about three pints of blood in her abdomen.

It was a ruptured ectopic pregnancy, a condition where the pregnancy develops in the ovary instead of the uterus. She was very unwell on the table but is improving at the moment though how long she will remain so, I don't know. Most interesting.

Today has been routine until lunchtime when I was called to see a woman in obstructed labour with twins I relieved the obstruction without difficulty and went on to deliver triplets. Everyone is very thrilled except the mother, three more boys. They are quite well at the moment, weighing 3-11, 3-10, 3-7, which is excellent for triplets. They are the first they have had to be born alive together here so it is quite a gala day. For lunch we had antelope, which was delicious and we had mint sauce with it! We also had sweet corn but I was not very struck with it. This afternoon was the antenatal clinic and now I am about to lecture to the nurses so will finish this on a future occasion.

It is now Sunday afternoon. My lecture to the nurses passed off well and without incident. On Saturday I removed part of the iris from a woman's eye that had been squashed out during an injury and later in the morning performed a Caesarean section for obstructed labour. In the afternoon we all went to the Salvation Army field where there was a Guide celebration by the local Guides. Enid Blake the Sister Tutor here is the District Commissioner so it was quite a big do. In the evening I went round to the sisters house for dinner but unfortunately had to go and attend to a girl whose father fell on her out of a kola tree and fractured her thigh. I was on duty during the nights of this week and last night was called to see a woman with rabies, a terrible sight. Fortunately she died this morning. A cup of water was brought for her and she evinced the most frightful terror of it. Hydrophobia.

Your letter posted on Monday arrived yesterday with its news. We have some very nice roses here and dahlias and a form of gladiolus but most of the flowers are imported.

This morning Andrew and I went to the Yoruba service but we did not understand any and after our return started the accounts which are still to finish, but are going well. There is a singsong tonight to which we shall go so I don't think I shall go along to church. Today has been frightfully wet. A tropical downpour at mid-day has continued in lighter rain but still a steady rainfall, and the place is flooded. I must cease. With much love, David

14.6.52

It is now Saturday night and as I type a praying mantis is sitting on the shutter a few feet away. It is about three inches long, green in colour and looks as if it is praying. At the beginning of the week too, Jacks' house had a rhinoceros beetle, a very fine specimen. I suggest that you look it up in a book to find out its details so as to save space here.

Last Monday I got the prints from Mr. Fashade, the local photographer. They are quite good but not as good as they would be in England. The negatives are fine but enlarging is not easy and he doesn't seem to have got it quite in focus. However I am sending them on by sea mail so they should be with you in about three weeks. On Tuesday our local paper, the Vanguard, (some copies of which I am also sending by boat), and which has only been going a month, said that our nurses were inefficient. This caused great concern and we called a meeting to thrash out their allegations. However all has blown over now.

On Wednesday I had an audience with the Owa of Ijeshaland who lives in Ilesha. He is called His Highness and one has to address him as such. I went with Jack who was to introduce me, and we were shown into the throne room at his palace. At one end of a rather dingy room is a big throne and on either side a smaller throne on which we sat. After fifteen minutes he came in and I was introduced through an interpreter of course. We exchanged salutations and so on and then combining business with pleasure we examined him as that was one reason for our invitation to meet him. After the examination a servant brought in some kola nuts, which are regarded as a great delicacy, but I did not enjoy it. Anyway the thing to do is to take the one nearest to him as he offers three in his hand that is the one he would have taken himself. As we were getting into the car some other of his relatives thrust a bottle of gin at us that we refused. Jack says that every time he goes the same thing happens. The Owa is a very important man in the country and has many wives. He is over 70 now but still is King of Ijeshaland.

Later in the afternoon Andrew and I went up to the new site to inspect the wells. Despondency reigns there because the third well has struck rock. This is most worrying because if we cannot get a good water supply then the hospital will suffer. It is now 11 o'clock so I will retire.

Sunday morning - It is nice and cool now much the best part of the day. The sky is overcast as we are now in the rainy season and so the heat is not as intense as it might be. After service however it will be scorching.

On Thursday I did a few minor operations in the morning, as it is one of our theatre days. The three doctors here agreed to write to Dr. Bolton (the Medical Secretary of the Mission House in London) about someone to supervise the work on the new hospital here, and so I wrote suggesting that Ken Parker might come here for one tour until the new hospital is built - that is what the letter was about. Anyway treat that information as confidential until we hear from the Mission House. It would be grand if he came out. He and I would share a bungalow and incidentally expenses! I have been discussing with Marion (Jack's wife) the staff problem and we have agreed that a cook and a trainee steward would be the best. Salaries including a washman would come to seven pounds a month and food to six pounds each month. In addition I am eligible for a living alone allowance, which brings my income to £330 so it looks as though I should knock along alright. Of course if Ken should manage to get out and live with me the living alone allowance (£40) would go but it would be more economical even so to share expenses.

Service in Yoruba is now over. It is a liturgical service with four hymns and two psalms, which are sung. We recite the creed. Two features are the notices, which are even longer than Father's! This is followed by a time for extempore prayer which are punctuated by long Amins the latter is Yoruba.

On Friday evening I went round to Jacks for supper. Two other guests were there, from the women's Training College up the road from here. After dinner we played Monopoly, just the same as ours except that it is the American version, the money being in dollars and places are streets in New York. Yesterday Jack went down to Lagos to meet Margaret Ingham who is arriving on Tuesday in a cargo boat. The voyage will have taken nearly four weeks, which seems a long time.

In addition to this I am sending off a letter with some prints in of this place, with brief descriptions of them on the back. Also a package of four of our local papers, which you should find amusing, they provide our laugh for the day. All the Europeans have sent some home for the same purpose.

The children here are flourishing and get on very well in the climate. I find it quite reasonable if you have a rest in the afternoon for an hour or so until three o'clock, but if there is something to do it is very hot. One or two days it has been 85 in the shade and with the high humidity on top you perspire if you remain still. All are keeping well despite the work we have to do. Yesterday Andrew and I must have done fourteen operations between us and in addition balanced the accounts, which takes some hours. I was hoping to have received some sea mail by this time but perhaps it is coming on the cargo boat. I am hoping mine goes on the mail boat next Thursday

Much love, David

22.6.52

It was good to get your letter at the beginning of the week, with all its news. It is nice to think that all the letters have arrived. I, too, this week received mail by the sea route. The Punches and Recorders have come and a packet of advertisements. Two things, firstly there is no need to send the Recorder or any of the publications of the Mission House as they are sent on to us automatically, I do not think it is wise to put on which ship you hope they will catch as most of the mail, I understand, comes by cargo boat and that is why it sometimes takes six weeks. However to time it for Elder Dempster boats is the thing and what we do here. Last Sunday I sent off a packet of prints and a few of our local news papers which should make humourous reading when they arrive, which may not be for a few weeks. Michael seems to be doing well re taxi - it should be excellent fun. Who are the other shareholders? The tree camp of Stanley's seems to be good fun I should like to see it - the silk worms too are a new venture for the Cannon family. Thank you very much, Henry for the letter, which I hope to answer in the fullness of time, whenever that may be. The Air Times is greatly looked forward to by the whole household here. I will send some copies home for you in a few weeks time so that you can see for yourselves. It has 24 pages.

Last Sunday evening I had a difficult maternity case, a complicated twin delivery, one baby having been born at home and then the woman had taken some native medicine that sent the uterus into spasm which would not let the other baby, now dead, be delivered. However by one means and another we extracted the baby and the mother is well.

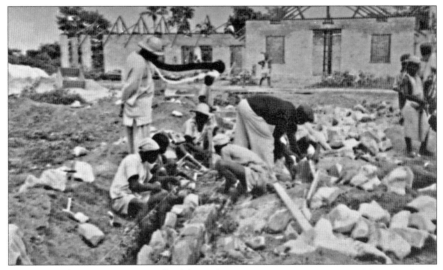

Building the new site

On Monday the editor of the local paper sent round some letters which criticised the hospital, and asked what we wanted done about them. We said we weren't keen on having them published and so they haven't been, which is a good thing.

On Tuesday morning Andrew and I had our photos taken by the local photographer for our driving licenses. Mine looks like a very sinister film star, and I will send on a spare one to you next time I send some photos. Afterwards I did a Caesar assisted entirely by the African staff, the anaesthetic given by our home trained dispenser. I got the baby out in exactly five minutes after making the first incision, which is excellent. Both mother and baby are doing well. Later in the evening I opened the abdomen of a woman who had the symptoms of intestinal obstruction. However the mass was a very enlarged gall bladder and liver, so we left it alone and she has made an uninterrupted recovery.

On Wednesday Andrew and family and I went up to the new site to see how work is progressing. We were pleasantly surprised at the amount done since our last visit, but there is still most of it to do. We haven't heard anything further about Ken coming out for one tour but may hear something by next week. Jack Souster went down to Lagos last weekend to meet Margaret Ingham, but her boat was delayed, so he returned on Wednesday.

On Thursday I was relieved of the ward work, so that I can look after the office work for a time. I started clearing up the office, which, has to be seen to be believed, but put in a good day at it. In the evening we had a night off work, language study, new site plans and so on and played a Chinese game called 'pick up sticks,' an excellent game depending entirely on steadiness of hand and eye - most enjoyable.

On Friday I realised that I had been in Ilesha for four weeks, and the time has flown past, it seems quite unbelievable. After prayers I learnt that Andrew was ill, with a touch of malaria we think, which is taking a gastro-intestinal form. I had therefore to abandon my work in the office and do his for him. Out patients was very hectic and then Jack, who is looking after the women at the moment, had one or two operations to perform. At the same time I had a strangulated hernia to do, with which Jack gave me a hand. This patient too is doing well. In the afternoon there was the antenatal clinic at which Jack and I saw over 100 patients between us. In the evening Jack and I had the most interesting case in the maternity department. I cannot go into the details suffice it to say that I doubt whether Jack or I will ever see a case like it again. For Henry's benefit it was a case of exomphalos in a breach delivery in a primigravida. The front of the abdomen is missing around the umbilicus. This allows the babies liver and intestines to present. The mother is fine. Also on Friday evening we heard that one of the hospital drivers crashed in the Austin taking one of the sisters (Enid Blake) to Oyo for a months language study. Neither of them was hurt but the car is damaged, the whole windscreen having fallen out. It is now in dock. The same driver went down to Lagos that night and brought up Margaret Ingham who arrived at Friday mid-day in Lagos and here last night.

Yesterday, Andrew was better and did one operation in theatre, which was as much as he could manage. I did a hernia and one or two other things that went quite well. In the afternoon we had to estimate how many light fittings we shall want in the new hospital. It is difficult trying to decide what will be required when only plans are available but we think it will be about 250 fittings.

In the evening I had to sew up a rather bad cutlass wound in the knee, which I hope will not get infected. Today Andrew is much better and I am just about to go to the Yoruba service and will go to the English service too if all's well.
Much love, David

Dear Michael,
You may be somewhat surprised at the speedy return or rather reply to your letter, but by the same mail I received a letter from Mrs. Booth of the Mission House requesting a photograph of me by the end of the month. This is both for the record and to have a block made. They suggest a postcard size but I think that the passport size, which are in a drawer in the spare room should be alright but a bit bigger. If they could make a copy and let us have it back again it would be a good thing as they cost about seven shillings each I think. If possible it might be as well if you took it up in person and explained. They want it by the end of June for the September issue of the Kingdom Overseas publication.

By the same post Mother's letter arrived, I am very sorry to hear of the boils, and hope that by this time they are better, whether with medical aid or by nature only. The garden seems to be flourishing though the mulberry tree seems a bit of a menace to the surrounding vegetation. In the Pearson enclosed garden we have lettuce, beans, tomatoes, corn, radish and ground nuts ready for eating. Carrots, cabbage and cauliflower will be ready soon, so we are not doing too badly either at the moment. Potatoes do not grow in this district and we have to get them sent down from Northern Nigeria once every six weeks. However yams are an excellent substitute when dished in certain ways. My seeds are as yet unopened, though I shall have to start planting them in the Souster's garden, which I shall take over when they leave. Regarding my establishment, the six pounds is for my food for the month, the boys all get their food in their own houses in their time off. I don't think I shall have my own establishment until August because the cook wants to go back to his family for a month, as he hasn't seen them for six years. They are very jealous about their kitchens and do not like anyone using it when they are away. For this reason I expect I shall be here for a further two months. My share of the food and servants comes to about seven pounds a month, which is of course most economic for all of us.

I am very interested in the taxi. It is - or should I say she - one year older than OW was, though it sounds to be in better condition if it will do 200 miles without blowing a big end or something. To which part of the continent are you thinking of going, and how much will your passage be and so on? It sounds fun.

It seems that the John Wesley Society in Oxford has flourished under your secretary-ship in the last term. Subscriptions must have been good to give such presents to Mr. and Mrs. Kissack. The retreat seems a bit of a do being in a Nuns Home for Incurables but no doubt most refreshing. John Wesley might have murmured a bit if he had been in a position to do so.

The tapestry ought to be good for the price paid, but I expect it will last a good time. Please give my congratulations to Ken and Valerie and to Winston. It is good to hear that the appeal for us here to have Ken for one tour hasn't been turned down out of hand. He would certainly make a great difference here. Only last evening I had to cycle up to the new site to check some wood that had been delivered and for which we are being asked £100. Bills, which we have had to pay in the last two weeks, have amounted to £1200 so you can see we have to be rather careful. All this is in addition to the medical work that has to be carried on. I have just finished operating in the theatre on the cases from the female ward and Andrew is doing the cases from the male ward. Jack is up country at the moment at the Ifaki dispensary so we are down to our basic two doctors.

I shall write on Sunday if all is well, and let you know our detailed news of the week. I have had some more photographs printed and will send some off when I have a few moments. Andrew and I have been taking some photos of the new site for the September issue of Youth, of which you must get some copies. The hospital is being boosted and we have supplied photos and Andrew has done a very good artists impression of the Hospital as it will be, when it is completed. We certainly need as much money as we can get hold of. Andrew and I are responsible for it all now.

Time moves on and I must close, please try and get the photo in soon. I will let them know that you are getting one.

I am keeping very well and life is far from dull.

Write again soon, much love, David

June 29th 1952

Sunday is here again and a very busy one too. At the moment I am waiting to be called to the theatre to operate on a woman who has an intestinal obstruction. I haven't been able to get to the morning service for the first time since I have been here, which is really quite good going. It was good to receive your letter midweek and you will have had another from me by this. I used my hat last Monday for the first time when I had to go out and supervise the work of the lorry in torrential rain. It was most effective and I must get photographs of myself dressed up for rain. The rest of my equipment is likewise excellent and so far as I know so far, complete. The mosquito boots I do not use much as they are very hot to wear in the evenings. The long trousers seem to discourage the mosquitoes just as well. Last Monday I again lectured to the nurses, and in the evening refilled one of the cassettes of the film that I have used with some film from a 5m. reel which Andrew has brought out with him.

Tuesday was the beginning of Ramadan the Muslim fast. It is a public holiday, though the hospital being a Christian institution does not observe it. Unfortunately I had already given two of the drivers the day off before I realised that they are not supposed to have it. However all is well. In the afternoon I had a lesson from Mr. Ajayi and then Andrew and I redesigned the maternity block. However the Sisters did not approve of our arrangements of the sterilising room so we have had to redo some of it.

On Wednesday evening those of us of our household spent some time in prayer about the problems of the hospital, which we found helpful.

Thursday I did one or two operations in the theatre, which are OK so far, though it is early to say yet. Pause - I have just had tea, that is some hours later. I was called up to the theatre and operated on the woman who had an intussusception. I used a spinal anaesthetic and the trouble reduced quite easily. I shall be going up to see her in a few minutes - however to return to Thursday. Later in the afternoon I had a lesson form Mr. Ajayi and then I performed a post mortem on a man brought in by the police having been found dead out in the bush, He died of starvation as far as I can tell there being no evidence of foul play here. I had to have a bath, wash my hair and a complete change of all clothing to remove the smell. These postmortems crop up about once a fortnight and we take them alternately.

Friday was a bad day, starting in the small hours with one of my maternity patients dying. She had come in perfectly well five days previously and had a normal delivery. Afterwards she went downhill very rapidly with what I think must be the galloping consumption of olden days and almost unseen in England with the modern treatment available. A second patient died later in the day with pulmonary embolus something over which here we have no control and might happen to anyone.

We had a letter from Dr. Bolton to Jack saying that he was seeing Ken on Friday so we are all agog to hear what if anything is happening. Later in the afternoon we went to the new site to see the contractor who was up on one of his flying visits. We found that they had reached the roof of the welfare department and had started putting the blocks on the foundations of the male ward. Unfortunately cement is getting short and we are having difficulty in getting a further permit. Cement in Lagos is 11 shillings a bag. In Abeokuta £1 and at home five shillings a bag. We get all ours from Lagos and bring it up from there with our own lorry that saves money but is time consuming.

Saturday was an interesting day. In the morning I removed a fatty tumour from the leg of one of my patients and then did the odd minor op. At mid-day Sister Louie Trott from Ikole brought a patient 80 miles in her car for a caesarean section; however when they arrived the baby was well on the way and the woman had a normal delivery a few hours later. In the evening I was called to see a woman who is pregnant but is deeply jaundiced and quite disturbed mentally. Jack has seen her at my request and we are both baffled by her, I have seen nothing like it at home so we are treating her expectantly. At the moment the drums are going and weird chants filling the air. There must be a funeral or some other rite going on somewhere. In the evening Andrew and I played Lexicon as it was Saturday night. I was winning however when I was called to a forceps delivery. However when I got there I found he baby almost delivered so all was well.

This morning as well as the woman with obstruction coming in there was a woman about seven months pregnant (28 weeks). She said she had diarrhoea but she was in labour and a few hours afterwards was delivered of what cannot be more than a three pound baby and a small sixteen week foetus which must be the second twin which had died three months ago.

We certainly see some odd things here! I didn't get to church this morning but I hope to get tonight although it is the Yoruba service. In the best of health, much love to all, David

Sunday 6.7.52

The two letters written last Sunday arrived on Friday and it was very good to hear from you both.

Glad to hear of George Bruce's success and especially pleased to hear of Ken's interview with Dr. Bolton and that he is willing to come out. I hope that Michael's piano accordion playing went well, by the time this arrives he will be on the continent if all is well. They should have a very good time if all goes well. Michael's letter was full of difficulties they had with preparation, but I expect it will be very much worthwhile. I expect Michael is thrilled to have a typewriter - this goes very well but as you see it needs a new ribbon, which I was hoping to get from Lagos sometime. Today I am sending this air letter and at the same time another air letter containing negatives which you can have enlarged. As the other letter might be too heavy for airmail I am sending this so you will be sure of hearing from me this week.

Last Sunday night was very hectic as a patient came in with severe abdominal pain - we made a tentative diagnosis of ruptured uterus, but could not get permission to operate. However on Monday morning we opened the abdomen and found the baby (dead of course) and the placenta under the diaphragm and the uterus ruptured from top to bottom. I removed the baby the uterus too as it was no good to her, but unfortunately she died later in the day. If we had had permission earlier we might have made a go of it.

Tuesday was much as usual except that my afternoon siesta was disturbed by the advent of a girl with a fractured tibia and fibula that I had to treat.

Wednesday was a busy day beginning with a difficult forceps delivery on an already dead baby. I had to perforate the skull in order to make it possible to deliver it. Later in the day there was a patient who came up with a dislocated shoulder that had been out for a month at least. It went back with difficulty but I am doubtful as to how long it will remain so. During the afternoon we all went up to the new site where the work is starting on the male ward. There seems to

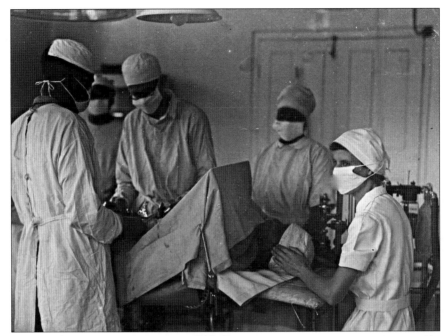

Old theatre

be great activity but we are going to be short of cement as we still need some 12,000 bags and all of it in Nigeria is going to the new University in Ibadan. The wells too are not doing anything but we have hopes of getting a well tester with which we can drill a small hole to see if we are going to strike rock or not. In the evening we again spent some time in prayer for the affairs of the hospital.

On Thursday we had quite a heavy operating list, Andrew's mainly, and I assisted with two rather difficult cases. The list lasted from 8.30 until 5pm and then we put the tennis net across the court and had a game although it was not marked out. It was most enjoyable to get some active exercise. In the evening Margaret Ingham came in for dinner and afterwards we played pick-a-sticks and I made a record score of 225, which I understand will take some beating.

Friday began with the news that there was a patient with retained placenta awaiting removal so I had that to do before beginning the work. I wrote to Bill Callender in the afternoon and invited him along to the hospital, though I learn from one of the hospital drivers that it is six days journey by road in the dry season and quite impossible in the wet season. In the evening I lectured to the nurses and really enjoyed it, making a commonplace subject most dramatic.

On Saturday, I attempted to excise a mass from a leg of a woman who had had it for four years. Jack assisted me but we found it was inoperable, and had to give up. It was very disappointing and the alternative treatment of amputation will not be agreeable to the patient I am sure. In the evening two of the Nigerian clerks came round by invitation after dinner to talk. This they did without trouble, and told of themselves and how the town regards the hospital. After they had gone we spent some time in attempting to draw plans of the staff houses, which have yet to be built. It is not very easy to get in all that we want to get in and yet keep within the budget.

Yesterday the sea mail began to arrive. It usually takes some days to come and it is pretty staggered. A BMJ arrived and MMH magazine. We were disturbed to read Dr. Bolton's article on Ilesha, which gives the impression that all the money needed was forthcoming and none to be found. In fact we need to postpone the building of some blocks until we have paid off some of the loans on the money borrowed, which will take years.

I think that at last it is settled that I move into the bungalow at the end of this month but for the first week continue to have my meals with Andrew and Jean. I am going to write soon to Mrs. Cooper (the wife of the Methodist District accountant in Lagos) to get some stores for me as our lorry is going down during this week for some cement, and can bring them back. All the folk here are being most helpful and telling me the sort of thing I must get from Lagos and what can be bought here. The weather here is much cooler, so cool in fact that two blankets are necessary at night, and a sweater in the evenings. The rain is terrific too and some of the roads very treacherous. It is my turn to go to the dispensaries this month, though not for a week or two. All is well here in Ilesha and time flying past. It seems no time at all since I was writing last week. Hoping that you are all well. Much love, David

Sunday, 13.7.52

This week has been a very good one for mail. Your letter and Michael's arrived on Thursday, but on most days of the week sea mail has been coming up in dribs and drabs, from the boat of ten days ago. I received the packet of letters and the magazines, which have been most enjoyable and read by the whole household. The weather in England is a main subject for conversation out here because it would seem that if anything it is cooler here. Some evenings I have put on a jacket to have my meal or sit about in because the night air is quite chilly. We all have two blankets on the beds at the moment. Anyway I hope it is cooler for you now at home! Very pleased to hear all the news from home I should think that you can guess how eagerly mail is awaited out here and as soon as it arrives all else is forgotten as we exchange items of news. You seem to have had a very busy week what with one thing and another. I am looking forward to hearing, and seeing for myself, Priors Court - it certainly seems a lovely spot. Also looking forward to hearing if Michael got off alright and how his companions got on in No. 1. If all is well they will have been in France for some days now and getting used to the French traffic regulations and so on. I wonder how his French is standing up to it. I am looking forward to hearing direct from him.

The Sunday school outing seems to have been a success, and Stanley to have acquired a few more pets. Michael's letter was full of his doings and of Madeleine, his vehicle. He too seems to have been very impressed with Priors Court.

Last Sunday evening I heard a cocoa plantation expert preach in the Methodist church. It was a very learned discourse, he is a fellow of Oxford. As I returned I had to go and see a patient with tetanus, who was very ill indeed, She died the next day.

On Monday I went to the local CMS bookshop and bought a new typewriter ribbon, which as you see has made a very marked improvement to the blackness of the type if not any change in the accuracy. However I think the accuracy is improving as the weeks go by and I get more practice. One of the travelling Hausa men came with some goods and as my bungalow to be requires some poufs. I bought three for two pounds, which is quite a bargain. I also bought a note-case made out of crocodile skin for three shillings, because the Nigerian pound notes are bigger than ours and won't fit into my other note-case. Also on Monday I lectured to the nurses and in the evening Jean cut my hair. We had a letter from Dr. Bolton to say that Ken is coming out!

On Tuesday I had a letter via slow mail from the Sunday school at Queens Hall, Hull asking me to prepare a paper on the hospital here for some Sunday evening or other. It is not until November so there is plenty of time though I shall have to make a start on it. It will also do for my talks when I come home on furlough.

On Wednesday I had a seriously ill obstetric patient who caused a bit of anxiety at the time but recovered eventually to my gratification. In the evening as is our wont we spent some time in prayer for the hospital and its needs.

On Thursday Jack went to Ibadan to take Phoebe to the dentist. I took prayers for him in the morning but was smitten with diarrhoea soon afterwards. This persisted for a day but soon passed with treatment. It was not sufficient to stop me going to the Ife hospital 20 miles away, which is run by the Seventh Day Adventists. They are all Americans and have plenty of money to plough into the work there. The doctor in charge is a very pleasant chap and he showed me round all the buildings. It is a bit bigger than our present hospital but not as big as the new one. On my return I slept well and on Friday did a full days work. We had a most unusual baby born - or rather part of a baby. It was what might have been a second twin, however I took a photo of it to record it for posterity.

Last night, I was invited round to the Women's Training College to dinner by the Principal, Miss Saunders. There were eight of us altogether, including Jack and Marion. It was a very pukka do with liqueurs and so on, which those of us from the compound passed by. It was quite pleasant, though a bit of a strain. We played rhyming consequences, a rather difficult game to play. It was after eleven when we managed to escape, which made one very tired this morning.

I went to Chapel. The service was in Yoruba and very long and after the service a Circuit Steward presented the quarterly meeting report, which lasted 35 minutes. The service until this point had taken two and a quarter hours so we did not stay to the Communion service which followed. The service this evening is being taken by Hezekiah one of our interpreters and an anaesthetist. He is a very good chap and will come with me round the dispensaries when the time comes. That brings us up to date with the news. I am very well and the work remains very interesting. I learn that Jack's wife Marion is the daughter of a minister named Nicholson who has travelled round Huddersfield, Halifax and so on and knows Denby Dale, Skelmanthorpe and so on very well. Its odd how one meets folk in rather out of the way places. My space is gone I see. Looking forward to hearing from you I hope Father is enjoying Preston.

Love David

Sunday 20th July 1952

It was grand to receive two letters from you this week the first containing news of Michael and the second the general news of the week. Glad to hear that you have received the prints and the negatives and the local newspaper. The papers you will find very amusing, as you say - it thinks much of itself. I read out to Andrew and Jean your vivid description of the taxi and its occupants. It must have been great fun for them, I often wonder how they are and what they are doing. I hope Father is enjoying Conference, glad to hear that he got there safely.

Could you tell Ken that we are writing to Dr. Bolton today to let him know that we have seen Mr. Jobling the contractor. We have had to wait such a time because he has not been near the place for a fortnight or more and only came up last Wednesday. We had them in to dinner on Thursday night and had a very pleasant time.

The silk worms seem very fearsome creatures, a roll call twice a day seems a necessity! I have been considering sending Stanley one of the large beetles we have out here which looks like a rhinoceros, but feel it would be wiser to wait until I can get home and introduce it myself as they are about four inches long at least and rather frightening. Garth seems to have redeemed himself, and there will be rejoicing in Abbots Langley. Our garden seems to be flourishing, out here, there are not a lot of flowers, though on the whole the trees are more beautiful, many of them having coloured flowers on them. Just now being the height of the wet season, things are at their greenest, but when the long hot weather comes everything turns brown, I believe.

The week has passed very quickly. The weather has remained cool, though

34

we have had a good many inches of rain. Monday was a busy day. In the morning Andrew and I put on a plaster jacket on a man who had a fractured spine. Some job but the patient was very good and co-operated well. In the afternoon I had to do a caesarean section and I did it under spinal, the operation going very well. The baby cried at once and both mother and baby are fine. In the evening we had a staff meeting to discuss recent demands on behalf of the nurses for more pay and more time off. I was elected secretary of the committee and Andrew will of course chair the meeting. On the night round, I have been on night duty this week, I had to see a patient who had had a miscarriage in the morning and had been bleeding heavily ever since. I have never seen anyone so bloodless. She died despite my endeavours as I knew she would, because here there is no blood transfusion service.

I received a letter from Ken and wrote a reply to him at the hostel, answering the questions he asks.

On Tuesday I was called in the middle of my language lesson to see a woman who had taken some soda crystals by mouth, in an attempt I think to commit suicide. As it happened she lived until last night when she died after rallying once or twice.

On Wednesday we went to the new site to see the Joblings and to see how things were going on. We found the male ward well on the way to completion and a pump down by the well to pump it out. In the evening we spent some time in prayer again. it is amazing how many of our prayers have been answered already, especially about cement because it looks as if we shall be able to get much more quite soon. Also, today, three Dutch Reform Church Missionaries rang up to say they would like accommodation for the night so we had to rally round and put them up.

On Thursday I performed a ventrisuspension operation on the mother or some relation of the editor of the Vanguard. It went quite well but the woman is a bit of a grumbler, and not easy to get on with. In my language lesson in the afternoon I have started learning the Lords Prayer in Yoruba. It is one of the set pieces for the language exam that is held next April, in addition I have recently learned the numbers up to 100, and more greetings. The Joblings came in to dinner in the evening and we discussed the houses for the new hospital. We are agreed on the Doctors houses but the Sisters, cannot agree on what they want. In the afternoon I went into our swimming pool, which is very pleasant. We have just had it cleaned out and as yet there is insufficient water in it to swim but there is enough to splash about in with the children. It was most refreshing.

On Friday there was a pause in the business of the week and I wrote a letter to Aunt Elizabeth. I haven't heard from her but Auntie A. mentioned her in a letter I had from her this week; so I thought that I would write.

On Saturday I performed a similar operation to the one on Thursday on another patient, which went well. In the afternoon Andrew and I went up to the new site and found that they had started the foundations for the third nurses home. This is a bit unfortunate because as they are at the moment there is much to be desired. Yesterday evening we went to chop with Jack and Marion and afterwards played 'Oh Hell' a favourite game with missionaries apparently. It is a mixture of Whist and Bridge in a way, but where the name comes from I don't know. Anyway it was very pleasant. We had roast pork and stuffing for the meal, with plum pie to follow - a very tasty meal and one that we might easily have had at home. There was a torrential downpour half way through and the approaching rain sounded like an express train approaching. If you are caught you are soaked to the skin in a few seconds and the rain hurts!

Much love, David

July 27th 1952

It was good to hear from both you and Father this week. Both letters were waiting for me when I returned from trek on Thursday evening. Glad to hear that you had a good weekend with the Wyatts and that the services went well. Michael seems to be having a whale of a time, it must be very nice to laze by the Mediterranean, even if their future itinerary is a bit vague. I suppose they were wondering whether to go to Spain or East to Switzerland and Italy. I am sorry my letters are taking longer - they have all been posted on Monday so I think it must be some delay in the air service. Yours usually reach me by Thursday or Friday, but then they are posted on Sunday.

By the same post I received letters from Alan Taylor, who tells me he has just got engaged and one from Mike Watson. They are all well and Mike is in the Air Force, and when he gets his final posting Doris and the baby will join them. At the moment they are in Belgium with her people. Father seems to be enjoying Conference but the Methodist finances seem to be in a very rocky state. I have also had a letter from Aunt Elizabeth, which must have crossed with mine. She seems to be failing rather from comparison of writing with previous letters. It is very good of her to write. The doctor seems rather a nebulous quantity, but if he does turn up show him one or two of the best negatives, and see what he says to them. The silk worms must be very interesting to watch at this stage, though to add gold fish to the community seems a bit much. What kind of moth or butterfly do silk worms turn into?

The week has flown past again almost without noticing it. Last Sunday evening I went to the church and heard a sermon in English by the local photographer. He preached for 45 minutes an average length out here. Afterwards we had hymn singing in the Sisters house.

Monday was made interesting by a man who came in having tried to operate on his own hernia, and arrived with some of his intestines hanging outside. He died later in the night.

Tuesday went quietly, with a language lesson, but Wednesday I had out on trek. One of the doctors each month has to visit two dispensaries out in the bush and this month it was my turn. We load up the kit car with instruments and medicines and set out with a driver and an interpreter, both Nigerians of course. We left about ten o'clock in the morning and travelled 60 miles along the mud tracks in the jungle. The tracks are very poor and it takes many hours. The scenery is marvellous as all the time we are climbing and getting closer to the

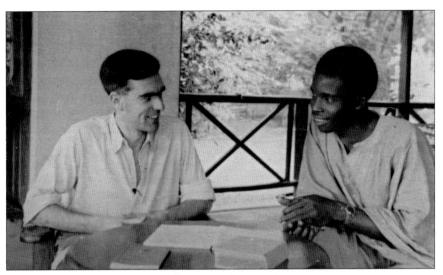

Language lesson

high land in the Northern Provinces. The bush gets thinner and the air drier as we go and at Ifaki (which you can find on the map) there is a good patch of short grass. I stayed in the home of the Revd. Jones who is on furlough at the moment, the individual Mr. Ajayi spoke so well about.

It is a terrific house and quite empty although his steward turns up to help. Jean had packed up some food for me, and they have a herd of cattle so there is fresh milk. The house was filthy and there were bats flying around the room all night as they nest between the walls and the ceiling. Very eerie. I took a sleeping bag and a rug so on the whole I was comfortable but it is not the best night I have ever had but then I was on trek! In the evening we went down to the village and I saw the patients who gather on the last Wednesday of the month to see the doctor. A very varied selection, normal antenatal patients, to a new case of leprosy, one of tuberculosis, yaws, a fractured arm and the usual coughs and colds. On my return to the training college where the house is I spent the night as described above. Early in the morning we set out for Ikole also on the map. Where the sister is Louis Trott. She has a small maternity ward and children's cots, which she manages herself. It is a very lonely job, but as she is an individualist she quite likes it and wouldn't change. I saw some patients which she wanted me to see and then went to her little dispensary and saw some outpatients. I operated on one boy from one of her wards on an ordinary table in a small room by the open window with anaesthetic, which we had brought up with us. Successfully incidentally. I had lunch with her and took many photos of her establishment. Unfortunately it was some old film and it was no good so none of them have come out which is most embarrassing. However there will be many opportunities to take more. We returned the 80 miles in the afternoon and evening bringing back a patient from Ifaki who I thought would benefit from hospital treatment. The journey back was good in so far as the roads will allow and the patient in the back on the floor seemed none the worse for his journey. It is a tiring trip but most interesting and it is good to get out of the compound and see new country.

On Friday I opened the abdomen of a patient and found that her ovarian tubes were greatly inflamed, thus proving the diagnosis. It went smoothly and the patient remains well. On Saturday we did not have much operating in theatre so I slipped up to the new site and saw that the roof is now on the male ward, and they have started on the foundations of the nursing school. It is getting on quite rapidly, but it is only the shells of the buildings, which are going up at the moment. Also yesterday, William who will be my cook came to me and said that he had found a small boy, a rarity these days and could he come on Monday that is tomorrow, and start in this house to learn how to serve at table and so on. Jean is willing so we have an addition to the staff, his wage will be one pound a month to begin with. I am keeping very fit and in excellent spirits. Hope you are better. Love, David

August, 3rd 1952

I am writing this in my new abode having moved in yesterday. At the moment William the cook is away and is going to take a holiday after he has seen the Sousters off in Lagos. Pius, the Souster's steward is here until he comes back, and is looking after me. However I am still eating over at the Pearson's, and they have my small boy, Samuel who has been here a week now and is learning from the Pearson's steward all the duties he will have to perform. He is a very bright boy who reached standard six at school, about school certificate standard. He is a Methodist and fourteen years old though about Stanley's size and he has a very cheerful grin. I think he will be a great asset. I have bought the Souster's wireless for twelve pounds, it cost £25 being a short wave set. It works very well and I listened to the news from London last night, which is quite a thrill and reduces the distances.

In addition I have acquired two cats, a mother and her kitten. One of the

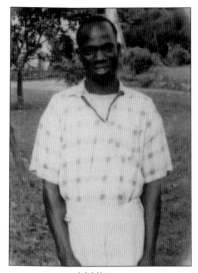

William

teachers at the Women's training College however is going to have the kitten when it is old enough, but judging from the past history of the mother she will have more kittens before long! The stewards feed them on scraps and porridge so they are not much trouble, although last night one of them caused quite a disturbance having just caught a field mouse somewhere and brought it into my room for me to examine it.

I had a letter from Michael just before he was about to start on the trip over the Alps. I trust he is home safely and he has had a good trip. It must have been a great adventure.

I am very sorry there is so much delay in the letters arriving. I have been faithful in sending them off by the same post each week, so the delay must be en route. Jean's mother too has not received the one which you mention as being very late so perhaps bad weather is delaying the planes at this end. The rain is sometimes very bad and the airfields probably get very soggy. Glad to hear that the mulberry tree is doing its stuff and you are acquiring a taste for them. Fruits such as strawberries, raspberries currant bushes are missing out here and if you want a pie you have to open a tin of plums for instance, which is rather expensive. Glad to hear of the good Sisterhood and that the Wyatt's enjoyed their weekend. Very sorry indeed to hear of Mary's brother, a tragic event. Please pass on my sympathy to Mary.

The week has passed very quickly as usual. It has been very busy and full of farewell meetings for Jack and Marion. Last Sunday afternoon I drove the Sisters up to the new site for a parley about the buildings. We took up our lunch, and had a very enjoyable time settling many points. The building is coming on quite well and the foundations of maternity and the theatre are going to be dug next week. Also we are putting in the foundation stones ready for unveiling at a suitable point.

Monday was much as usual except that some of my pupil midwives had a preliminary test and came out very well.

Tuesday however was a very busy day. I had two very difficult obstetric cases in the morning meeting one condition for the first time. There was no chance for the baby but the mother stood it quite well and is going home tomorrow. In the afternoon whilst I was having my lesson from Mr. Ajayi there was a phone message to say that there was a woman bleeding to death in a house in the town.

I set off in the kit-car with a nurse and driven by one of our drivers. The woman was pretty ill but after giving her an injection we brought her back and I operated on her half an hour later. However she has done quite well, although we are not out of the woods yet. It turns out she is quite a prominent woman in the town and the other day a deputation of her relatives called at my house and thanked me for the care that she had received.

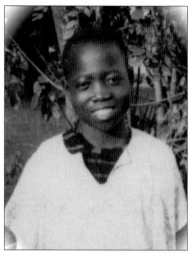

Samuel

Wednesday was a very straightforward day but Thursday was very busy. In the morning we had several operations, and then in the afternoon there was a farewell in the church for Jack and Marion. The farewell was attended by the church members, and most of us managed to get to it. A great feature of all such occasions, which the Nigerians love, is a group photo on which we are all portrayed. It is quite good, but they are very careful in arranging them so that everyone is in the order of precedence. The other feature was the Methodist School band, which has to be heard, to be believed. The individual instruments sound like pan lids but the rhythm is terrific and they are only very small boys that are playing. I was most impressed and would have liked a recording. If you were to come out we must certainly arrange for you to hear them. After this there was a farewell for the Sousters from the Hospital Week committee in the waiting room here. Not only was it a farewell but a welcome to Andrew and myself. It is fully recorded in the Vanguard. In the evening the staff had a farewell party for them in the Sisters house. Food was provided by each of us in some way. Turkey was the main item carved by Andrew and me. There were thirteen of us altogether, and afterwards we played beetle in the form of a drive. It went very well and we presented them with a very beautifully carved nest of tables Actually they are made by only one man in Lagos so they are ordered for the boat and will be put on board to save being carried.

Friday was settling the last things, and Andrew and I got stuck in the kit-car so that I had to get out in the torrential rain to push. No ill effects however. Sad farewell yesterday, but we shall soon get used to being completely responsible.

Very fit, much love, David

August 10th 1952

Dear Mother and Michael,
Sunday is here again and this week I am writing on a shilling letter because there

is much news and also because there are many things which I should like Ken to bring out with him when he comes. They are expensive items I am afraid but now we are settled in the house I can see the deficiencies.

I received Mother's letter on Monday and Michael's yesterday. It was good to hear that Michael arrived home safely after such a trip. It must have been a great experience and at the back of my mind is the query as to whether we could do the same when I am on furlough for a fortnight or so, say Spain and Italy. However that is some time ahead yet and there are more important problems to be dealt with. Glad to hear that Cousin Nan enjoyed her stay and I hope the tempo of things has speeded up since she left. Your trip with the Goddards seems to have been most enjoyable- very nice of them to take you out. I trust Henry is enjoying his week on duty at the Royal Free and having his first taste perhaps of having to get up at night.

I hope the holiday in the Wye Valley is going well and you are having better weather than we are. The weather here is very dull and humid with frequent showers. The garden is flourishing but so is the mould on all the leather things especially the trunk. It has to be cleaned every day otherwise it gets covered in mould and shoes have to be polished daily to prevent them from following suit. My garden is flourishing and I have something of everything in it. The seeds from Sutton's have come up well and Alfred, my gardener, is busy transplanting them. The cucumbers have a good start although Marion has had difficulty in growing them. However I hope that I am more successful. I have over 50 tomato plants bedded out at the moment so should have a good crop.

Glad to hear that you are sending some photos to that spot for enlarging. The negatives are good aren't they? I have just learnt that I have been paid £1.13.0 for the eleven negatives which the Mission House have bought from me of the new site. Quite a profitable business! I am hoping to take some more of the new site this afternoon as we have been invited up to tea at the Joblings who are there this weekend. Could you send on the Old Boys register I shall be interested to see where my contemporaries have gone?

It would be rather interesting to set up a silkworm farm and sell them for Stanley's pocket money if Mother can put up with them. No doubt he would get quite a sale at Priors Court. I suppose it is not long now before he goes.

I have had quite an interesting week here. On Monday we had a visit from Dr. Davey the leprosy expert who is now in charge of all the leprosy work in Nigeria He looked over the inhabitants of our village for the leprosy patients and found several with active disease, for which he is going to send us the new treatment. We were hoping that they would not be active so that we could close it down, but it looks as if we shall have to keep it up for the time being. It will mean one doctor has to spend one morning a week at it when we get to the new site some three miles away.

On Monday evening just as I was getting into bed the phone rang and it was some visitors to the Women's Training College up the road. One of the children had a temperature and wanted advice. I gave some and Andrew went up the next morning to see them. Since then we have had two further unnecessary calls from them so we are going to make out a bill and send it up.

Tuesday was a routine sort of day with outpatients and the odd operation, nothing out of the ordinary. However being on duty I was up twice in the night.

Wednesday I opened the abdomen of a woman in the ward and removed an ovarian cyst and her appendix. She also had a mass higher up but it was fixed and I was not able to get it away. I fear it was malignant.

William, the cook, returned from seeing off the Sousters and I interviewed him but found he wants more money than I think is right to give him comparing it with other cooks on the compound. He has gone on holiday and is thinking it over but it is a bit unsettling to think that I may have to find another cook. In the evening I had to see a girl who had cut off one and a half fingers in a machine for cutting corn. I have attempted to save the tip of one finger although it was practically off, whether I have done the right thing or not I don't know, anyway we shall see.

Thursday I had a rather tricky maternity case in which I thought it necessary to open her up to see if her uterus was normal. I found everything as it should be and she delivered normally two days ago, which is a relief. In the evening Jean cut my hair very well, the best so far. She manages very well considering the chaff she has to put up with during the performance.

On Friday we had word that the cold store food had come up from Lagos to the local European type shop. I went with Jean and Michael to meet the man in charge as I shall have to get many things through him in a week or twos time. I also heard that there was sugar at one of the other shops so we set forth and bought 50 pounds. Twenty for the Pearsons', 20 for my store and ten for the sisters, as they had some left. We get it in bulk like this because it may be months before there is any more sugar in the town. Unfortunately it all has to be weighed out in pound dollops and in all we were there about half an hour just buying sugar.

Yesterday we did not have much operating to do so spent some of the time writing the business letters of the hospital. This is an incredible job, and takes much time. At midday we went, Andrew and I, to the new site to see the Joblings and see how the work is progressing. The pump from our shallow wells does not seem strong enough to me and they are having trouble with it. We have been invited up to tea this afternoon so we shall see how they are getting on with it. Yesterday evening a man asked to see me and it turns out to be the husband of the woman whom I fetched up from the town in response to a phone call. She is the headmistress of the local CMS school. Anyway the husband said he was sorry he did not live in the town and could not invite me to his house and would

I accept this gift. It turned out to be a length of material out of which tropical suits are made. There is sufficient for a pair of trousers I believe, so I shall have it made up when I find someone to do it.

I am settling in well in the new house. It is very nice and peaceful, quiet after having the two Pearson children around all the time. The boy Samuel is doing very well and I should be very sorry to loose him. The house is clean but I have got three cats or rather two cats and a kitten. I promised to have one cat, which is a good thing for keeping down mice, rats and lizards and other undesirable visitors. However the cat which Jean was going to take will not leave the house and if put across the way just comes back again, and my cat's kitten which was to go up to the WTC is not yet weaned so I am stuck with three of them. Last night, when I went to bed they were all in my bedroom chewing a rat they had caught and brought to present to me. I had great difficulty in clearing them out. During the night too I was called to a shoulder presentation in a patient who had taken twelve hours to get here after the arm of the baby had presented - not a very easy task but the mother will be all right I think.

In my vegetable garden I have the following things growing, tomatoes, cabbage, cauliflowers, lettuce, yams, mint, parsley, pepper, sweet potatoes, carrots, long beans, butter beans, beet, cucumbers, so there is quite a bit of work to do. The other flowers are chiefly dahlias and if you have any spare roots or can pick any up cheaply, they will be very welcome out here where we have competition between bungalows as to the best dahlias

Now there are various things I should like Ken to bring out with him if possible. A small trowel for the garden, a cruet with a salt cellar of the open variety with spoon as salt won't pour. Six forks, and six teaspoons. A set of carvers and two sets of double sheets. There are none in the house although there is double bed. Two white tablecloths, the table is 2'6' x 4' and dressing table mats, please. I realise this is a tall order. There is a house allowance of £22 but I shall spend that on crockery, a dinner and tea service in Lagos when I meet Ken. I find that most of the utensils here were Marion's and have of course gone. The sheets and cutlery will be easier to cart about and more useful. In addition there are some instruments I would like Ken to bring out but if Michael could get them for me I should be most grateful. They are on the enclosed form. They will be rather expensive but they are necessary for the treks we have to do.

Well time has gone and I must cease. Hope you are all well, and refreshed after your various holidays. Much love, David

17.8.52

I have just finished a round and it is Andrew's turn for chapel this morning. I expect you will be getting ready for chapel in the Wye valley although you will have left when you receive this. How had Henry enjoyed his living in? Glad

Stanley had a good Birthday, I'm afraid I forgot it again. The top of the Derry and Toms sounds very nice, I didn't know there was anything like that up there. The mulberries seem to be doing well. I had my first crop of runner beans the other day, very tender. The tomato plants and the cucumbers doing well but at the moment are not bearing fruit. Glad to hear that you all arrived safely. I hope it did not disturb Uncle's leg too much. Your journey would seem to be a bit unfortunate, but you arrived intact evidently. Stanley seems to be well set up with playmates fortunately otherwise he would be a bit of a handful. 'Madeleine' seems to be a bit of a problem. I hope Michael is able to sell it, I should not have thought it would be very difficult. The pears from next door sound very nice. Apples, pears, plums and currants we miss very much, and although other fruits are plentiful you cannot make pies from them. Glad the tomatoes are doing well, it has been a good year for them evidently, with the sun.

The week here has been fairly quiet without any very startling events. Monday and Tuesday were much as usual but on Wednesday Mr. Mellanby came over to see us and stayed the day. He is a man from Ibadan who is manager of an engineering works there and who has the contract for the engineering on the new site. We went over the building with him and decided on equipment and so on. He is a very nice chap though a wee bit unusual in some way. He is a nephew of Sir Edward Mellanby, the chairman of the Medical Research Council, a very notable person in the medical world. His brother is professor of Medicine at one of the Universities. He showed me how to synchronise the two generators in our engine room. A most complicated business the noise of the two engines running together, and the mass of dials and lights to watch making confusion. However I mastered it.

On Thursday I did two big operations, one on the thyroid and one in the pelvis. The first was difficult because one is working very near the big vessels and nerves going up to the head. However she is well and it seems to have been successful. At the moment I have the wards full and with some very interesting problems. There is a school girl with typhoid, who is very ill I fear and an old lady with tuberculosis in addition to several operation cases who are recovering.

On Friday, Stanley Hall who is a teacher at Igbobi College came up to stay for a week's holiday. He was at the same candidates committee as I was and was at St. Andrews the term before I was. He is a very nice chap, very tall and thin, and as he is an accountant before he took up teaching, he helped me with the accounts and we got them done in record time yesterday.

Friday was a very busy heavy day with clinic and a whole mass of injections, still we managed to get through them, and yesterday was a little easier, so we managed to get some time in the office clearing up some papers.

Last evening the two Margarets came in to supper, at the Pearsons that is. I haven't got my establishment going yet. We had a very nice time and after the

44

meal played *Oh Hell* a favourite game of missionaries. We finished in good time and I got to bed early. This last week I have been taking the prayers and so tonight I start on night duty, which is not so good. With Jack gone it seems to come round much more quickly. This is one thing that Ken will not be able to help with, though we have a list of things for him to get his teeth into when he has had time to settle down. I wrote to him during the week, putting in the letter one or two things which I should like him to bring out if he would. It is not nearly such a formidable one as the one I sent to you.

William returns from holiday on Tuesday and then comes the moment to see if he is willing to stay or not. I think that he may decide to do so and in that case I shall start living in here. I have got a number of stores in and am about ready to start. All I need is flour, except for the things like butter, meat, eggs and so on, which William buys in the market. Samuel the small boy is doing well, and is very much attached to the Pearson children. I hope he will stay even if William goes. William found Samuel so has considerable say in what he does. However I hope it all works out for the best. Sister Elsie Ludlow (Matron for two decades) goes off for a fortnight's holiday in two days time so the Sisters will be a bit short staffed. In addition Andrew is going on trek this week so I shall be left to hold the fort.

The weather remains temperate, never dropping below 70F and never going above 80F. It rains s pretty regularly and the sky is usually overcast. I have taken some more photographs recently though I haven't finished the roll yet. The photographer is away so I couldn't get them developed yet anyway. In the August issue of *Youth* you will find a small word about yours truly. I should be glad if you could find a few copies and file them for deputation purposes in the future. The September issue should have more in. Boat mail came yesterday. Thank you for the *Punches* etc. Much love, David

August 23rd 1952

I have done very well for letters this week, receiving two from Michael and one from the Wye Valley. At the moment I am writing on my verandah and the Chairman of the District and his wife Rev. and Mrs. Angus are also typing and writing letters respectively. I will go into why they are here soon. Concerning my subscription for the Old Boys. I cannot remember if I have or not but suggest you write and find out, and also if it is reduced for missionaries as it is for ministers. Glad to hear that the films of France have come out and I look forward to seeing them in the fullness of time. I have another reel in my camera, which ought to be quite good. I expect to finish it today. Sorry to hear that the weather in the Wye Valley is not good. Odd news has filtered through about the tragedy at Lynmouth, which you know quite well. Sorry to hear too that the car is cracking up but glad to know that it was not more serious.

In Ilesha much has happened this week. Last Sunday evening I went to the chapel and heard Enid, the Sister Tutor here, speak on temperance. It was the usual type of sermon but did not go down very well here. On Sunday night I was on duty and had to get up to see seven patients so the night was very broken - the worst I have had. On Monday we had to cope with some car trouble on the new site. Mr. Jobling's car having broken down some miles away, so our lorry went out and brought it back again. In the evening we had the Super in to evening chop. He is a Nigerian of course. Things were not too easy at first though we soon settled down. He feels that there should be another class for nurses, but it is difficult to see when it could be fitted in. Again I was up in the night but since then it has been easier and now I have finished my week of night duty.

On Tuesday I got rid of the kitten to one of the teachers at the WTC but have heard since that it still eats a great deal and they are thinking of getting rid of it. Its mother too has gone to a Nigerian family so my family is down to one cat and it is very friendly and an asset in the house catching all the lizards and creepy crawlies. The monkey also, we all found a bit of a problem as no-one really wanted it - has gone to a Nigerian. On Tuesday I got in some stores, including flour, butter and so on. Otherwise it was a quiet day with nothing outstanding.

On Wednesday however, William returned and now I am established in my own house with my own staff and am entertaining my first guests who are perhaps the most important possible. Things are going quite well however. On Wednesday Andrew went off on trek, leaving the hospital in my hands. It was an extraordinary busy time and I didn't finish operating until 9.30 in the evening. In addition to all the normal work I had some proofs to read and the nurses to inject with T A B. Also the District Officer, Mr. Isles, came in with very severe reaction to some poison ivy that he had handled. It took me an hour to treat him and he came again next day. On Friday however he wasn't better so we admitted him and he is staying in the room in the Pearson house, which I had had. He is better now. The District Officer is the man in charge of the district, in the Colonial Service and assists the Nigerians in the government of the place. He is the most senior man in the district.

The nurses who had been injected had painful arms and some difficulties have arisen in their management and the relationships of one of the Sisters with the nurses, so Revd. Angus has come up to arbitrate. On Thursday I had another very busy day, operating in the morning and managing to start up my own household. I had breakfast in the Pearsons' and then moved over here for my meals, and since then have been here the whole time. In the afternoon a woman who had been injured in a motor accident came in with severe shock and terrible lacerations to her buttock. However despite all my efforts she died later in the evening In addition a boy came in with a fish hook through his finger that I had to remove under anaesthetic. Andrew returned from trek having had a good time and safe journeys.

Saturday we operated in the morning, and unfortunately had a patient die on the table. He was a very old man and had some trouble in his chest as well. In the afternoon I started the accounts, which I have since finished this morning. At the moment Mr. and Mrs. Angus are resting so I am getting this written. We are hoping to get to service this evening after our meetings. I forgot to say the other week that we have had a chameleon in the houses and have tried to get it to change different colours. Various shades of green and brown are easy to produce but when we put him on a union jack he couldn't make it! On the red part he just remained greenish brown so red isn't in his repertoire evidently. It is a very slow moving creature normally and depends on prey approaching it rather than he approaching the prey.

My household is settling down, and both William and Samuel being very good. I am keeping very fit and in good spirits - looking forward to your letters.

Love, David.

Sunday 31st August 1952

You seem to have had a most enjoyable holiday, despite poor weather though by now it is but a distant memory. I hope Madeleine (Michael's car) is settled for by now and off Michael's hands. She must be something of a liability. I should have thought that you could have found someone to let it to for five years and the rent would have paid for its upkeep and some over I should have thought. There must be someone in Methodism who would like it, and look after the property well. However you have thought it over thoroughly no doubt. Very pleased to hear of Shelagh's recovery, she has done very well. Stanley will be getting very excited I expect looking forward to his new life. He will find it very strange at first but no doubt will soon settle down.

Here I have had a most interesting week. As you will remember we had an urgent staff problem last weekend, which with the help of Mr. and Mrs. Angus we have managed to get settled satisfactorily I think. The Angus's left on Monday morning after leaving me one of the chickens with which they are showered when on tour. It was live so I kept it until last night when we had it for evening chop. During Monday morning I had to do an emergency caesarean section on a woman who I thought would die during the operation but she survived and is doing very well. The baby was dead before I operated, and it was a case of saving the mother. We ran out of cement on Monday and we have had to buy some locally in order to keep the work going. It is almost twice as much as in Lagos due to the cost of getting it up country.

On Tuesday I did not feel very fit, but kept going and did the usual things that needed doing. It wasn't very much but I just felt I did not want much to eat. However on Wednesday I was quite recovered again.

On Wednesday however Andrew developed a fever. This was very difficult

47

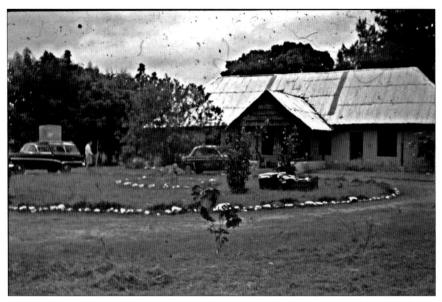

Afon

because he was going on trek up north to a part where we had never been before. Andrew was going to assess the situation, for future work. In the evening the Sisters and I had chop together over there and afterwards adjourned to the bedroom for coffee and prayer. Andrew felt that he was not fit to go and asked me to go instead which I very gladly did. I set off with Hezekiah and a driver in the kit-car about 9.30 in the morning. Our first stop was Offa, where I called in at the Methodist School and saw the manager who is looking after the circuit accounts while the Rev. Raymond Rowlands is at home on account of some illness in the family. The manager, Mr. Ogunsanya seemed very glad to see me but there was nothing I could do for him. However whilst there I saw the van which the Ludlows used when they were out here. It is out in the open and deteriorating rapidly. They are wanting £150 for it but no-one will offer anything like that sum. It is frightfully expensive to run I believe. Evidently it is more well known at home than it is out here! We pressed on from there to Ajasse-po where I inspected the dispensary, which we supervise for the NA. I was most impressed by the amount of work done, and the efficiency of the nurse who works there. The type of countryside changed considerably and there were vast stretches of open land with short scrub rather than the thick forest with which Ilesha is surrounded. It was grand to be able to see for miles and feel the breeze. We then went on to Ilorin to pick up petrol and to look at one of the large towns on the edge of the more civilised part of Nigeria.

North of Ilorin the population gets much sparser and there are fewer white people comparatively. Ilorin is a disappointing place for being so well known in

Nigeria. It is much the same as any other Nigerian town. The difference is that is the most southerly of the great Muslim strongholds, over 90 per cent of the people being Muslims and in the north they are virtually all Muslims. I saw the Emirs palace through the guarded gates of the compound and attempted to photograph it, but it was some distance away. We then retraced our footsteps some of the way to Afon the main place on our visit, the place where the Ludlows worked for ten years. The compound where I stayed the night is a lovely place with marvellous views though the house having been empty for some time was a bit odd. I had taken oil lamps and food so I was well set up, the driver and interpreter were in a room in the same house. I saw the in-patients there were five of them three being babies and then I went down into the village as a message had been brought up to say that the chief had heard of my arrival and wished to see me. I went down in the kit-car with the interpreter and we were introduced and had a palaver for about half an hour, which is a long time for these chiefs. He was surrounded by his councillors, and his wives hovered in the background. We discussed medical work in the district and he apologised for the lack of patients it being the eve of a great Muslim feast in remembrance of Isaac being willing to sacrifice his son. They will kill rams tomorrow and there will be no work done throughout the land until the festival is over.

On Friday morning I examined the weaving school, and then we returned home via Ogbomosho and Oshogbo All these places are marked on the map. Saw two ostriches and a peacock. The rest of Friday and Saturday were very busy and this morning we had a two hour service in the church, in Yoruba. It hadn't finished when we came out but we felt we had had enough! I have got my diary up to date and am going to continue my paper on Ilesha. I am on duty tonight Andrew is preaching and I spoke to the Nurses class on Friday. I am very fit and my household is running smoothly. The cucumbers growing well!

Love to you all, David

Sunday, Sept. 7th 1952

Your letter and Michael's arrived by the same post on Thursday so I had a happy lunchtime reading them. My letter would reach you in good time because the Angus' took it down to Lagos when they went down by car on the Monday and it only takes a few days from there. I am afraid my letter last week would be very late because there was no collection of mail last Monday because of the Muslim holiday, which is a bank holiday here. However this should arrive as usual.

Glad to hear you had a good time at Adwick and to hear all the news of our relations there and at Hooton. I hope to write to Auntie Sarah after I have finished this. Sorry to hear that Henry has been under the weather. Glandular fever is common with medics and there are one or two episodes of it during a medical course. By this time the conference at Sheffield will be over, I hope

Michael and Winston have had a good time. Thank you very much for getting the things ready for Ken to bring. It is good news that he is coming early, we heard last Wednesday. It means though that I shall not be able to meet him unless we are very lucky. With cargo boats such as the 'Mary Kingsley', the time of arrival here depends very much on the weather and how many boats in the queue before it waiting to unload. Margaret Ingham came on the same boat three months ago and it took almost a month. However Len Cooper will be meeting it and if the port authorities give him enough warning he will ring me and I will go down. I shall be going down to bring him up in any case, of course. Thank you for the instruments they seem to be just right.

This week has been varied with the routine work and with a further visit from the Chairman, who stayed in my house again. He was here on Circuit business this time and was going on tour of the Oyo district. He seemed very fit and all went well. The week after this I am having Len Cooper, the district accountant and his wife up for a few days whilst he goes through our books, so we are kept pretty busy entertaining. Andrew and Jean have some folk up next weekend.

Yesterday I went down to Ibadan on our diesel lorry which was on its way to Lagos to pick up some cement. The journey of 72 miles took three hours and the noise is terrific. However I got there OK and went to the C.F.A.O garage, a French company who keep spare parts for International trucks. I bought a new diaphragm for the petrol pump of our kit car, which has broken. After buying this I went to the Austin dealers there, S.C.O.A another French company. As you know one of our Nigerian drivers turned our Austin Countryman over completely with one of our Sisters inside. Fortunately no one was hurt, but it might have been very serious. Anyway the estimates are out and the manager says that it would be about £600 to mend and the pre-accident value was £400 and he advises the company to pay. We hadn't realised that the damage was so great, and it is a disappointment that it is no use. However if the insurance company pays up, we shall be able to buy a new vehicle.

I had lunch in Ibadan with the Boys Brigade man and his wife Mr. and Mrs. McMillan, two Scots folk, who are very charming. They live in the new reservation, a lovely spot just out the town. I came back to Ilesha by the local bus. It took four hours and cost five shillings. A cheap form of transport but a costly experience! When I say that the bus which is designed to hold about 30, had 61 on it and that it was a broiling day you have a slight idea of what it was like. However a good nights rest and all is well. Needless to say I had a bath as soon as I got in!

Last night we had some torrential rain and Elsie who has been out here over 20 years has not seen anything like it. We must have had many inches. It has rained consistently today too. This morning I went to chapel but we came out after the first two hours, as we were getting restive. It was Hospital Sunday and the praises of the hospital and its staff were sung and then there was a memorial service for one of the church members who died last month. He was a young man who had been in the hospital and we had transferred him to Adeoyo Hospital, Ibadan. For all these occasions they make up special hymns giving a biography of the dead man and set to a local lyric. They are most quaint.

I hope to send on some more negatives next week. Now these will be in two lots. One lot I want to get copies of and keep. The other lot I want some copies of and sending back out here and the negatives sending on to Dr. Bolton for money raising purposes. But I will explain further when I send them next week.

My garden is flourishing and my first cucumber is almost ready for picking. Tomatoes and lettuces are ready and cauliflower and cabbage flourishing though they still have some way to go. You ask about the house. There is a large enclosed verandah that acts as a lounge and dining room. There is a small dining room that is too dark to use. Behind this is the pantry and servery. Behind that, is the bathroom, and the boot room. Behind these the two bedrooms. One of these has a double bed in it (my room) and the other two single beds (Ken's room to be). When we have guests we shall either put them in the old dining room or I shall go into the other single bed in Ken's room if he is agreeable. We have to be pretty accommodating out here as you can see. Am keeping very fit, looking forward to hearing from you. Much love, David

Sunday 14th September 1952

It was good to get your letter on Friday and Michael's on Saturday and read all the news. Sea mail came also and I received the parcel of magazines that you sent from the Wye Valley and in addition a Methodist Recorder with the weddings of both the Sangster children, Margaret's being in Medek Cathedral. I also heard from Keith who has asked me to be Godfather to his newly born son Matthew. It will give me great pleasure to stand in loco parentis. Could you get me a serviette ring for him and send it on I will let you know what the initials are when I get hold of them.

Glad to hear that Ken got away well, I am looking forward to seeing him in about a fortnight's time. Stanley will be almost off now leaving the house very quiet I expect.

It hardly seems any time at all since he came to us. I must remember to write to him soon after he gets there. Most interesting to hear of David Swarbrick's activities, it must be quite fun on their boat. Re the cucumbers - I had the first myself and have given the second to the Pearsons'. There will be half a dozen more at least. I hope they last until Ken arrives I can make a complete salad out of the garden just now and all my vegetables are home grown.

John Wesley would turn in his grave if he knew that Skinner said that it was a good thing that the class meeting had died. He is on the S.C.M. staff or was.

Sorry to hear about the depreciation in second hand cars. It is most unfortunate to have happened at this time, but it looks as though you will have to sell for what you can get and cut your losses. Glad to hear of your jaunt to the theatre. That is something we have not got, but it is surprising how used one gets to being without these amenities.

The week has not been as varied one as last but the main item of news is the severe criticism that we have had in the local paper. Each day for the last seven days there has been a letter or an editorial complaining of various things in the organisation and running of the hospital. The two main points, they are attacking are the fact that in the government hospital in Ibadan there is free medical treatment as the place is run by taxation. Therefore why cannot the people of Ilesha have it? The other point is the fact that they are complaining that the nurses treat the visitors and patients badly. Nigerian nurses don't display the sympathy in quite the way which European nurses do but there is no call for the local folk to criticise their own people because most of our nurses are of the same tribe as the people of Ilesha. The hospital replied in a mild way yesterday and if necessary we shall write further. We are fighting for the nurses who are remarkably good tempered over it. It would not surprise us if they all went on strike because of it. That would be a natural reaction in a non-Christian hospital. Anyway I think the worst is now over.

On Monday I had a very heavy day in the theatre with three most interesting cases, all of which are doing well fortunately. Otherwise the week has been fairly quiet. Mr. and Mrs. Angus stayed with me again on Thursday night on their way home again. They seem to have been here quite a lot recently. The District Officer said the other day that the Lieut. Governor of the Western Province was coming to look round the new hospital tomorrow but we have since heard that he is not. It would be quite an event and we should all have to be on our best behaviour. Next week I am due to go to Ikole and Andrew to go to Afon so we have a busy week ahead. Then the following week Ken should come though it is doubtful if he will be to time. There is a memorial church being opened in Badagry to commemorate the landing of the first Christian Missionary 110 years ago. It is on the 24th September, the day before Ken is due so with any luck I should be able to get. The way to the church is a four hour trip by launch from Lagos through the lagoons which sounds most attractive. I should like to go very much if it can be arranged. My garden flourishes and all is well with it except the tomatoes. The very heavy rain has spoilt some of the leaves and Alfred the garden boy says it is unlikely that they will grow properly. This is a misfortune because I have over 50 plants in all with their first truss. However I can soon grow some more I suppose. It is necessary to wait until nearer the end of the wet season so that there is less chance of them spoiling. I am keeping well and *enjoying life very much. I trust all is well at home and the Connectional year got away to a good start. Much love, David*

Sunday 21-9-52

Your letter arrived on Thursday as usual this week and Michael's on Saturday. I look forward to these letters more than I can say and relish the time spent reading them. Stanley seems to have had a good time the last week or two before his going away, no doubt very excited. By now he will be at Priors Court and settling down, and feeling that he had been there a very long time.

I had a letter from Ken yesterday posted in the Canary Islands saying that the Captain of the boat had calculated that he would arrive in Lagos on the 21st.which is today. This arrived when there was no transport so I have not been able to get down to Lagos. However I think it most unlikely that the boat would get there before its expected time by so much. Anyway we rang the Chairman in Lagos and he is going to ring up the port and should the boat in fact come, meet it and let us know so then I can get to Lagos tomorrow. I am sorry it has worked out this way but as soon as we knew he was coming on a merchant vessel we knew that this difficulty would arise. It is very good to know that he is so near.

You seemed to have a busy Sunday a fortnight ago, I expect Betty is now on her way on the high seas, a year learning the language must be a bit putting off. Glad you enjoyed the valedictory service, and interested to hear of Bob Cundall's appearance. The visit to the Woodfords seems to have been an interesting experience. I was very distressed to hear of James' illness. It sounds a rather rare condition if they are operating on a fat disorder of the intestine. I should be interested to hear more details - I hope he is recovering after the operation.

Glad to hear that the photos arrived safely and they are taken in hand. I think some of them are rather good don't you? The camera does very well and I am getting used to it. It's range is from five feet to infinity and speed of one second to 300ths, with of course a time stop. There is a delayed action gadget which allows seven seconds to elapse after releasing the shutter till the photo is taken to allow one to get into the photo oneself. The diaphragm stops are from two to sixteen which all shows a good range of exposures. Very interested to hear of the prune maker and also of the forthcoming lecture. I should be most interested to see an official programme and to see any press cuttings that may be available. Interested to hear of Woodfords start in the great I.C.I. I hope he settles down well.

About negatives - If you can find some way of keeping them I shall be very pleased, as I intend to send most of them home as they keep better there than here. I have some cellophane envelopes here that I am using but the difficulty is that they tend to curl up.

The week has gone as quickly here as it has at home I expect. There have been the usual routine things to do though none of the very spectacular operations. Last Tuesday the Coopers from Lagos came up and I had them and the Pearson's in to chop in the evening. They were very late coming across but we had time to play Lexicon afterwards. Whilst we were playing a car came and the Johnson's of East Nigeria came on their way to the east. The Coopers were staying at Andrews having borrowed one of my single beds. The sudden advent of these folk meant I had to turn out of my bed and let them have it. I had a camp bed borrowed from the Sisters in the room that is going to be Kens. They stayed to breakfast and then set out on their next day's journey, which took them as far as Benin. I did not have a very good night - what with a cough in the next room, a hard bed and calls to the hospital.

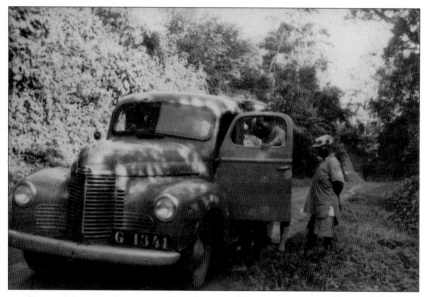

Battery trouble

On Wednesday it was my turn for the Ifaki to Ikole trip so I set off with a driver and interpreter about 10.30. We had quite a good run except for some battery trouble. I saw 37 patients at the dispensary at Ifaki and in the evening I went on to Ikole and stayed the night there rather than at the house of bats at Ifaki! I slept very well, and after rising at a more reasonable hour than usual I saw the in-patients there and then saw the outpatients. After this I had to reduce a fractured femur in the ward and then after lunch we set off back home. The journey back was very bad taking five hours instead of three. There had been a lot of rain and the roads were in places just slushy mud. At one place where there was no obvious fault in the surface we skidded for about 30 yards and ended up in a shallow ditch full of water and a few inches from a palm tree. It took us about half an hour to get on the road again. We travelled back very slowly and noticed the many skid marks on the roads which denoted previous trouble. In addition the road was lined with many lorries that had conked out.

On Friday afternoon Andrew arrived up at Afon doing the trek, which I did last month. Once again there was not much work do but there was a very fine sunset, which made up for it, over the plain.

Last evening the Coopers returned and we are going to go through the accounts with him today and tomorrow. I did our accounts yesterday and they came out first time. The amount in our safe is about £1600 so it wasn't bad. I have had a cold this week but it has gone now.

Much love, David.

Sunday, September 28th 1952

Your letter arrived on Friday of this week, and as usual was very welcome. The most important fact this week is that Ken is here and in fact is sitting reading Punch a few feet from me on the verandah here.

Criticism is continuing but we are getting immune to it and not letting it worry us although Elsie Ludlow is upset by it very much.

Stanley will be at school now and settling down, you will have received his first letters home if all is well and I look forward to seeing some of them in due course. I hope to write to him today. Glad to hear that he went off well, no doubt he and Shaun are both up to mischief already.

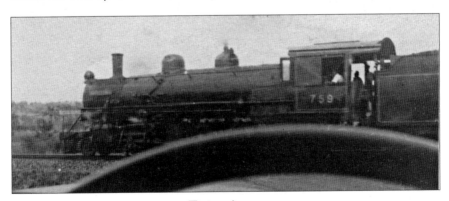

Train - Lagos

I was most distressed to hear of the tumour in Ernest's baby. I am afraid that it is only forlorn hope with radium, which can but postpone the evil day. There is a chance if they are caught early and removed entirely, but if they have already spread the damage is done. I worked for Mr. Donald for a time (at the London Hospital) and he is a most capable surgeon especially with children, who are his specialty.

55

It has been a very busy week here beginning last Sunday evening during our hymn singing. Jean stayed in with the children, and she rushed across to say that Ken was on the phone, so he arrived before the time stated by Elder Dempster which was most awkward. However I

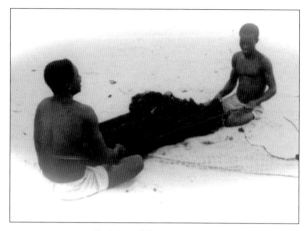

Folding Nets - Lagos

had rung Mr. Angus and let him know that he was due to arrive and they rang up the port, which said he would dock between five and six. However he was in by four and had to ring the Mission House to fetch him from the customs shed. Such is the penalty of coming on a half empty cargo vessel. However Ken survived the ordeal and I said on the phone that I would go down and fetch him up.

On Monday I had to do a Caesarean first thing and then I set off in the International with Samuel who had asked me if he could come with me. It was a very wet day but we made good time only stopping a few minutes for lunch on the way. I left Ilesha at 10.45am and arrived in Lagos at 4.30pm the kit-car running very well, despite floods I had to go through just outside Lagos on the very low lying road. Samuel had never been further than 20 miles from Ilesha and had never seen a railway engine and to his delight we were stopped twice at level crossings. Still more he had never seen the sea or a boat, so when we crossed the Carter Bridge near Lagos which crosses over a large lagoon his cry of wonder was very moving. We were made welcome by Mrs. Angus and then I went upstairs and met Ken who looked very well and had had a very good voyage. In the evening we played Chinese Chequers with the Anguses and then retired to bed, and believe me I was ready for it. On the Tuesday we went out shopping and spent our household allowance on crockery and Ironware for the house, including some electrical fittings. I bought some drugs for the hospital and some odds and ends for other people. This took most of the day, but after tea we managed to take Samuel up to the sea at Victoria Beach so that he could see the sea properly. He was most impressed and has returned to Ilesha a travelled boy.

Again on Tuesday night we were tired but were up at 5.15 the next morning to go to the opening of the new church at Badagry. We left Lagos at 7am in two launches. There were six Europeans, the Anguses, us and a lady from the Y.W.C.A.

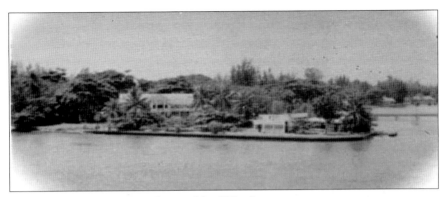

Lagos, May '52 - Lagoon

Lagos and one of the members of the Methodist church, Lagos. The first launch was called Toil and about a 100 Nigerians crowded into this. The second launch was called Labour and we went on this with about 60 Nigerians so it was much less crowded. There was a native band on each so the noise was terrific and got very wearing. The lagoons are lovely and I hope to have some photos of them in time, but after the first few miles they were much the same. It took over five hours and we were stuck off Badagry at midday with a seized engine when the service should have started. The heat and the crowds were terrific and we were practically trodden underfoot by the mass of people all trying to get into the church. Government Officials and all the local Europeans were there. Eventually, we were escorted into the church by the police. The church was built by Mr.

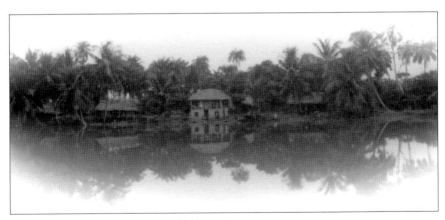

Badagry Lagoon

Jobling, who is building our hospital. He has made a very good job of it. We had tea after the service and then embarked for the return journey about half past six. Unfortunately we stuck on the mud as we were leaving the small quay and didn't get off for some minutes. However we set off home and the journey

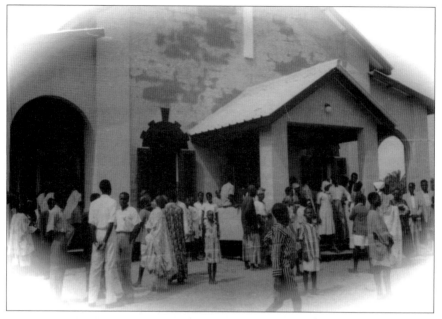

Badagry Church

seemed interminable as we didn't get into Lagos until 11.10pm feeling very tired.

On Thursday we finished the shopping and set off for Ilesha in the mid-morning. We made good time until we were nearly at Ibadan when one of the tyres went down. We hadn't a spare wheel so we had to go into Ibadan, Ken and the Interpreter went on the bus. We brought the latter back from Badagry. It took three and a half hours to get going again and so it was just after seven when we got into Ilesha. Arches of welcome had been rigged up for Ken and he was made very much at home. He brought me many things from you, which are just right and will be very useful. Thank you very much indeed.

When we got back, we have been settling down and doing odd jobs in the house, Ken already proving his worth. Yesterday there were the odd operations and we went up to the new site. We had a visitor on Friday night, a parson of the Dutch Reform Church. The guest who stayed with Andrew was a diviner and he has found water for us on the new site.

Am very fit, much love, David

Sunday, 5th October 1952

This week I have heard twice from Michael who will by this time have returned to Oxford for the first time and be going up tomorrow for the first term of his final year, unless he gets an additional year to do further work. I was most interested to hear of Stanley's letters home and to see copies of them yesterday. Somehow they seem to be very like the William books almost too good to be true.

No doubt his spelling will improve in time and become less of a drawback. Interested to hear of the assault on the stamps of Nigeria. Next time I send some negatives home I will send some stamps with them so that a collection can be made. I have tried to get all the lower denomination stamps but there are not a full set in our post office here, the 3d and 4d being absent. I will ask some of the folk who live in Lagos to try to get some for me, and I will do it soon as the new stamps will soon be coming in I expect.

Glad to hear of the successful Anniversary and that Morgan did very well, though sorry to hear of the mother claiming damages, but I expect it has blown over by now. Glad to hear that there is some improvement in James Sansom, though I cannot help thinking it is just a temporary remission. Interested in the prune problem. Ken remarked that it seemed to him to be a retrograde step to turn plums into prunes but if Michael could turn prunes into plums? The slump in second hand cars seems to be very real. I wish it would take effect out here because our transport is a very real problem at the moment though Ken has spent the week overhauling our diesel lorry. We really ought to buy another kit-car but we haven't enough money.

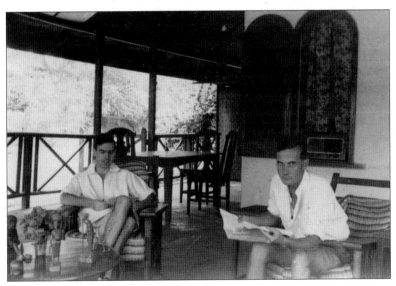

Ken and David on verander

At the moment you will be at Sunderland and I am hoping to hear soon how you have been getting on. It must be interesting to see all the old friends again and see how the place is flourishing. Is Mr. Hubury still there? I hear that Revd. Skelding is leaving - who is taking his place?

Compared with last week this week has been very quiet and a good thing too. Andrew and family are going to Umuahia in the east of Nigeria on Tuesday of this week to a committee about the new combined hospital all at the same place. Andrew is the representative from the west. It is a big undertaking to take his family because it is two days journey each way and the roads are very bad just now. I think he would have been much wiser to leave the family behind. They will have opportunity to travel about when the children are bigger. However there it is. Anyway I shall be very busy whilst he is away but Ken is here to do all the odd jobs which otherwise I should have to do in addition. I received a subpoena to attend the magistrates court in Ilesha on a manslaughter case, the victim of which died in our female ward. I went on Monday at the time appointed and the officer in charge said that he would call me when the case came but I have not heard anything so far. The court is sitting for three weeks so it may be any time in that. It is a bit disturbing to have it held over one's head all the time.

On Tuesday we had a party here to celebrate Ken's arrival and house warming. All the Sisters came and the Pearsons' so we had quite a do. Afterwards we played drawing games and consequences which went quite well and on the whole I think that people enjoyed it. We had ground nut stew as the main dish which is two chickens dismembered and done in a stew with rice and hard boiled eggs floating about a bit in it. It sounds pretty messy but it is quite nice. This was followed by jellies and cream, coffee and so on. On the whole a good do.

On Wednesday we had a fellowship meeting in the evening during which Mr. Jones of Ifaki who has just returned from furlough turned up and stayed the night in the Pearson's house. We had a hospital committee afterwards and discussed the houses on the new site, and I am glad to say that we are finally agreed on the new house for the Sisters. There has been much discussion about this house, but they seem to have made their minds up at last about it.

Thursday was a quiet day and in the evening Ken tried to mend Margaret's wireless without success I am afraid. He hasn't the equipment with him for the testing of the component parts.

On Friday evening we continued our Hospital committee and decided that there should be a more representative committee composed of representatives from all branches of the staff so that we can obtain their advice.

Yesterday I spent quite a time in the theatre and opened an abscess in the upper end of the tibia of one of the patients. It was not easy to do but I think she will be better afterwards. I was watched throughout by Joy Bathem of the Gold Coast who is now at Shagamu and is a friend of Margaret Ingham's. She has been up for a few days holiday during their half term.

In the afternoon we had a meeting of the Hospital Week Committee which is composed of the influential members of the town, who are in an advisory capacity and are to help us with our relations with the town. They said we were to ignore the attacks in the paper and to use the N.A. levy about which there is said to be much feeling in the town. On the whole a long but useful time was spent. After *evening chop we went up to the new site to see Mr. Jobling who has arrived after five weeks. We are going up shortly. This morning I had to introduce Ken to the church and altogether the service took over two hours even though we did not stay to the bitter end! One day last week I saw a cobra in one of our garden beds. I flung some wood at it but by the time the boys brought sticks it had gone. Ken has spent the week servicing the diesel lorry and will spend next week on the new site.*

I am very fit, much love, David.

October 12th 1952

Enclosed there should be some used and unused stamps for the various collections, primarily Stanley's. It is not easy to get the unusual denomination in a place like this but I hope to be able to get them through the folk in Lagos. There are a few negatives too and instructions about these are on a separate sheet.

Your letter arrived on Thursday this week and was very warmly received as usual. Glad to hear the Anniversary was good and that Mr Sangster did well for you. I expect the WW at Guildford went very well despite your natural reluctance to air your wisdom before BDs and such. I hope the weekend with the Bolams has gone off well and not caused too much disturbance. Glad to hear that Michael's rooms at Oxford will be suitable and that he is still with Michael Bennet, who seemed to be a very nice sort of chap. Glad too, to hear that James is holding his own. The radium treatment may take it out of him a bit though and put him off his food.

Your Sunderland trip will be over now and you will have met very old friends I expect. I should like to go to Sunderland sometime and see the place again and see the folk who I knew at one time though could not recognise now.

This week has been pretty hectic as Andrew and family have been away the whole time, getting back late last night.

Last Monday Ken and I had in the Joblings to dinner and in the course of conversation I found that she comes from the West Riding, Shelley, is it near Skelmanthorpe? He comes from near Beverley so that we found we had a lot in common. They are looking for a small holding to retire to and have had their eye on the Wye Valley and know the places you have been to very well. They probably know the forbidden cottage! We had a very pleasant evening discussing plans and so on. We have fixed the site of the residences though we are having to redraw them and get them properly drawn so that they can come up before the November Committee which do all the preparatory work before Synod in January of next year.

The Pearsons' left first thing Tuesday morning for Eastern Nigeria for a committee at Umuahia. I found that a patient with an intussusception had been left in Andrews ward so I had to do that operation in addition to the work of the day. In the afternoon I found a meeting going on in the hall of outpatients being led by the secretary of the National Union of Nurses. He had called this meeting against the wishes of Andrew and without the knowledge of the staff. I dismissed the nurses and sent the chap away after explaining that he was trespassing on our land. He has not returned for which I am very grateful.

On Wednesday I did Outpatients and then went up to the new site to meet the Public Works Chief who came up to see about our water supply. He is a very sound man though does not appreciate the economics of the situation suggesting that we should depend on the town supply which will cost about 6/- per 1000 gallons and we use about 3-4000 gals per day. We will have to dig more wells therefore and rely on them for our water throughout the year.

In the afternoon I had to operate on one of our nurses and then on a hernia that had strangulated, so on the whole a busy day. In the evening I worked on the lists for our yearly order to Allen and Hanbury's and Thackery's which is a very tedious business typing out all the catalogue numbers and the prices of each commodity. The total will come to about £500 I should think.

On Thursday I had a phone call from the Headmaster of the Ilesha Grammar School asking for an appointment to be seen. This I had to fit in with the operations for the day and a visit from A. & H. representative. Mr. Mellanby, who came again to see about the wiring of the new hospital. The firm for which he was the Managing Director had gone bankrupt, and some of the things are in the hands of the liquidators but I think we should be able to get it back alright, but it does not increase ones faith in the man. We are getting another estimate from a Nigerian to see if his costs would be about the same as Mr. Mellanbys so that we have some check on what is going on. At mid-day whilst the others were having chop (they both stayed to lunch) I had a forceps delivery with happy result to both mother and child and therefore to me. They are both doing very well.

On Friday the work was very heavy. I saw about 80 people in the morning giving about 20 intravenous injections and in the afternoon we had about 145 patients at the antenatal clinic, of which I saw 70, so as you can see, it was a busy day. Ken went down to Ibadan on our lorry to get some spares for it and came back by bus having much the same sort of thing as I had. He has settled down very well and of course is a great benefit to the hospital and it is good to have someone about the house all the time.

Yesterday it was again an operating day and I did another hernia who had come in for the operation. There were one or two other things to be done and then I dealt with the correspondence which arrived for the M.O. In the afternoon we did the accounts and then went up to the new site to see how things were getting on. We took up four nurses who wanted to go but unfortunately we had a very bad tornado, which kept us stuck in the buildings for about an hour so that we did not get back as soon as we should otherwise have done. The lightning was magnificent, I have never seen anything like it. Although night fell during the storm you could almost have read a book there was so much light. Never before have I seen the actual discharge from the cloud to the earth, zigzagging down. The thunder was deafening and it was impossible to be heard. We must have had many inches of rain in that hour.

The Pearsons' and Sister Ludlow arrived back last night about 10.30pm very tired after their journey. I haven't heard the full story yet but I know they almost missed the committee and had to go by train for part of the way, which seems a bit of a commotion.

I forgot to say that last week I had a letter from Mr. Patterson from Uganda. He is moving about so I haven't ben able to reply to him but it was most thoughtful of him to write from what is his nearest point to me although 1600 miles away.

The weather here is getting warmer in the afternoons and I believe the rainy season is nearly over. Then we shall have several months with no rain and our supplies get low. We have storage for 73,000 gals on this compound, so we have a little in hand to keep us going if we are all economic in our usage, though it gets very brown and dirties all the white clothes turning them a sort of brown. I am told though that when we get them home again the brownness comes out after one or two washes. My white socks have proved most unsatisfactory two pairs having shrunk out of all wearability. Time runs on I must close. Despite the extra work I have kept remarkably fit and in the best of spirits.

Much love, David.

25th October 1952

It was good to receive two letters from you this week. The first early and the second one last evening after my return from Afon. I also had one from Michael and one from John Tester in Nazareth so I have had a good week from this angle. I am glad to hear that you had a good week at Sunderland.

It must have been heavy driving for father all that way. Interested to hear that Michael went to Worthing for the day before he returned to Oxford. Sorry to hear of Stanley's little note, but I should think he is feeling better by now. I trust his head hasn't suffered any permanent damage. Glad you like the photo of self and Mr Ajayi at our lesson. It is taken by the automatic delayed release on the camera as there were only the two of us there at the time.

I didn't know whether you would receive my last weeks letter as it had stamps and negatives in and was just half an ounce overweight. If they are very strict it might have been sent by sea mail which would delay it but I should think it would be OK. Anyway I hope it arrived safely.

I was pleased to hear of your successful function at Westminster. Interesting how these things get around. It is a saying in the mission field that parents know what is happening to their missionary children before they have happened because somehow all the news seems to get home remarkably quickly from one source or another. Glad to hear that James Sansom is sticking the radium treatment well, it must be a sore trial to his parents all this messing about and not being too hopeful of the result. Michael's letter seemed a bit low as if he found it a bit cut off from the busy life of the university such as he had during the last year. I expect he will settle down to it but one can see that the continual eating out will consume a considerable amount of time. I am sorry to hear of Dr. Bolton's illness. I trust he is soon better and that it is not too serious.

This week has been our week of treks, and so a busy one. After Andrew's return from the east there was much to talk about and get up to date with. They seem to have had a most interesting time and a very busy one.

Monday was a normal day except that we have been offered a new vehicle, a Standard estate car for £400, which is the sum of our insurance of the Austin which crashed. In addition we were offered a Ford kit-car for £250, which was a bargain but it has fallen through unfortunately. We are getting the Standard from the 'Economic Survey' which is closing down.

Tuesday I had my lesson with Mr. Ajayi and afterwards lectured to the nurses. During the lecture we had a terrific storm with very much lightening. The lightning does not seem to be so dangerous as it is at home because the village for the leprosy patients was struck a few yards away without any damage being done. The noise was terrific and I had to abandon my lecture because I could not speak against the noise.

On Wednesday Andrew went to Ifaki and Ikole so I had the hospital to look after once again. During the morning the town clerk came with the money that the Owa owes to us for treatment. The Owa although the king is very bad about paying his bills and we have to go to the town clerk to deduct it from his salary before it is given to the Owa. An odd way of going on! Anyway we now have the £22 which was owing. That night we had an urgent call from a patient who was bleeding very badly near the hospital. Ken went out at midnight to fetch her and then I had to raise her from the dead almost. However she is improving now, I'm glad to say, though when she came in she was very ill.

On Thursday I had another difficult case but she died whilst I was away at Afon on Friday evening. Andrew returned on Thursday evening. On Friday morning I did the outpatients whilst Ken got together the tins of food which we were going to take to Afon. We had an early lunch and set off about 1.00pm. We called at the station in Oshogbo on the way through but the baggage clerk was away at the time. We went on to Offa where we looked at the van, which Joyce Ludlow used to use. It is quite unuseable and not worth £50 as scrap. I understand it never went well and was very expensive to run. Somehow Joyce Ludlow seemed to go about doing many things, starting many dispensaries and so on but there is precious little to see for it now, though one cannot judge on outward things of course. We then called at Ajassi Po to see the nurse in charge there. The native court was also sitting opposite the dispensary and the chief, when he knew we were there asked us to go in and greet him. This we did and exchanged salutations, in front of all the people gathered there. After that we went on to Afon where I was warmly welcomed in the compound.

I saw a few patients that had waited for me and in the meanwhile Ken got the lamps out and got the baked beans on toast made, so that when I got back to the house I had a bath and the chop. We read in the evening on the verandah by the light of the kerosene lamps. As we talked we thought that if anyone had said that we should be thus situated about last Christmas we should not have believed them. We both slept very well and after seeing the patients the next morning the chief of Afon came up on horseback with red trappings. He looked a magnificent figure and a white and dark brown horse with red trappings. I hope to send photos at a later date. We had a good journey back (it is about 95 miles) despite the poor roads. We drove ourselves not taking a driver, only an interpreter. Now Sunday again, and another letter full.

Am keeping very well and fit, love David

Sunday, 26th October 1952

It was good to receive your letter on Friday this week. As you surmised, Michael did not have time to write so I have only had one letter this week, from home, but I also had one from Alan Taylor telling me of events at Selly Oak. I was sorry to hear of the death in Michael's household but by now I expect it has settled down to normal again, though as you say not conducive to hard work. Eating out continually must be disturbing and I should think that one does not feel so much part of the university as when living in college. Re Christmas, Ken and I were interested to hear of discussions on this topic It is difficult to get things home from this end so I'm afraid that gifts brought back personally by me will have to be waited for. If possible I should like a bedside lamp. I should probably have to pay some duty on it, perhaps about 20 percent so it wants to be cheap but substantial. However if you make enquiries and find that duty is more than that a book would be most acceptable.

Glad to hear that you are having some bright and sunny weather and that the garden is looking well. Mine is getting better again after the holiday of the gardener, in whose absence it had become almost unrecognisable and practically back to bush again.

The rains are still with us but I believe that very soon they will stop and the 'harmattan' will be upon us. At this time the mornings and nights are very cold *but midday is very hot and dry, all the woodwork cracking and everything becoming covered with red dust which comes up from all the roads. The last rains last year were on 11 November. It seems odd to be able to know the exact day on which rain stopped for some months. You seem to have had a busy week with one thing and another. Father too seems to have got about a bit. Interested to*

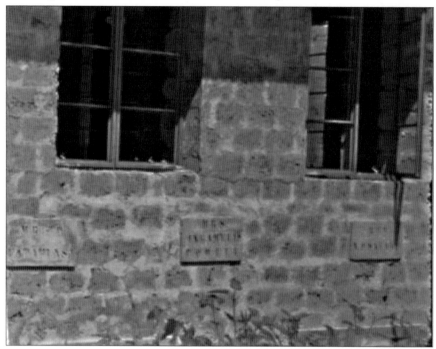

Foundation stones

note that there is an old 'London' nurse at the bible college. I should not have thought there were many nurses there who remembered me. I don't understand the reference to Uncle K's nurse. Why has he got a nurse at all? It sounds as if it might be Nurse Cross from your description of her. Glad to hear your class started the season well, and that Stanley's letter was more cheerful. How was he when you went down? No doubt up to mischief. Sorry to hear that the stove proved refractory in Fathers' absence.

The week here has not been very eventful. My wards are very full at the moment and Andrew's are empty, so he is preparing the statements for the November committees, which take place in Ibadan next month. We have to get a lot of decisions made at these meetings so they want careful planning. Mr. Mellor (see prayer manual) came up to see how the building was going on the middle of this week. He seemed quite impressed with it, and in discussion with Mr. Jobling we felt that it was possible that we could move in in May next year. This is much earlier than we expected but is only possible if the work goes on as it has been during the last few months. As you know a third doctor is coming in May to relieve Andrew and myself for furlough, so that we shall move in whilst he is here and there are three of us, and in addition Ken. Mr. Jobling is due for furlough in March but he would be willing to stay on and see it through. This means that Andrew will be home next summer and autumn (he is due first as he was out first) and I should be home about Christmas time, Andrew will have a shortened furlough I think. Needless to say we are all very thrilled to think that we shall be moving in so soon though it means much hard work to be done.

Thursday was a very hard day in the theatre. I had three major cases in the morning and then being on duty at night I had an emergency to do at eleven o'clock. It was a woman whose pregnancy was in one of her fallopian tubes and not in the uterus. It had grown to the size of a grapefruit and had then burst. That was a week before she came in and so you can imagine the state of the inside when I got into it. However she is holding her own to date and seems to be going to pull through.

Ken has had some fever this week and has been quite off colour with it. He has had about three days indoors with it but is getting better now. I have been very free from fever (due to malaria) and seem to be lucky in that direction though no doubt I shall have a touch sometime.

Yesterday evening we went up to the new site to see how the maternity ward is getting on. They are putting in all the small foundation stones into it and on looking round we found one that was upside down. This will have to be remedied first thing on Monday morning otherwise there will be a riot if the giver finds out. It is one of the chiefs of the town. We did the accounts yesterday afternoon and found them to be ten shilling out which was a bit mystifying. However with some adjustment we got them to balance correctly. Yesterday evening Ken and I went to the Sisters for chop. The Salvation Army couple the Bonnets were there too so we had quite a nice do, playing darts afterwards, which was good fun and very relaxing. Fortunately I had a quiet night and come off night duty now which is a relief. Somehow I don't seem to sleep so soundly when I know that I am going to be wakened up at odd times.

It is nearly time for morning service, always a marathon do. Then this afternoon at five, I am taking the service for those with leprosy. It was thrust on me last night, so I must think of something to say This I shall do during the sermon (in Yoruba) this morning, Am keeping very fit

Much love, David.

Sunday November 2nd 1952

Thank you very much for the two letters which I received this week, one on Thursday and one on Friday. In addition I had one from Mike Watson, enclosing a photo of my Godson who is getting quite a big boy now it seems. Glad to hear that you had a good day on Young Peoples Day and the services went well. I have been this morning to the Junior Harvest at Otapete (that is the name of the church). I took Michael Pearson and brought him out at the notices, that is after an hour and ten minutes, but the rest of the service will have gone on for another two hours. The church is decorated with palm and banana leaves, which gives it a very beautiful appearance. The altar is a mass of produce and there must have been nearly a thousand people there, many sitting in the aisles and in a palm shelter outside.

The hymns are chiefly lyrics and the music is provided by the equivalent of a percussion band, which sounds very African. The people sway in time to the music and at one point the tempo is rumba and when you take gifts up to the altar you have to do it in rumba time. Unfortunately we all came out before this was billed so I don't know what it looked like. In addition I am a chairman's supporter, which means I have to go to the bazaar tomorrow and make a substantial donation, in addition to buying something. The Senior Harvest is in about four weeks time and at that I shall have to go up with the other members of the hospital to make my contribution. In addition as a class member we shall have to go up again as part of that, so as you can see it is a very expensive occasion. They hope to make about £800 out of it. They have a different system of giving here, a penny or three pence on Sunday and then several pounds at times like harvest, Easter, Christmas festivities. It seems quite a wrong thing to us as we keep accounts but they prefer giving in a lump sum.

Henry's friend seemed to have good qualifications for being a ships surgeon! Glad you enjoyed the play, the cast seems to have been a very good one. That is one of the things which is definitely lacking out here but it is surprising how one manages without the frills of life. The wireless is going again and other members of staff who hear it say how nice it is to hear some English music again! Your round trip seems to have been very successful, but I am very sorry Michael's isn't more comfortable. I suppose too that by now the term is half over or will he stay on a bit do some reading before he comes home. Glad to hear that Stanley is happy enough but somewhat dismayed that he is so quiet, I think, though, that he was perhaps a little overawed at having his people come up to see him. It is always a bit of an ordeal to the boy! He no doubt will recover at home.

I hope Chris Smith's wife is better now and that they have removed the offending organ, inflamed or otherwise. You underline a bit about a picture from the Hull Sunday School. I received one about four months ago which I acknowledged at once through Gladys. They sent the one of Jesus with the children of all colours round about him, but as I pointed out to Gladys to be explained gently to those responsible, the Nigerians loathe it and will not have it on show for two reasons. First the dark skinned boy is the only one not in arms of Jesus and two he has not got any clothes on. The Yoruba people especially are some of the best-dressed people in the world, I expect and none of more than two years goes out without clothes. That letter which I sent was replied to, but that is the only picture that I have received from Queens Hall Hull Sunday School.

Could you send out the advertisement and I will get them to change the address and then they will come out here and not bother you at home.

Last Sunday evening I took the service over in the leprosy settlement. It is a very short service about 35 minutes, taken chiefly by the nurse who goes across to interpret. It is sad to see the men, many hobbling in, some unable to read, some unable to speak well, none who understand English, but they are pathetically grateful to one for going across to speak to them. It would be a good test to many preachers to have to talk to them through an interpreter because it makes you think clearly, simply and briefly! One has to be extraordinarily simple with one main truth and make it story like. There were seventeen of us altogether. The hymns have to be pitched by the nurse and she chose the tune of While Shepherds watched for one of them, which sounded very strange on a hot summer afternoon.

The rest of the week has been much as usual. Ken went to Ibadan on Tuesday to get some spare parts for the engine of the lorry, but he was unsuccessful, although he had a good day. On Wednesday after prayers we each picked the name of someone else out of a hat and that is the one for whom we buy a Christmas present as from the whole compound so that we all get one on our tree. We have fixed the price at 10/- and the Pearson's who have tried it in China say it works very well. On Thursday I did a Caesarean, which Ken watched. He seemed very interested and no doubt has filled part of his letter with it. Have swum several times in our pool this week. Very pleasant and cooling. It is about five and a half feet in the deep end. Had the Pearson's to chop and a game last night.

Love David

November 9th 1952

It was good to receive two letters from you this week. In addition I had a letter from Michael. Aunt Sarah also wrote to me in reply to a letter some time ago. I am afraid it will be some time before I get round to answering it as there are several to answer before that. One of the questions she asks was about Christmas present, I think the best thing really is not to send her usual gift out as she suggests, but have it paid into my account at the bank. I understand that Father should be able to endorse any cheque for me and have it paid in. English money is not recognised here and there is customs duty on any gifts sent out.

I was very glad to hear all your news especially about Michael's lecture. He did not tell me about the congratulations from the Secretary of the festival, he must have done very well. I should love to have heard it.

We are very grateful to Aunt Elizabeth for the gift and when I get the OK from you I will write and thank her for it. When we get official notification from the accountant Andrew will write as well, on behalf of the hospital. We will certainly buy a specific piece of equipment with it and I will photograph it and send her a copy. However that will be a little way off yet. Sorry to hear about Sam Oni. Ken too is upset, as he was quite friendly with him.

This week has been particularly hectic. Last Monday Andrew, I and some of the Sisters were asked along to the church as chairman's supporters at the Junior harvest, the sole object of which is to make money. They have these special events at the church at Easter and Harvest and try to make enough to run the church for the rest of the year. The Sunday collections are minimal because of this. There is no idea of steady giving. Anyway we met together and decided that as we should have to give at the senior harvest in a months time that ten shillings apiece would be satisfactory. As none of us had done it before we even went as far as to ask the minister what we should do, and he agreed that ten bob would be alright and in any case no-one would know what we had given. Full of bright hopes we set forth. We were all arrayed behind the chairman who when he gave his donation counted out eight guineas in full view of all the people.

The organisers rang hand bells and waving the money in the air shouted 'eight guineas', the shout being taken up by the crowd and echoed around. The hospital staff looked at each other in anguish! The next person called upon gave four guineas and the fourth two guineas. Then we began! There was hardly any shouting a few mild claps. A perfectly horrible situation all in open competition and if one knows that ones name is going to be read out then one gives more. Another side to it is the fact that they feel unable trust one another and it is called out in public as a sort of check. All the first four were given chickens as a reward but we had not the face to accept ours and returned them for auction. Somehow the whole idea of a harvest is absent. One of our nurses, also a chairman's supporter gave ten and six pence, which made us all feel rather bad.

On Monday, but in the morning, the Resident of the Western Province came to visit. Only Andrew saw him and he did not introduce him to anyone, about which we were all displeased.

On Tuesday I had my lesson and then went into the swimming pool, which is really refreshing as the temperature now is over 80 in the shade and metal in the shade is too hot to touch. On a hot day it is impossible to go under the roofs of the houses here on account of the heat under the metal roofs.

On Wednesday we had our time of fellowship together and we all find it most refreshing and hopeful. In the evening Snowball (the cat) was most restless and I predicted that she was going into labour. Sure enough when we woke on Thursday morning there were three kittens in the box. We found homes for them so we did not have to dispose any of them. Unfortunately the next night some animal ate them, we think, very distressing indeed. It was probably a bush rat which is about the size of a rabbit and when hungry will enter houses for food. We are all very upset except the cat which seems to have got over it already.

Also on Thursday I wrote to Mr. Gunn (the consultant gynaecologist for whom I worked in Bromley) sending him a photograph of a patient that I had taken. I hope he appreciated it. I shall be rather intrigued to see if he replies.

On Friday all went well until after the nurses class in the evening when they refused to sing and afterwards refused to leave the room. Evidently they were dissatisfied about the soup that night and the food in general. They made a frightful noise and refused to listen to Andrew. Sister Ludlow told them that if their attitude did not change, as we had promised to look into the food situation, they need not stay. They took her at her word and no nurses came on duty yesterday morning, they packed their bags and left. Fortunately news of the strike had reached the minister, Rev. Salako, who stopped their transport leaving in the nick of time and persuaded them to return to the Nurses Home. The hospital week committee was hurriedly called and after three hours of negotiations the nurses resumed work at four pm yesterday afternoon. Meanwhile we all had to remain looking after the patients, assisted by the ward boys, kitchen maids and so on. It was quite an experience. We were all very tired in the evening but I had asked the Joblings and Pearson's in to chop to discuss the finances of the new hospital in view of the November Committee next Thursday to which we are all going. We had quite a good time but went to bed in good time. In addition to all these I have had several forceps deliveries and the hospital is full to over flowing and last night we had to turn away some patients and send them to Ife 20 miles away. As you can see a busy time is being had by all.

The weather here is getting warmer still, and the gardens are getting exhausted. The last two lots of kidney beans I have put in have not come up. I fear that the heat and moisture spoiled them. I don't think the broad beans either are doing anything.

I have just been up to see a patient who is very ill. The parents belong to the Apostolic Church and refuse to let him stay, as they do not believe in hospitals. I have tried my best but they are adamant. It's a terrible position to be in.

Time has gone and I must close, much love, David

Sunday November 16th 1952

It was good to receive two letters from you this week and to know that things are going well at home. I was especially interested to hear that Jack Souster had been in to see you, it was very good of him. I am sorry to hear that he has not yet got fixed up anywhere, I do hope he does so soon as it must be very unsettling. Glad to hear the photos have come back and are good. I am looking forward to seeing them sometime. I will do as you say about the cheque and when I receive it, and I'll I will write to Aunt Elizabeth. Glad to hear that Stanley is in good form. I have received a letter from him this week which came by slow mail. It was written on the 2nd October so has taken some time. It is very quaint and contains the news about his two first games of rugger and the facts about the rabbits and moles, which occurred at the beginning of term. At the bottom he wrote a note saying that there were some stamps in for any boy or girl who might want them but he has crossed it out having changed his mind when it came down to it. In fact no one out here amongst the local children do collect stamps so they would not have been any use.

I didn't realise that Mr. West had anything to do with the picture as it came direct from the Sunday School, however if it is necessary I will try and find time to write though at the moment I have many letters to write as it is time to get them off by slow mail to reach England about Christmas time.

This week has slipped by here much as usual, time certainly has wings as Stanley so rightly says.

On Monday we had much palaver about the nurses at our hospital week committee. They are going to interview the nurses and point out to them the error of their ways - this is much better than we doing it as they tend to disbelieve anything we tell them. The committee were very sympathetic but have sifted all the complaints carefully so that justice will be done. Meanwhile the nurses have gone on as if nothing had ever happened and it is difficult to imagine they are the same set of girls that behaved so hysterically a week ago. Butter would not melt in their mouths at the moment.

On Tuesday we had a local man in the house who is doing an estimate for the electrical work on the new site. He had only just left when in walked Mr. Mellanby who has given us the other estimate, a very near squeak because the fur would certainly have flown if they had met. It turns out that the Nigerians' estimate is about £300 more than that of Mr. Melanby, so that he will get the contract. He stayed to chop again and we had quite a nice time. He was collected by a friend of his who is a tyre vulcaniser in Ibadan. He came too late for chop so all I could offer him was coffee. In the afternoon we had a session cleaning out the swimming pool, which we are using more as the heat increases. Andrew, Jean, Ken, Margaret and I tied string to the corners of three sheets which is not easy. Then having swum in it and stirred up all the dirt and scraped the bottom with specially designed scoops, we have to sink these sheets which is not easy. We have to sink them in the shallow end and then walk them down to the deep end. The dirt is precipitated by adding alum and copper sulphate, which also to some extent purifies the water. On Wednesday we pulled up the sheets with all the dirt and it certainly makes quite a difference. The pool is certainly a great asset and we hope that we shall be able to have one on the new site. After *this effort I had a lesson from Mr. Ajayi.*

Wednesday we spent preparing for the November Committee on Thursday, by typing out the agenda and balance sheets and so forth, quite an effort. Andrew is secretary of the medical committee of Synod. On Thursday Louie Trott from Ikole, Andrew, Jean and a driver set off at eight o'clock for Ibadan having left the children with the Salvation Army people. Jean had an appointment with the dentist and then they all went shopping for Christmas, as this is one of the few opportunities of getting anything. They bought me some items for Christmas and my present for the member of staff that I drew out of the hat, under strict vow of secrecy. In the afternoon I drove three Sisters to Ibadan and we arrived in time to have tea and then go into the committee. It was a good drive taking five minutes over the two hours it being 80 miles. The committee went quite well except for the point that we made that there will be no profit this year for the paying off of loans. This caused consternation because the whole plan depends on us being able to pay off loans at the rate of £1600 for ten or so years.

A sub-committee has been formed to look into this so Mr. Mann (see prayer manual) is coming up at the beginning of next month to look into it. If only the church at home would support the scheme it would be plain sailing. All the English church has done is the Wesley Guild £2000 and the Women's Work £1000. The Mission House has lent £3500 at interest but not given any extra. All it needs is 1600 people giving a pound a year to Ilesha for ten years which is not a very crippling thing to do. We returned at night and this time I drove back the Pearsons' and one of the Chiefs of Ilesha who is a member of the committee. We had a gentle race with the other car but at a crucial point our chief began making queer noises and I hurriedly stopped and he was sick! This set us back a bit and then to cap it all we had a puncture just outside Ilesha but it only took ten minutes to change the wheel.

Yesterday, Saturday The Rev. Charles Day and wife, Margaret arrived and are staying temporarily in the Pearson's house until they can collect a compliment of boys. They are an expectant couple and will be a great asset over Christmas. We are all well here. Much love as always, David

Sunday November 23rd 1952

Both your letters to hand in good time this week, the first being written in Shepherds Bush Road. It is good to have someone to bring things out such as Mr. Ajayi though I don't think he will be here till after Christmas as he is coming by cargo boat and calling at every port round the coast. Raymond Roland will be here sooner I am sure. Interested to hear of Henry's escapades, and of the visitors that dropped in at home.

I cannot imagine Michael as a teacher somehow. I think he ought undertake something more original and where there is more scope for initiative. However it all depends on whether he gets a second or third I suppose.

Here it's getting really warm the thermometer going up rapidly. The mornings and evenings are cool but mid-day is very hot indeed and it is a great effort to walk the hundred yards to the hospital from my house. Yesterday was scorching so Andrew, Jean, Ken and I went to the pool and swam, really refreshing. The pool is really a very good institution. We are hoping to get one on the new site if funds allow.

The week has flown past as usual and it does not seem long since I was writing last week's letter. Last Sunday night was a very bad one as I had to get up five times. Some towns people had eaten some so called fresh fish and three came in with very severe food poisoning. One of them was one of our staff so we have been short handed during this week in that direction. On Monday evening we had the Pearsons' and Days in to chop and had a very good evening. He was last working at the Seaman's Mission in Poplar and before that in Bristol, and he has some good stories to tell.

On Tuesday I had one or two operations to do in the evening and then gave the class I teach obstetrics to a test rather than a lecture, so I had some papers to mark in the evening. They did quite well considering and I was pleasantly surprised. On Wednesday, Ken and I with Hezekiah set out for Ikole and Ifaki. We had lunch with Mr. Jones at Ifaki and then in the afternoon I saw the patients at the dispensary in the village whilst Ken had a restful afternoon. In the evening we pressed on to Ikole and stayed at Sister Trott's where we were made very welcome. In the morning I saw her patients and then the outpatients. Meanwhile Ken mended some lights for her for which she was most grateful. Just before lunch we went to a nearby village to see a church which is one of the most elaborate I have seen, and it is a small village of about 100 people I suppose. It looks very well and they are very proud of it. We were introduced to the pastor in charge of it. After lunch we set out for Ilesha again and arrived having had a very good trek. On Friday Andrew set off for Afon leaving me in charge of the place once more. I was kept pretty busy with people coming and the routine work to be done.

On Saturday I had eight cases in the theatre and in the midst of all this i had a message to say that our lorry had had an accident in the bush with another lorry and although none were injured, the lorries were in the stream upside down. After Andrews return at midday, we went to investigate this - at least Andrew and Ken did and found the other lorry as stated but ours was partly on the road and partly in the ditch, but at least the right way up. I had to go at this time to fetch Sister Blake from Oshogbo so I was unable to go out and see it. In the evening the Pearsons' came round to chop and afterwards we played 'Oh Hell' having a very pleasant evening. We were all very tired after the weeks work so we retired early.

This morning I have been to church taking Michael so I had an excuse to come out at the notices, that is after an hour and ten minutes. They are a real ordeal, but unfortunately I was sitting next to Margaret Day and our equilibrium was upset to a violent degree so it was a good job that I came out half way through.

I heard this week from Gordon and Barbara Cooper, a young couple who were at St. Andrews but are now teaching in Lagos,(see Prayer Manual). I have invited them up for Christmas as the custom is to have a big party here as we are unable to get away from the work as teachers are. I had also invited Pat Norcross who Michael will know but he is getting married soon and has been moved to Kano so he is unable to come. I had a very nice letter from him, saying how much he appreciated being asked. I have been trying to get some letters written for Christmas by slow mail but it is very difficult to find the time with all the affairs of the hospital and the new building at the moment. I am afraid the typing is worse than usual this week as I am trying to write more quickly.

Am keeping very fit, much love, David

Sunday, November 30th 1952

It was good to receive your two letters this week. Unfortunately at the moment I cannot just put my hand on the first one to answer so it will have to wait. At the moment the thought of the three hour service to which I have to go in about five minutes is a bit off putting. It is the senior harvest and as the hospital representative I shall have to stick it out. It so happens it is my turn for morning service otherwise it would have been Andrews job!

Sorry to hear that it so cold at home. Here it is getting pretty hot, and there will be no more rain until next March. Already the green of the grass is not so bright and it is not growing as much as it was and soon it will wither and fade and just the earth will be left with much dust which will fly about anytime a vehicle comes down the drive in the compound.

Here our transport is still in a state of flux, and we are going to sell our lorry, the one that was damaged in the accident last week and are buying a tipping four ton Austin lorry so it looks as if it will turn out well in the end. I hope this one is more reliable than the last one we had, it ran on diesel which is unreliable. The driver who piled it up comes before the court tomorrow for dangerous driving and driving with an expired license. Ken will go with him to do what he can but it does not look too hopeful. Sorry to hear that the prints are not sufficiently good for the photogravure process. I should have thought that if they were glossy prints then they should be OK. I think the negatives themselves are satisfactory. However it will be interesting to see the ones they put in.

We have just received the magazines and Punches, two lots and have been looking at the new cars portrayed therein. The three and a half litre Jaguar took my fancy it would be possible to get it here for £1200. Compared with many of the smaller ones it is relatively cheap.

This week has been one of the common round and daily task, with nothing outstanding happening. Monday I had a mild attack of diarrhoea, but a day in bed or rather a few hours in bed put it right and I was up for the evening meal again, and have been very fit since. Samuel used water from the well unboiled for our orange squash and I think that that did it. He was severely reprimanded by William who was greatly disturbed. Tuesday was very hectic. In the afternoon I had a difficult forceps delivery to perform on a woman who was brought many miles by car from the Akure hospital where their doctor was on trek. She had previously been to a native ju ju man with disastrous results so it was not an easy task, but the mother is recovering well.

In the evening we had three emergency cases brought in upon all of which we had to operate and it was after midnight when we finished.

On Wednesday we had our usual fellowship class and afterwards a Christmas committee. There are a great number of things to be done at Xmas time for the patients and nurses, and it looks like a time of hard work for everyone. On Christmas day for instance we start with a Communion service for the entire compound at 6.30, services in the wards, distribution of presents to all the patients and nurses, and a special trip to the leprosy patients. Mid day meal is in our house and it is to be a cold buffet for nineteen of us plus the two children. This is going to take some planning but I am going to ask the Coopers who are coming up to spend Christmas with me to bring up a piece of ham from Lagos and some tins of salmon with which to make sandwiches. In addition chipolata sausages on sticks. Fortunately it will be a take and eat meal and not a sit down one. In the afternoon we are distributing the Christmas presents which we have given each other. They are to be placed in a sack which will be hung up on our verandah so that the anonymity will be maintained to the end. In the evening our Christmas dinner proper is in the Sisters house followed by as many games of which we are capable. The numbers come from all those on the compound, plus guests plus Rev. and Mrs. Day who are here till synod and the two Salvation Army people, the Bennetts. We should have a good time.

Thursday was again busy with twelve cases in theatre but we got through them in about five hours. In the evening the Pearsons went to the District Officer's for dinner but did not have a very good time as there were several business men there who were hitting the bottle pretty hard and I think they were very glad to get away.

Friday was another day of hard work but in the evening we went over to the Sisters and had a gramophone recital. The records were well used and the needles steel ones but it made a very pleasant change. Enid Blake who ran it is very particular and we are not allowed to read whilst listening. I picked up a magazine whilst the record was being changed and she would not start until I put it down! Much grace is needed at times!

It made a very pleasant change. Saturday was again a long theatre morning and it was followed by paying the men. In the afternoon we did the accounts and then went for a swim in the pool, which is evaporating slowly. In the evening Andrew and Jean came round to chop and afterwards we had a committee with the Sisters. Space gone; we are all well, I am very fit, much love, David

December 7th 1952
Your midweek letter of November 27th has arrived with the first batch of photographs but the second has not yet put in an appearance. However, on Friday Mr. Ajayi arrived with the Chairman, who is going up to Ifaki. He gave me the parcels which you have sent out. The biscuits look very nice on the outside and will be saved for Christmas. To obtain such a tin in Lagos would cost about twice the amount with out transport. The letter and photographs arrived safely. Also on Tuesday the Rowlands' arrived in Lagos but have not called in here. I shall however be going to supervise their dispensary on the nineteenth so I shall be able to get the parcel then. They said on the telephone that they had brought it safely.

I see from your letter that it is still very cold, and that Henry had a nightmare. Let him come here and then he might have some real ones! The night before last there was a strange man walking around the compound armed with an antique rifle and a machete. The night nurses were somewhat alarmed and insisted on having a guard the next night. Two constables therefore came and mounted guard at the gate and this seemed to have the desired effect because he was not seen again.

Glad to hear that they had a successful Ilesha evening at Queens, we need all the help we can get. I have received the scrapbooks from Queens so I will write to Mr. West and thank him for them and he can pass on the thanks to whoever is responsible. They are full of pictures of the Royal Family and I have given one of the Queen to William who cannot read but does appreciate pictures. In addition I have heard from Stanley who wrote a priceless letter which I must answer today if possible. It was one of those air letter things which he must have purchased from the post office. He has also written to his grandpa he says.

The week has gone with the usual rapidity with the usual amount of work. On Tuesday Andrew and I had to interview many nurses and to examine the candidates for next year. This took some doing but we are both dismayed to learn that we have no say in the choice of candidates. It is left entirely to the Sisters and really some of the nurses which we have at the moment any one with half an eye could see that they will be unsuitable. However we cannot change every thing at once. In addition Mr. Mellanby the man who is undertaking the electrical work on the New Hospital came and wanted to look at the buildings so that he could get out the wiring diagrams.

On most evenings this week at the church there has been the harvest bazaar, but we haven't been. However we have given our subscription of 30 shillings. Thursday was memorable for the fact that Andrew undertook to give Jean a Toni perm in the evening. It was the first one he had tried although he started just after six it was nearly midnight when he finished so he is hoping that it lasts the full six months that it is supposed to do.

Friday, Ken went to Ibadan to collect some electrical equipment. He had a good day and managed to get all he needed. The same day we got our new car, a Standard Vanguard Estate car that will do what we want very well indeed. It takes six people very comfortably and leaves room for boxes in the back. If necessary it is possible to put the back seat down get more things in though then it only seats three. We have got it for £400 in hand which is the sum we received from the insurance for the old car which was smashed up. At the moment also we are thinking of buying a new lorry but there are divergent opinions in the district as to the best thing to do. At the moment the situation is that if we do not get some transport quickly we shall have to delay the opening of the new hospital another year. Anyway no doubt it will work out.

On Friday the Chairman turned up and with him Mr. Ajayi. It was good to see them both again. Mr. Ajayi looked very well after his voyage and seemed in good spirits. The Chairman had a very acrimonious discussion with the local church and was disturbed at the spirit of the place. He looked in on his way down again and had chop with the Pearsons', and saw M. G. who is doing her last tour here

Dr. Harry Haig and his wife stayed the night last night on their way home to Ituk Mbang. They seem very knowledgeable and very efficient. He is doing

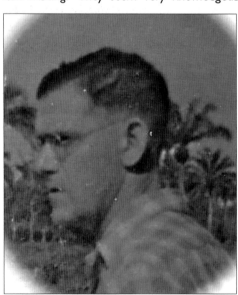

Harry Haigh

deputation and lives in Ilkley, so the Aunts in Yorkshire might be able to get hold of him to speak. He is in charge of the United Hospital which is to be built in Umuahia in the East, and was most interested in the new site which we went up to see this morning.

Christmas approaches quickly, we are arranging all the activities which are needful in a hospital where we have the welfare of the patients and nurses to think of. We are going to have a very happy crowd of folk and we are all looking forward to it immensely.

This afternoon we are going to a Carol Service in the Women's

Training College up the road which will be the first sign of Advent so to speak. It is almost unbelievable that with the heat we have now that Christmas is less than three weeks away.

It is not possible to send things home from here for Christmas to any great extent so my curios which I am slowly collecting will have to wait till I come home. I have dispatched odd Christmas cards by the last boat which I hope will arrive in good time. One or two I will send by Airmail nearer the time.

Enclosed is a 2/6 stamp from a parcel and some negatives with explanatory words. It is the Nigerian Census tomorrow and the District Officer is coming for tea to tell us how to complete the forms for all who sleep on the compound tomorrow night. Much love to you all, David

Sunday, 14th December 1952

I was very sorry to hear about James Sansom, it must be a very trying time for Ernest and Vivian, and the next six months will be very difficult indeed. They will need all our prayers.

Mail is a thing to be looked forward to out here and everyone knows when sea mail is due and looks forward to it with undisguised anticipation. Glad the prayer meeting went well and there were so many there.

The weather seems to have been most unsatisfactory at home, we are all remarking about it here as it forms the solid core of letters written to all of us. It is mentioned with a slightly superior smile as we think of you all huddled in front of the fire, heavy clothes, overcoats, hacking coughs and all the paraphernalia of bottles of medicine etc. Here we are delightfully warm in the minimum of clothing, and as I type this on the verandah I can see the early morning mist rising and know it will be a lovely warm (Jolly Hot) day with a cloudless blue sky with no chance of rain or fog. In fact we have arranged a picnic on the new site this afternoon.

Interesting to hear of your activities in opening stalls and so forth and appreciate all you are doing to raise money for the Hospital.

It is quite unbelievable that Christmas is but ten days away, and here we are in the heat, it doesn't feel Christmassy at all. No holly, no shops decorated or in fact shops to decorate, no Father Christmases around the place. The people do not understand Father Christmas, he hasn't entered into their folklore. In fact to the majority it is just a Christmas festival which results in a Public Holiday. Our guests are beginning to roll up, the first a Church Missionary Society sister from a hospital in the East has arrived at the Sisters house, and others are expected in about a weeks time. I have had some stores sent up from Lagos including a tin of boneless cooked ham weighing two pounds which cost sixteen shillings so it should be good. Ideas are beginning to dawn about our buffet lunch so I hope that it will go smoothly. Mrs. Cooper, one of my guests should be able to give a *spot of advice when the time comes.*

The week has been a very busy one with visitors. Last Sunday afternoon seven of us went up by invitation to the Women's Training Centre where the students presented a service of nine lessons and carols and it went very well indeed. It was very pleasant to hear all the familiar carols in English when one is in an unfamiliar place and it makes a strong link with home. In the evening I went to church but it was a Yoruba service, so it should be English tonight. Afterwards Ken and I went round to the Days for coffee as there was no hymn singing here and then Andrew and I went into the Sisters to help in the final choosing of candidates for our new nursing year, not an easy task. On Monday the deputy Director of Medical Services for the Region came in to look round and to see the new hospital. He and his wife were very nice folk although obviously in government service and used to having large dinner parties and so forth. He seemed quite pleased with both the present site and the new one. He stayed at the other house to lunch and went back to Ibadan in the afternoon.

On Tuesday we went up to the new site to see how the houses are getting on and found them putting in the foundations of Andrews and were digging out mine. As they come on I hope I shall be able to send some photos of them going up. Unfortunately the Joblings weren't in too great frame of mind so we didn't get anything very concrete done and couldn't arrange the windows in the living rooms of the houses. We hope to have more suggestions ready when they come back again. In the evening Mr. and Mrs. Mann arrived from Lagos (see Prayer Manual) to look into the finances of the hospital and see if we are going to make enough money to be able to pay off the loans over the next 20 years. They are a very nice couple and as you will see have been out for a good number of years. They have a boy at Kingswood School about fourteen-years-old. I think in Upper House. Mr. Mann has a yacht in Lagos and once caught a 165 lb fish in the lagoon single handed on a fine line.

On Wednesday we took him up to the new site, but he wasn't so impressed with it as he might have been. Still he felt the building had gone on quite well and later after examining the books thought that we should be able to manage it. We shall have to put up prices a bit in order increase our revenue.

On Thursday I had a difficult hernia to do, one that had been done before. It had became infected and had recurred. Unfortunately although the operation went very well she has a frightful cough, which nothing touches so she may well cough it down again quite soon. Friday we had 165 patients to the antenatal clinic in the afternoon a very large number.

Did out annual numerical returns yesterday. All up!

Much love, David

Sunday December 21st 1952

Christmas is almost upon us and by the time you receive this it will be over. Thank you very much for the parcels, which I have received but not opened. One came by post and is about the shape of a book. I got Andrew to open it and he says it is for Christmas so as yet I have not seen it. Yesterday, I returned from my visit to the Rowlands at Afon and they gave me the three parcels which you gave them to bring out. I have only opened the cake and find that it is in perfect condition so Ken and I have sealed it up again. We were having a small party for Ken's Birthday which is today and the guests admired it very much indeed, especially the almond paste which is very difficult to get out here, and the cherries which are unobtainable. The other parcels I shall leave until Christmas Day. I have heard from the Gordon Coopers and they arrive tomorrow, so we shall really feel that Christmas is coming because at the moment it does not feel like it at all.

I was interested to hear of Fathers' visit to Dunstable. Mr. Longley is super of the Oyo circuit here and I met him at the November committees and shall again at Synod I should think. I hadn't connected the two families up. I don't actually recall Len Dickenson though the name is familiar.

Arrangements here are in hand for the buffet lunch I have to provide for 20 folk, and the Coopers have made me some mincemeat, which they will bring up with them. We have as yet made no arrangements for the nurses Christmas party so we shall have to think of that though Ken has the lighting in hand. Carol and play practices occur spasmodically trained by a variety of people but we are all looking forward immensely to it.

The week has been as busy as usual. Mr. and Mrs. Mann returned from Ifaki on Monday having found an error of £100 in our accounts. This is a trifle disconcerting but we have an idea where it is. Otherwise it is all pretty straight. Learnt that there are some tigers about seven miles away amongst the rocks. In addition the lagoons at Badagry where we went some time ago and of which the photo was taken are full of crocodiles. I was sorry about the print and will try to find some typically African scene to photograph and send in for competition,

On Wednesday Andrew and family set off on trek to Ikole and found Sister Trott well. They had a good but uninteresting time returning the next day. Meanwhile I had several big operations to do, which so far are recovering well, though in the nature of them, it is early to tell just yet.

Friday I did Outpatients in the morning and then after an early lunch set off in our new Standard for Afon, with Abe one of our interpreters. The car went very well and we had no trouble, taking just three hours to do the hundred miles including visits to the dispensary at Ajassi-po I found the Rowlands in good health, though she is tired as she is expecting a baby early next year so she is staying in Lagos after Synod in order that she shall be on the spot.

We talked about the land north of Ilorin (better get out the map). A new road has been made from Kaiama to Bussa and then on further north. This had opened up great tracts of unexplored land where no missionaries have ever been, and to which the Muslims have not yet penetrated. Raymond has been up once *or twice and says that the people are still living in the stone and iron age and hide behind trees when a white man appears. The thing the people ask for is medicine and Raymond feels that the work could be opened up via that route. A commission is investigating the situation early next year. The Chairman, Raymond, an African minister and I suggested a Doctor might go too, the idea appealing to Raymond. There are many hippos, leopards, panthers, crocodiles, and so on in the river nearby, and as you will see the district is unmapped. The road is cut by the rivers Oli and Menai so that it is only passable from February until May. Anyway it depends of course on what Mr. Angus says but it would be rather fun to go. Think of the photos one could take!*

I do hope you will have a very Happy Christmas with warm weather and not too much work. Love, David,

Sunday, 28.12.52

It is Sunday morning, Christmas is over but has many happy memories and we are all in need of a rest! Thank you very much indeed for the lovely dispatch case that you sent me via the Rowlands. It is a super one. I opened it on Christmas morning and had a lovely surprise- it is magnificent. The lamp stand too is very nice and just what is required a most useful gift, and the cake is of course also lovely.

I was glad to hear of Stanley and his metamorphosis into a publicly minded individual. It must be quite a change! I expect he is very thrilled with his watch, one that really works. Here we have been experiencing the real harmattan with the very cold mornings (about 65f) and the very hot afternoons about 85-90f. There is a thick mist in the early morning which lasts until about 9.30 and a very heavy dew which dampens everything.

The week has been very full and busy and seems to have flown past. Last Monday Gordon and Barbara Cooper arrived about ten p.m. after a good but slow journey up. They were in good form and very pleased to come up I think.

Tuesday was a busy day medically but fortunately since then we have not had much to do, There only being one operation which was on Christmas Day. Barbara brought up a tree bear, which is about three weeks old a lovely furry little thing. It has soft paws without claws and makes a very good pet, I believe. Unfortunately the climate here did not suit it and it died three days ago, or rather it was dying and I helped it out of its misery. It was a very attractive little beast. On Tuesday, Monica Humble, (who played the piano for the services on the ship), one of the Sisters guests arrived and also John Boshier, the Pearson's guest and Dr. and Mrs. Winston of Lagos arrived as the guests of the Days, so our personnel increased rapidly. Many people dropped in for a chat and coffee that evening so we were kept busy.

Wednesday, Christmas Eve was pretty hectic, most of us thinking about the

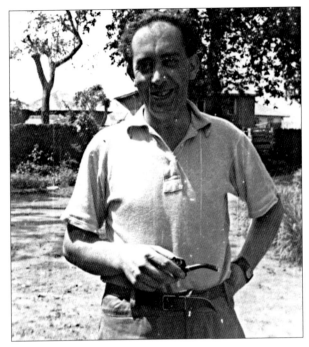

Charles Day

meals they had to prepare for the morrow. Barbara had brought up some ham in a tin and some cocktail sausages so we made many jellies and mince pies. As well as making small ones, and William made a large one and we had it for lunch today. Sure enough it arrived for the first course with chips and we had custard for sweet. We never turned a hair and ate it with relish, it makes a most unusual dish! Evidently William thought it was meat mincemeat. In the evening we went Carol Singing by the light of hurricane lamps, first round the wards and then round the leprosy village and then finally to prominent Methodists in the town. The carols were mainly in Yoruba and in between houses they sang their own lyrics to which we danced along a sort of rumba step, which is the foundation step of all their dances. The lyrics were far more interesting than the carols, more joyful and natural somehow. Anyway it was a very good though hot performance. In one house all 40 of us were invited in for drinks and biscuits - some crush. Most of the guests came too and really enjoyed, what is to them, their first glimpse of the real Africa, Lagos being so Europeanised. We were really tired when we got back having danced several miles.

On Christmas Day I was up at 5.40am and arranged the things for the Communion Service at 6.30. Mr. Day took it very nicely in our hospital chapel. After breakfast we distributed the gifts of five shillings to all the labourers on the staff, and then the guests took the ward services at ten o'clock. After this we distributed the Christmas presents to all the patients and, after a cup of coffee, to all the leprosy patients as well. It was a very happy time and all the patients enjoyed it very much indeed.

In our house we had a bran tub and during the day we put in all the gifts for the compound. Then we provided lunch for 20, ham, sausage, salad, jelly and mince pies and coffee as a sort of running buffet, Barbara Cooper helped greatly and William and Samuel did very well. After food we had the giving out of presents by Elsie - the most senior present. My gift from the others in the compound was a pair of Yoruba slippers, very nice. After the opening of the gifts some had a rest whilst the children made whoopee on my verandah. Then at four o'clock by our time, we gathered round the wireless and heard the Queen. The reception was perfect and equally as good as at home. We used a newish car battery, for the occasion. Afterwards we went en masse to the Pearsons' house for tea.

After tea the nurses did a Nativity play in the male ward which they have been learning and it went very well. After we had seen this we began getting ready for the dinner at night. We all put on our best bibs and tuckers and the ladies wore their very lovely evening dresses. The Sisters house was got up to represent a ship and we all had sailor type fancy hats. Grapefruit, soup, turkey, five vegetables, plum pudding and apricots, coffee followed by charades, a few carols, prayers and bed. A lovely day!! In the morning of Boxing Day I had to go to a village dispensary and so took many guests. It was a good trip to a lovely village in some hills fourteen miles away. In the evening the nurses gave a concert for the patients, including a dramatisation of the healing of the blind beggar at the well, which was very well done. In the evening six of us played Oh hell! Last night was the nurses party, more about it in my next. I hope you had a lovely time as we did here. Much love, David

Sunday, January 4th 1953

A Happy New Year to you all. I saw the New Year in, in the operating theatre working on a very ill man who unfortunately died later in the day.

I received your letter and card on Monday and Michael's letter yesterday.

Last Sunday afternoon we went on a picnic to the river about nine miles from here. It was rather smelly but it made a pleasant change to get away from the place. The guests were quite intrigued to be really into the bush away from civilisation as we know it in Ilesha. In the evening we had a play reading, the first of D. L. Sayers in 'Man Born to be King'. I took the part of King Herod and on the whole we had a most enjoyable time, there were fifteen of us taking part. It lasted just over an hour.

On Monday all the guests departed leaving us very quiet, but work quickly absorbed the time as we had to cope with all the patients who had waited until *after the holiday to come to the hospital.*

Tuesday was a busy day and then on Wednesday Andrew, Jean and I took our first language exam. There are four of these exams for laymen with set books and so forth. There was a two hour paper, dictation and reading. The syllabus includes memorising two benedictions and the Lords Prayer, numbers up to 100, greetings, 20 pages of a grammar book and an 80 page reading book in Yoruba which starts very simply such as 'I see a man' up to quite complex constructions. We all three passed and the report sent to Synod recommends that we are put into the next grade. Andrew and Jean got 80 per cent and I got about 60. The marking was exceptionally strict. I made the same mistake four times in the dictation and had four marks taken off. Mr. Salako, the super took the exam, though Mr. Longley of Oyo is the District language man.

New Years Eve I spent in the theatre after we had had a Watch-night Service in the prayer room taken by Mr. Day. In the morning there were one or two operations and in the afternoon we went for a picnic on the new site. Friday I had to do a caesarean on a very small hunch-backed woman who had had old tuberculosis of the spine, which had now healed but left her with a terrible deformity. The baby was not very big but it is well, I only hope that she keeps it well and looks after it. It is grim the way the babies die as soon as they are taken out of the hospital, due to lack of cleanliness and knowledge in artificial feeding.

On Friday afternoon there was an antenatal clinic followed in the evening by a staff committee. Am keeping very fit. Much love, David

Sunday, 11th January 1953

I have just been interviewed by two members of the Nigerian C.I.D. about a post mortem I performed sometime ago. They now want to know if it could have been murder. A very tricky point. However I have stated that in my opinion it could not have been so. I suppose that will be a sign for the accused to confess. Such are the thrills of being a missionary!

My Christmas presents continue to give great pleasure, especially the dispatch case which is a lovely one and has caused much envious comment here. I used it with great effect last Thursday of which more anon.

On Monday I was to go to the court according to my subpoena. I went and the Assistant Inspector of Police said that he was very sorry I had turned up and that I was not to come until I was called. The same applied to Andrew, so we got on with the days work. Our District Officer is leaving tomorrow and the new one came round last Monday and seems quite a nice chap, he has two children much the same age as the Pearsons', Michael incidentally is three today. On Tuesday Ken took the engine out of the Morris Minor and got it back the next day having adjusted the clutch plate. He is really fantastically good at his job and has settled down remarkably well and is invaluable.

Wednesday Andrew and family went to the dentist in Oshogbo in the morning, leaving me to cope with the outpatients. However Wednesday is not a bad day but next week for ten days Andrew will be in Lagos at Synod so I shall have a great deal of work to do. However no doubt we shall pull through, so long as we do not have any staff disturbances. Also on Wednesday whilst our driver was carrying a load of stone about five and a half tons, two back wheels of the lorry came off and passed him, a most frightening experience. However Ken has put in some time on it and got them back in running order again ready to start tomorrow! However he too is appearing in court at Ife to support our driver who is still on this charge for dangerous driving.

On Thursday Andrew and I were both operating and we were called to the court to give evidence on two cases of manslaughter and both together on one case of a woman, one of the wives of the Owa, assaulting three policemen. However, we waited for half an hour, and then I came away to get on with the next operation. However just as I left they called me evidently and Andrew had to say I had gone away. Consternation in Court - Inspector of police getting very flustered - policeman sent on bicycle to fetch me. However by that time I had completed the next operation so when I returned to the court I gave my evidence, and everything in the garden was lovely. Unfortunately I have to go again tomorrow for the second case.

On Thursday Ken went to Ibadan to see if he could get some parts for the lorry wheel. He was not successful but had a good day otherwise getting us some much needed custard powder and a few potatoes to see us on until our supply comes from the north.

Friday was a busy day with many outpatients in the morning and large antenatal clinic in the afternoon. However a supply of instruments and things came from England in large parcels so we had fun opening these.

Saturday, yesterday, was busy with eleven operations in the morning. Andrew had an emergency at six and then I carried on with a hernia. Andrew followed with another hernia whilst I did six abscesses. We had a rest in the afternoon and then went to the new site to see how things are progressing there. Things are going quite well but there is a great deal still to do.

Keeping very fit, much love, David

Sunday, January 18th 1953

I hope all is well at home. We have been consulted by the nurses, who would like some pen friends in England. Thus we are each asking our churches at home to see if there are any girls of secondary school age who would like to correspond. If you can find any at Rivercourt would you send the names and addresses to me and I will choose one of the nurses who would like to write. We require 30 altogether.

This week has been pretty hectic, as Andrew went away last Tuesday. Last Sunday evening Jean was preaching at Otapete and it pretty well knocked her up so that she was in bed for the whole of Monday and part of Tuesday but is now quite well again. On Monday we had a visit from the District Officer who brought round a man from the Education department to look at our old buildings to see if they would be suitable for a Teacher Training College. It is good to have this enquiry because it will give us a lever over the local Methodists who want to purchase but do not think will be able to raise the £10,000 we are asking. I was up four times that night, on one occasion, having to admit a patient from the hospital at Ife. She was a maternity case, as they did not have a Doctor in that night. A Cockney Sister brought in the patient. The Sister, has picked up the American intonation from her colleagues who are all American. Her letter began 'Sorry Folks, No Doctor on board' and continued in that vein all through. It was not particularly funny at 4am. The patient had a normal delivery next day, so I wrote a very polite and professional letter back just to show how it should be done!

On Tuesday Charles and Margaret Day wanted to see the Owa and as Andrew was busy I rang up and took them along. It was much the same palaver as it was when I was introduced, except that it went on much longer. Andrew left in the afternoon for Ibadan where he was attending a committee of Mission and Government doctors to discuss affairs between them, such as free treatment for under eighteens. He was to go down to Lagos on Wednesday and broadcast the ten-minute religious service at ten to seven. We listened on my wireless and though reception was poor we could hear his voice though it did not sound like him at all. He did it again on Friday and we heard perfectly having rigged up a stronger battery and new earth.

On Wednesday a Plymouth Brother named Ross blew in and stayed with us for the night. He is an American and on his way to the East. He told us many stories of big game he had shot and all his most marvellous equipment. Obviously no shortage of money there. For some reason I slept very badly that night and woke tired however the day passed without undue incident, except for a manual removal in a shocked woman in the evening. At about nine o'clock three missionaries of the Church Missionary Society turned up unannounced, and asked to stay the night. We put up the Rev. Ross and Jean put up the two women, one a Sister and one a Doctor. We had to rustle up a meal by opening tins but it was very good. A late night, therefore. It was a frightful night, as I had to get up four times and also do a manual removal of the placenta. The day was hectic but is over now thank goodness. It is the busiest day of the week.

We had a letter that day from the man whose lorry our driver ran into. He is suing us for £262. A bit of a headache. I rang up Andrew in the evening to find out about the Medical Synod committee but he was very tired and could not marshal an answer. He said he would drop a note however. Friday night was grand, eight and a half hours sound sleep. Yesterday was busy with outpatients and two difficult obstetric cases. One operation was a hernia on a two and a half year old boy, a very pleasant and restful change from my usual work! Am keeping very fit but will welcome Andrews return!

Much love, David

PS. Could you send out 'Forensic Medicine' by Simpson and 'Medical Psychology' by Fred Gold from my bookshelves.

January 26th 1953

Here my fortnight of overwork is at an end and it has been quite enjoyable, to have been acting Superintendent for this time. Things have gone smoothly and work has not been excessive though it has been busy.

Last Sunday was quiet but on Monday I had a visit from the barrister who was defending a patient I had seen in the hospital and about whom I had to give evidence. He came to warn me that I would be cross - examined, which didn't increase my sense of well-being. Anyway I rushed through the work and then waited for the phone call to go to court. It never came however, so I had waited all this time to no avail. The rest of the day passed uneventfully.

Tuesday much the same happened but eventually the call came and I went to the court where I remained for about two hours. I gave my evidence and had a difference of opinion with the barrister and raised the odd laugh, which was immediately silenced by the many police there with the cry of 'order in court.' On the whole it was a very amusing experience. At one point the defendant, whilst I was speaking, tried to butt in and say something but was dragged back by the police and silenced. On reflection it was quite fun though at the time not so funny. I rather fear that there may be many such incidents to face because we are getting a great number of people to examine for the police.

Friday was very busy with a large outpatient number as judged by the fact that I took £27 in outpatient fees in the morning and £10 in the afternoon at the antenatal clinic.

Andrew returned at 6.45pm having had a good ride up and after my evening lecture I went across with Ken to coffee after chop and heard all the news.(I must just go up to the ward where a new patient has just come in). Evidently the medical committee was pretty stormy, and a new ceiling was fixed of £60,000 for the new hospital, which really means that we have to sell these present buildings as soon as possible. We went to the D.O. yesterday and he didn't seem too hopeful about it. He says the central government fund is too pushed to be able to produce the money so really the outlook is not too good unless we can find someone who has the money to put down on the nail as they purchase it. The local Methodist Church has no possibility of buying it.

Another item that came out of the Missionary meeting, was that it recommends that there is a rise of salary in this District - £50 married couples and £30 for single people. This would be very useful, if it was agreed by the Mission House. Mr. Angus has been elected chairman for the coming year 53/54 though he was run close by Mr. Mellor who would I am sure, be most unsatisfactory as chairman as he is too stuck in the past. He will be retiring soon.

Yesterday we got through some accumulated correspondence in the office and I did the accounts, which balance exactly again for the third week running. We have a balance of about £1500 in the safe at the moment. In the evening Andrew and Jean came round for chop and we played a game afterwards - a very pleasant evening.

The weather is warming up for the middle of the dry season. It is nearly ten weeks now since we had any rain, and the grass is brown and the ground very dusty. Last Tuesday the temperature in the sun was 117 degrees F which is warmish if you have to do much walking about, it does not encourage one to hurry. If I go to sleep after lunch as we sometimes have the opportunity of doing the perspiration pours off and one wakes, soaking wet. However despite these drawbacks it is very pleasant though occasionally one wishes that it was cool enough to have to get warm when getting into bed instead of not having any clothes at all.

Am keeping very fit and well. Furloughs will have to be changed again as we cannot move into the new buildings until October. Andrew thinks I may be coming home first after all, but we shall have to see rather than raise any false hopes.

Much love to you all, David

Sunday, 1.2.53

One thing will be immediately obvious and that is that I have a new typewriter ribbon in, and the second may become so that occasional patches of oil appear in the print.

Incidentally I am not sure if my note on one of the letters was legible. It was a request for Treadgold's Textbook of Medical Psychiatry and Simpson's book of Forensic medicine to be sent out, as there seems to be quite a bit of both!

My Birthday last Monday was spent in the common round and daily task, though I had a restful afternoon for the most part. Your telegram of greeting arrived at four o'clock and as I gather it was sent that morning, though early, it was very good indeed. Jean made me some peppermint creams, which she sent over at breakfast time, which were very delicious.

Monday, besides being my birthday was otherwise routine except that at four o'clock I had to go to the D.O.'s Office and certify a man who had gone quite mad. He was irrational and manic. I wrote out that I thought he should be detained for further observation and he was put in a cell for the night. Next morning the attacks were over and he was able to go home to the relief of us all. The affair has blown over now though it was unpleasant whilst it lasted. I have never travelled in a car with a manic before.

Tuesday was much as usual except that a very seriously injured man came in and we had to operate in the evening. I gave the anaesthetic and Andrew patched him up. He lasted for a further 24 hours and then died unfortunately.

Wednesday too was much as usual. I have a gynaecological clinic now on these mornings and it seems to get larger each week. However it all means more revenue so we do not grumble. In the evening we went to chop in the Pearson's house and then spent time in prayer. Lagos then rang up to say that Sister Cutler had returned from furlough and would be coming up on Friday.

Thursday was a busy day - Andrew woke up with a septic finger which meant he could not do any operating, but instead he went to Oshogbo to take one of our nurses to the dentist.

I had to do a removal of ovarian cyst, a large hernia, two D&C's, and various odd things, and finally remove half of Andrews nail under local. It hurt me as much as it hurt him, I think. It is most unpleasant to have to operate on one's friends. I finished all these operations at one o'clock having started at eight, which was very good going. In the afternoon Andrew, James (dispenser) Margaret and I cleared out the dispensary as we are sailing very near the wind with it at the moment. We took out all the dangerous drugs, which should not be there and about a 100 empty bottles.

During Thursday night a strangulated hernia came in which I had to get up for because Andrew's finger prevented him doing it, though as he was on duty. It went quite well on the whole I think the patient is OK now, but I haven't seen him since. Jonah, from Ifaki, came in to chop on Friday and we heard yet another angle on Synod. He is a most likable man, most sympathetic. The back axle of the lorry broke again, so Ken went to Akure to get another yesterday.

Yesterday I had another full day operating doing a transplantation of a ureter for the first time. It took me two hours. I then had another hernia and a tumour of the parotid. Quite enough! After this we had the male staff to pay, which took us until three. Last night the Pearsons' came in to chop. Lovely food. Real crackling on pork!

I am keeping very fit. The cat is having kittens I think, somewhere. Love David.

Sunday 8/2/53

Another week has swept by and Sunday morning is here again. I have just finished a round of my patients with Sister Gregory, and because maternity was busy, supervised a delivery by one of the pupil midwives for her book.

The days have not been too hectic but on Wednesday afternoon we went up to the new site en masse and planned the entrance to it. At the moment it is all scrub, so we took up a machete and mallet and drove stakes into the ground to mark the limit of our drive, gate, and then we designed a roundabout outside for the heavy traffic. We have been in touch with the local road committee of the N.A. and they have agreed to tar the road to the new site from the present main road to the Hospital. It cost £1000 per mile and it is about 8/10ths of a mile .We have a slight hope too, that they will tar part of the road inside the site too. In addition we thought over the water again and have decided to buy a 10,000 gallon tank which we shall raise up fourteen feet and will hold two days supply of water. It sounds a big tank but we shall need it. It will be filled from our wells primarily and topped up by the town water supply when it arrives which should be in six months time.

Last Sunday evening Andrew and I went to see Mr. Fadahunsi who is one of the leaders in the Western Region and is in the Western House of Assembly, the equivalent of our parliament. He says that it is pretty essential that the place here is evacuated by September so that the place can be renovated by the authorities if they are going to purchase it for educational purposes. This then would fix the date of moving more accurately - if it can be ready in time. Harry Jobling has been up for a few days this week and has got on well with the foundations of the Sister's house and has begun the foundations of my house. They have started to build Andrews now, so it looks as though things are moving more quickly again.

Mrs. Salako, the minister's wife has just come in to have a baby. The head is still rather high even though she has had four before, so I am not frightfully happy about it, and will be glad when she has been delivered. She is not really in labour yet. I also have another woman who is, I fear, going to die. She has pushed herself into a frightful mess, and on top has taken native medicine,b which is pretty poisonous and is very ill at the moment. I am trying to keep her alive but I fear there is little hope.

Andrew is preaching tonight at church but it is my turn to stay in at night, so I shall not be able to hear him. He spoke very well over the wireless during Synod and no doubt Ken will let me know how it goes. I will leave a little place to put in a plan of my house now started. It is a bungalow of course.

Much love, David

Sunday, 15th Feb., 1953

It was very nice to receive two letters from you this week and to hear that all is well at home, though the floods seem to have been pretty bad from what we read in the paper and what we have heard on the wireless. By now I should think the worst is over but there must be many thousands of people who have lost goods and money over it. A fund has been started in Lagos for British Relief which is most interesting.

Andrew and I have both exposed one reel of film, which together make a picture of the hospital and the work we do. We shall have them made into little slides and then let the Mission House have them for deputation purposes

During the night Andrew delivered a woman, as he was on duty, but unfortunately the baby was dead and the woman died the next day. She had a ruptured uterus.

On Tuesday we received a telegram from the Education Department saying that they were coming to look at our premises with a view to purchase of same. This was very encouraging but it meant that Andrew could not go on trek to Ifaki and Ikole as planned so I had to do it.

Thus on Wednesday I set out and called at a village called Ijeda which had written to say that they wanted a dispensary, to which we replied that the doctor would call to see any patients and assess the need. I was greeted by the chief and his court and then had to see 75 patients and afterwards dispense all the medicine. This made it difficult to get to Ifaki on time. As I left they presented me with two hens, one of which we ate the other day, a very tough bird even for here.

I had lunch with Jonah at the Ifaki college and then saw the patients there - 37 altogether. In the evening Jonah asked me to see some of his students to certify that they were fit for training. On the whole a busy day as I drove myself, 70 miles along roads that at home we would call cart tracks, with grass down the centre in places and where to meet or pass anything is a major driving manoeuvre.

I stayed the night at Ifaki and then went on to Ikole the next day and saw Sister Trott who is gong on furlough, shortly. She is thinking of going across the desert in the bus service, to Algiers and then boat to Marseille and then train to the Channel and so home. Several missionaries have done it and say how interesting it is, though one has to take food for ten days in the bus and cook your own at the stops. Nights are spent at oases and foreign legion posts. Ken and I are considering it!!! On my way home from Ikole I went to Ado Ekiti (see map) which is south of the usual road and called at the Church Missionary Society school there which is run by Donald Mason, a very charming man. They gave me tea and invited me down for a night anytime if I wanted a change. It has a most glorious view, that is, you can see forested hills in the distance.

Friday was a busy day with the usual clinics and so on. In the evening I gave a medical lecture, the second out of 24 to the second year, and just afterwards it began to rain, the first we have seen for three months! It made the ground damp and there was a wonderful smell of earth. They say that there will not be any more for a little while. Yesterday I operated for five hours continuously, patients well.

On Tuesday I go north with the Chairman for ten days so my next letter will be late without cause for alarm. I shall write it whilst away but post it on my return. Am very fit, Love David

Sunday, 22nd February 1953

I am writing this on a very bush table by the light of a lantern under the stars, some hundreds of miles from Ilesha. I am going to ask the Chairman to take this letter down to Lagos when we return so that it is not too late, though I expect it will be considerably later than usual this week.

Monday was much as usual except that I spent most of the afternoon preparing my things.

On Tuesday I did the routine work of the morning and then after lunch William and I set off for Afon, in the Standard Vanguard. We packed in camp bed, nets, drugs and my revelation case and quite heavily laden made good time to Afon where we were warmly welcomed by Raymond Rowland. (I am afraid it will be badly typed but conditions are not very good). Daisy Rowland has just had a baby and my projected date of arrival was most accurate whilst the doctor in the Lagos hospital was well out, so my credibility in that line is high at the moment.

On Wednesday I did the clinic in the morning and then had a rest in the afternoon as well as helping Raymond to service his car in preparation. About 4.30 the Chairman – Mr. Angus arrived with a driver and steward and learned that he had to leave the fourth member of the committee because his wife is

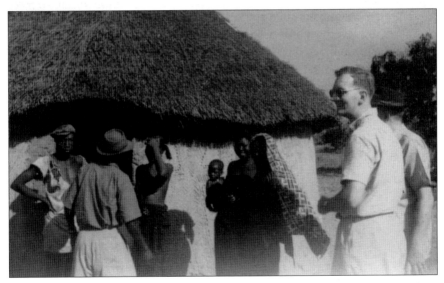

Raymond Rowland

seriously ill and so he could not leave Ibadan.

We had an interesting talk in the evening about missionary work and I brought him up to date with the work of the hospital. It had been arranged that if the fourth member had arrived he and I were to share a bed, but it worked out very well and I stuck to my divan bed in the sitting room.

Early on Thursday morning we packed up the two cars and set off. I drove the Chairman and William and Ali, the Chairman's steward. The two house boys come from the same tribe as the catechist at Afon who went in Ray's car so they have all got on very well together fortunately.

We drove to Ilorin where we filled up with petrol and took 30 gallons in tins because this was the last place we could purchase it. The road was very good to Kaiama, our first destination 126 miles away. Part of the way was through the Mushi forest which is a game reserve and is full of wild beasts, though as we went through at mid-day they were all asleep. It is most unwise to stay the night by the roadside. The character of the houses alters as we get further north. Here they are round with grass roofs, the walls being made of mud. In Yoruba land the houses are rectangular.

We went to the Rest House which is built in the same style, one large circular room, with a verandah round the outside, a smaller edition as the kitchen and bathroom. The only furniture was a chair and table. However we had two camp stools with us as well as full kitchen equipment so all was well. We saw the

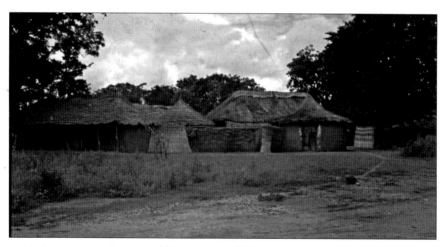

Kaiama round houses

Assistant District Officer who has a very lonely job here being the only white man in the district. He invited us round to chop in the evening that we gratefully accepted. He enjoyed having someone to talk to I think.

In the evening we returned to our camp beds arranged in the large circular room and after ablutions and prayers retired to bed.

The next morning we went to the village and after a short service in the school I saw some patients and ministered to 35 of them. They had the usual minor illnesses.

After midday meal we set off for Wawa, a very nice village. It has a very

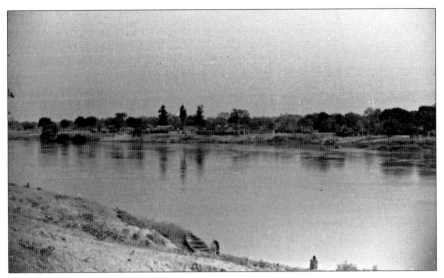

River Niger

progressive District Head who, speaks English. He has got his village well planned out and has planted some small trees which are just growing. It has a wall round it, a relic of the end of the last century, which is most interesting. Here the rest house was much the same though much smaller. The night was very warm so we slept out of doors under our nets. The cook, William and the steward did very well considering that all they have is an open fire, a few fire bricks and for baking a kerosene tin. Pots and pans and cutlery we brought with us. After looking round the village the next morning, we went to a small village on the banks of the Niger, where I got my first glimpse of that great river, which at that point is about half a mile wide.

The people in these parts have bows and arrows and spears and I bought a bow and three poisoned arrows in a quiver of bamboo for 2/6d from one of them, so I shall have some relics to show when I return to Ilesha. Whether I shall be able to get them home I don't know, I am trying to buy a spear but I don't know whether I shall be successful. In the afternoon of Saturday we came on to Bussa another town on the river, not a very nice place. The rest house is broken here so Ray was fixed up at the Mission Compound and Mr. Angus and I in the Emir's palace. This was a bit disturbing to think that we were to be separated but without causing great offense we could not get out of it. Anyway we are still OK!

Will continue in my next. Love, David

24th now at Afon

It was good to get home on Wednesday morning after a very good and safe trip.

If I remember rightly I finished the last letter at Bussa where Mr. Angus and I were in the Emirs palace trying to sleep. Although it sounds very fine it is not so really and it is just a glorified mud house such as we slept in the whole time, except that it had some reception rooms. It was exceptionally hot even for Africa, and neither the Chairman nor I slept very well, certainly he woke early.

On the Sunday morning we had a small service in the grass and bamboo church and then motored the 45 miles north to Agwarra over a very poor sort of path that could hardly be called a road. However we got there slowly and safely, and found the mud rest house on a hill overlooking the Niger and it turned out to be quite cool though Ray and I slept out of doors. There was no furniture in it so we had to rely on the camp stools. Throughout this part of the trek, for water, we went down to the Niger got a bucket full, boiled it and then drank it. Sometimes it was thin mud, sometimes thick. We all kept surprisingly well and suffered no ill effects beyond a few bites from insects. William managed very well under difficult conditions, having to cook in the open with an old kerosene tin as an oven. However he managed baked custard, roast chicken - very tough- and so on. His omelets were especially good

On the Monday we returned to Bussa and then on Tuesday the long 196 miles trip to Afon. I came back to Ilesha early the next morning arriving at 10.30. Here I found that Andrew had had an attack of malaria and had not been too well. However he is better now and back on form. He was glad to see me back! Ken had been to Ifaki to install a deep well pump for Jonah and he only arrived back this morning. He has had a good time and got the pump working.

Work here is very heavy again, we had a long day in theatre yesterday and expect a long one tomorrow (I am actually writing this on Friday night). One of the Sisters from Uzuakoli is staying with the Pearsons', a Miss Robinson, who was out in China previously as were Andrew and Jean.

From the trip we made we feel that there is no point in attempting any medical work up there of any magnitude. The shortage of staff, and the difficulty of supervision so far from Ilesha make it impossible to entertain the idea, though I fear that Ray will be disappointed, as he had thought that he and his wife might go up. However the Chairman wants him to continue at his language and get Afon on its feet rather than go on extending into new parts that we cannot cover properly. Dr. and Rev. Ludlow of course, pioneered this area but they did not, in any place they were in, do any consolidation and there is little left of their work. Afon, where they were for their latter time is only just on its feet and the medical work has to be subsidised rather heavily. This I have submitted in a report to the Chairman, which he will receive on Monday if all is well.

Much love; David

Sunday, 8th March 1953
This week here has been remarkable only for the illness of Andrew, (Monday to Thursday) and Ken (Thursday to Saturday) but they are both now better and back at work. As you will see it has been rather heavy for me but not unduly so.

Last Sunday was rather hectic with two difficult maternity cases. In the afternoon I wrote to Bob Cundall and in the evening went to the Yoruba service. There was no sing-song as a girl came in with Status Epilepticus which took a bit of stopping. However she is well now and full of beans. She is one of the pupils from our Methodist Girls School in the town here.

The kittens by the way are most attractive just now playing together. I have christened them Toboggan and Sledge, as their mother is Snowball.

Recently we were discussing flowers and vegetables. All the seeds which we have had so far, have either been used or gone off as they do not keep out here in the moist heat even if they are not opened. They ought really to be kept in a fridge I think and we will try to do so this time. In addition we have been wondering if we could grow some of those white and blue flowers for the Coronation, and put them in the form of a scheme with ER in it or something of that nature. Anyway I shall order a small quantity of alyssum, lobelia and petunias. I don't know if they will remain small, probably not but it is worth trying. In addition I am ordering small quantities of some vegetables, but only the ones which I know will grow out here. Unfortunately our enclosed garden bamboo fence has come down but the garden boys will soon have it up again.

On Tuesday night I had a difficult hernia to operate upon which had strangulated. Twelve feet of the bowel were gangrenous and unfortunately the man died three days later.

On the new site the work is going well and Andrew's house has the roof on. I personally am not very struck on the design and I think that now they have seen

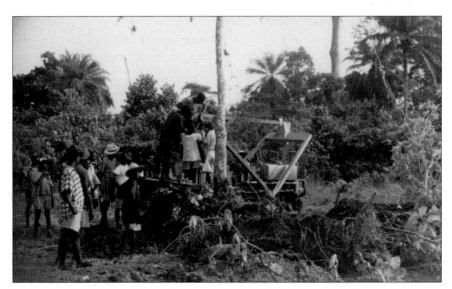

Ken with bulldozer

it they are not too pleased with it. It is a long house and more complicated than mine, which is simple and straight forward. The French windows for mine have come but it looks as if the others will have to be wooden rather than steel framed as we had hoped as we have run out of the steel kind.

Yesterday we had a visit from a Doctor from the University, Ibadan, who wished to see us here and learn what the hospital was like. He and his wife are both doctors. They have three children who also came and the entire family was very nice, and he seemed quite well pleased with the place and the work done. Some aspects seemed better than at his hospital at Adeoyo.

We have had an occasional rain here, enough to start the grass going back to green though it is still very hot. Ken has got the bulldozer going and it is levelling the ground on the new site well. We hope we can keep it for some time. I hope that you are all well. I am very fit, much love, David

Sunday, 15th March 1953

.During this last week there has been a standing committee and it agreed unanimously that we should withdraw from the work in the Borgu area, as it was too far from our area, and there is a missionary society that specialises in that district. In addition it would mean putting into the area another man and about £500 pa.which we have not got. It will be a blow to the Ludlows but their work as you say was spectacular rather than solid.

We have heard that the Philipson Grant has arrived at the treasury Oshogbo - so one or other of us has to go with a suitcase and bring back £3,100, which we shall have to stow away somewhere, I suppose, rather a responsibility. This grant is from the government to mission hospitals to enable them to raise the salaries of nurses, and lower fees. However with our rebuilding scheme we shall have to give the building fund £2000 to start with, which makes rather a hole in it. The rest we shall have to spend on equipment, new beds, and so forth for the new hospital.

The week has been rather busy as Andrew and family went away Wednesday morning and have not returned. It is the Ikole trek and they were going to have one or two extra days and return last night. However they have not turned up so perhaps Sister Trott has persuaded them to stay over the weekend. Communication is very difficult as a telegram takes a week to get through.

On Monday evening I went up to see how my house is getting on. The walls were up to window level and the windows in place. I have two windows in the living room and one in the large bedroom, which look very well. I much prefer the design to that of Andrew's house, as do other people I think. Theirs is a real hotch potch, whilst mine, though smaller, is much cheaper and simpler. I discussed and designed some built in wardrobes which will be fitted later. In addition I am having a small dining table which enlarges, some small book shelves made to measure for the corners and a low table for the wireless. In addition I am going to have all the beds (two) made lower so that they are more of a divan type, and do not look so big in a small room. I think that Ken and I will be going up there to live in May when the Wrights come out as there will be no other house for them to live in.

It will be most convenient for Ken but not for me. I shall have a bed down here also so that I shall be able to sleep here during my week of night duty. Otherwise it will be rather fun to have a new house! I am also thinking of having new curtains when I see what colour the walls are going to be. I have £10 of last years housing allowance left and shall have £27 this year which will cover everything well, as furniture and cloth out here are quite cheap. Jean is, I think, quite envious that we shall be able to get settled before the move. I should like my pictures sent out too. I am gong to have a picture rail put round the rooms, something that is quite lacking in the houses I have been in so far. I will think out how to get them out, but I should think that it would be good if someone who is coming out could put them in their luggage. Enid Blake for instance, or our new Sister if she is coming out first.

On Tuesday our order from Allen and Hanbury's came, in five large crates, which would not go in our office. I had to unpack them outside and take the stuff in by hand. It has all arrived except three pairs of scissors.

On Friday afternoon amidst much work, as Friday is our heaviest day, I had to interview a man for the post of dispenser here. He seemed a good man who has had 11 years experience in the army. He has said that he will start on the first of next month but out here one has to wait to see if he comes.

Yesterday was a usual sort of day, except that we expected Andrew back and he didn't arrive. I only hope he has not got stuck on one of the more remote bits of road which do not have much traffic.

Mr. Ajayi of Ifaki, who was at the International House, London, has just bought a car. With his added experience in England he will be getting now between £500 and £800 p.a. which is very good. The salaries of teachers and lecturers here is out of proportion with the labourers who get between £3 to £10 per month. Mr. Ajanaku, the lorry and bus king of is said to have income of about £10,000 per month according to the District Officer. That is a bit of a shock as he could easily solve our financial problems for us without difficulty. I fear that with such great disparity in income, with corruption as rife as it is, that when 1956 comes, to which they all look forward as a golden year of liberation, it will bring with it much misery and poverty. Despite the many problems we face I am still very fit, much love, David

Sunday, 22nd March 1953

I was most interested to hear of the talk of the Nigerian on Christianity in Nigeria. A lot he said is true but no one would say that Nigeria, before the coming of

Christianity, was not pagan, it most certainly was and in some places still is.

This week has been one of interest and tragedy. On Saturday night last our hospital washman came in with severe abdominal pain having been at work in the morning. I watched him carefully over Sunday and last Monday decided that I had to look inside so opened his abdomen. Just as I started Andrew returned from his break so we finished together. The patient had a perforated typhoid ulcer and died two days later. This event greatly upset the compound, quite naturally, because he had been at work on the Saturday morning apparently quite well. He must have had typhoid for three weeks.

On Wednesday evening Andrew began to feel unwell and by next morning he was feverish and he is still in bed. His temperature is down this morning for the first time and I wonder if he has not got typhoid, which is largely suppressed by the injection of TAB, which we all have before coming out. Anyway I am treating him for it and he is much better this morning, though it will be some days before he is up again. This has meant that I have had a lot to do again, but despite the heavy work I am very fit and keeping very cheerful.

On Tuesday Andrew and I went to Oshogbo to get the grant but after a lot of humming and hawing only got a cheque and we still haven't cashed it, as we haven't got a bank account here. We are thinking of opening one.

Thursday was a busy morning in theatre, as I had to do all the surgery. I did three hernias before the break for coffee at 11.15am which was good going as I only started at 9am afterwards there were three other cases so I felt to have done a good mornings work. On Friday I had a great deal to do with outpatients and the injection clinic but managed to get the work done. In the evening I had to take the nurses class! This was followed by chop with the Sisters. By the time bedtime came I was very tired but fortunately had a good night with only one interruption.

Yesterday I operated again in the morning and did the accounts in the afternoon. Just as I was getting down to them the District Officer limped down the drive having had a serious car accident 30 miles away and he had just been brought in. I patched him up and admitted his clerk, saw to the District Engineer and the chairman of the NA who were also in the car and then balanced the accounts at £1700.

Also yesterday was the big sports event of the year so I took Jean and the children for a couple of hours at four o'clock. It was most interesting, especially the pole vault. At one point a man, very well dressed, pranced in front of the spot where the District Officer and all the Europeans were sitting, followed closely by three young and beautiful wives all dressed identically. Many amused glances on our faces!

Much love to all, David

Palm Sunday, 29th March 1953
Here the work has been very heavy as Andrew has been in hospital in Ibadan for the week with amoebic hepatitis, and is not likely to be out before next weekend

and after that there will have to be a period of convalescence. However the work here should be easier next weekend being Easter and the Hospital closed as far as outpatients are concerned on Friday and Monday. I shall be very glad when he is back again, needless to say. Jean has not been too well the last few days and I have had to attend to her, but she is a bit better today. She hasn't had to go to bed but has had vague pain in the stomach.

On Monday last I was called to see Mr.Passman - a gold miner who lives on the hill just outside the town. It is a lovely situation, cool with a magnificent view. I sent some medicine up and find he is much better when he called in at the hospital to see me yesterday.

On Tuesday the Rev Arthur Banks from Gold Coast came to stay for two days as he is touring the West Africa District in preparation for a literature job at the Mission House. He stayed here as Ken was not back from his stay at Abeokuta and was a very pleasant guest indeed. He is interesting to talk to having been there for seventeen years. His wife and family are in the Missionary guest flats at Selly Oak though I didn't meet her whilst I was there so far as I know.

Andrew went down to Ibadan by car on Monday morning and on Wednesday Ken returned from his week end at Abeokuta having had an enjoyable and useful time with the Joblings putting several of their machines in order.

On Wednesday I learned that there is a further 1,000 bags of cement in the lagoon at Lagos and we wanted another certificate from the provisional engineer to get it duty free. This meant that we had to send in one of our men to see him, but he got it without difficulty. He saw Andrew too who was looking better and putting on weight. He quite enjoys the rest and the food I think though he does not like being in bed.

Friday was as hectic as usual with a vast number of patients and injections to see and give. However it passed off successfully and without untoward incident.

Yesterday was busy as I had to fit in a visit to the local treasury to get our grant from the NA towards the upkeep of three leprosy patients in our village. However it did not take as long as I expected and there was no difficulty. I did the odd hernia in the morning as well as the odds and ends. In the afternoon we went up to the new site where I found work on my new house progressing, they are plastering it now and Ken is fixing up the rainwater tank. Water is being laid on too, to the roof tank being put up so it will be well equipped. I am beginning to think about furniture and whether to have curtains by the French windows. It is really rather fun having a house to furnish using all the old furniture we can of course but remodelling it to fit the much smaller surroundings.

When we returned I found a patient with a strangulated hernia waiting so I had to set too and operate at eight o'clock despite the fact that I had the Joblings and Jean round to chop. However Ken kept them amused during my absence.

This afternoon the Rowlands from Afon are coming to have their baby circumcised. . I am very sorry that Andrew is away as I am not keen on the operation though I have done quite a number. We are all surprised that they are travelling on Sunday, but I suppose it cannot be helped. Tomorrow Jean and the children are going to Ibadan to stay until Andrew is able to come out, and will get some shopping and so forth done. It will make the compound feel empty as Margaret G is going down to Lagos too for a short break before going up to Ikole to take over there. We are both keeping very well despite the work. The rains have started and it is cooler, the earth being green again.

Much love, David

Easter Sunday, 5.4.53
I don't know whether you have read of the resignation of some of the ministers of the Nigerian Government during the last week? There has been rather a lot of unpleasantness in the papers about it and the Government has had to broadcast in an attempt to put matters straight. There is quite a bit of anti-British sentiment expressed in the Daily Times, the big paper of Nigeria, some of it written by a lecturer of Ibadan University. Elsie, who as you know has been here for 23 years has not known anything like it in the past.

Andrew is still away though he is out of hospital now. Unfortunately Jean and the children, who went down to join him last Monday are themselves ill, and when I rang up on Friday last Andrew was wondering if he should not put them into hospital if they did not improve. It is very difficult for them as they were staying for a night or two with a high government official, the Deputy Director of Medical Services for the Western Region when they became ill in their house, which I gather is not adapted for such emergencies. He was hoping that he might get back tomorrow, but I shall find out when I ring this evening. As you can imagine work is rather hard just now, as Andrew has done only three days in the hospital during the last month. However, if all is well he should be back soon and take his share of the work again. Throughout it all though I have kept very fit and on top of it all, though last night when I had to get up for an emergency maternity case I felt very tired and not much like rising.

We only have two sisters here at the moment as Margaret G is having a week in Lagos and then she is going to relieve Louie Trott at Ikole during her furlough.

By the way would you tell the girl who sends my BRF notes that she has sent Jan-March instead of April/June.

I wasn't looking forward very much to pay day but it passed off without any untoward disturbances except that Augustus, the carpenter asked for a rise. He is a hopeless chap who we only keep on because he is a staunch member of the Methodist Church, so I told him he must first show that he can work harder, and produce better work. The only effect it has had, is to give him an attack of fever which has taken him off work completely!

My house progresses, they are now plastering the walls outside and in, and have got the floor down in the bathroom ready to for the basin and bath. It begins to look very well, though the next task is to plant about an acre of grass in front of this house and the Pearson's which is next door so that we look out onto what will be lawns in the future. However, it is a frightful task but one which must be attempted if we are going to have pleasant surroundings to the house.

On Good Friday afternoon Ken and I felt in need of a change so in the terrific heat we climbed to the top of the local hill, which is called Mount Imor. The first half is easy but towards the top it is untamed bush which we had to fight through to reach the summit. There was no view because of the thick forest on the top, but from the way down we looked way over Ilesha, very nice indeed. This evening we are going out to supper with the Principal of the Women's Training College, which will be a pleasant change. Love, David.

Sunday, April 12th 1953

Sorry to hear of the coal shortage. I hope it has been resolved now, and warmth once more permeates the Cannon household. It would be rather nice if I could send some from here, as it is the hottest part of the year. The temperature rises up to 90 odd in the afternoons, though mornings at seven are really delightful. In the afternoon we do as little as possible and rest from lunchtime at 1.30 till 3.30 unless called to the wards.

Andrew returned from Ibadan last Monday but he still is very jaundiced and is not fit to work. He did a little on Friday last, and hopes to do more next week, but again I have had to undertake most of it. I have been on night duty now for over a month which is heavy going. However despite the extra work I am very fit and well, though as soon as Andrew is really fit I shall take a few days off and get away from the place, as I am really weary with medicine temporarily!! Unfortunately Jean has been in bed during the last week and the children have had fever off and on. I think that the whole family has had infective hepatitis, an unpleasant disorder in which one feels very unwell and have no appetite at all.

It was good to get a letter from the branch of the family in the West Indies and to hear that they are all well.

Soon I suppose Michael will be going up to Oxford for the final term, and all too soon finals will be upon him. Stanley too will be going back and soon have finished his first year, which seems very soon, though it will soon be the year that I have been here.

Dr. Wright is due out in May, coming out on the same boat as I did I think, at the same time anyway, and we are all looking forward to his advent. He has two children and another due in July. It looks as if the hospital will not be ready before the end of the year so Andrew will probably be coming home in December, before Christmas I think. We shall then move into the new hospital and then I shall come home as will Ken, I expect in the early part of next year

Last Monday evening I went to a dance in the town hall run by the District Officer's wife in aid of the library. Margaret Ingham wanted to go so I went with her. The Pearsons' went to bed at seven. It was an odd do, with the well-to-do Nigerians in immaculate evening dress, people like myself in not too immaculate lounge suits and then the other Nigerians in native costume, a most interesting set up. We only stayed for 40 minutes, as we were both on duty! Ken fixed up an engine for them for lights and was there too for a short time. Most of the Europeans of the town turned up to show willing. The evening before, Ken and I went to dinner with the principal of the Women's Training College after evening service. We had a good time though the food was not anything out of the ordinary.

On Wednesday evening we had Fellowship in the Pearson house, and it was good to be united again in this way. On Thursday evening Harry and Nellie Jobling came in to chop and afterwards we discussed the plumbing fittings which will have to be ordered. They are sailing next Friday so this is the last time that they will be here, thus leaving all the work in our hands, especially in Ken's hands. Our house is progressing, the interior decorating is now finished and the outside being done, The verandahs were made in the last few days and set the house off well. The bath is in and the sink in the kitchen, the wall has been plugged for the basin. The locks are on all the doors and the glass being put in the windows. I am now thinking of things like towel rails and curtains. I think I shall ask Jean if she could run up a few curtains when she is better. We are going to put up railways with pelmets to finish them off. When it is completed I will photograph it from every angle and send the film home. It is now beginning to look like a house fit for habitation.

The political situation does not ease. The Action Group is determined to have self-government in 1956 even if it means the disruption of Nigeria and the Governor puts the unity of Nigeria first, hence the crisis. If there is disunity in the country it would mean that it would be broken down into its original states, about eight, not just into north and south.

Many people think that if the situation is not eased and some compromise agreed upon there will be civil war between the north and south or between the east and west or between the labouring classes and the ruling classes, but that will not be for some years I think. Hope that all is well at home, flourishing here! Much love, David.

Sunday, April 19th 1953

As a change from the usual routine I am writing this freehand, mainly because I am in bed at the moment. Not that I am ill but Andrew, who is now back to work, *suggested that a day in bed would be a 'good thing', so I am happy to acquiesce. As it happens I have a bit of a headache and slight temperature (99.) no doubt due to an attack of suppressed malaria, which comes in this way and lasts for a few hours. Otherwise I am well and enjoying the relaxation.*

Sorry to hear the Easter weekend wasn't very fine - a pity you could not have had some if not all our heat! Just now the heat is at its worst, the rains have not really started yet, just occasional storms.

Interesting that young Banks and Stanley know each other. I am glad Enid Blake will stay the night, you will find her a good speaker I think. She is a Sister Tutor of general nursing.

If Mr. Angus comes, you will find him rather brusque at first, but as you get to know him, a most fatherly and human man. His eyesight is very poor and he has contact lenses, which he wears for so many hours a day. Without them everything is blurred and he can only distinguish folk when they are close to him. With them in, his sight is good enough to drive though he doesn't. I do hope he comes I should like you to know him.

This week has had one or two incidents. On Monday afternoon I did a Caesarean section on a woman who had a Caesarean Section in 1948, in 1950 she did not come in until her uterus had ruptured, so this time I got her in before the baby was due. All went well and she has a fine baby boy. The tragedy is, that it may well die when she takes it into her mud house.

On Monday afternoon Andrew and Ken went down to Lagos to see Mr. Mann and Mr. Jobling about our new building money, which would seem to be satisfactory. They had car trouble on the way down, which delayed them. They returned on Wednesday. Andrew and his family are all much better, and are sailing August 4th which will soon come. The Wrights will be here in five weeks.

Our house is now decorated and plumbing completed except for paint in the bathroom and the window frames - in three or four weeks we shall move up. The Joblings have sailed and return in October and we now expect to move in over the Christmas holidays with our guests to help!

Much love to you all, David.

Thursday, 23.4.53

At the moment I am staying at Ifaki with Jonah having a few days rest. It is a lovely restful place, with a fine view over the forest and a very delightful compound, which looks like the playing fields of an English school. It is as you know, an elementary teachers training centre, a two year course which qualifies the boys to teach in Junior Schools.

After my day in bed on Sunday I rose refreshed on Monday and did a full days work, and then as the week seemed straight forward I decided with Andrews consent to come up here for the rest of the week, so on Tuesday morning after doing my outpatients, I packed a bag, filled a small car with petrol and set off, arriving here about two hours later, after a good run. It was marred at one point where they were mending a bridge, such as they are, and had taken all the planks off leaving a twelve foot gap in the road. However some men around put back a few planks and I went across hoping for the best.

Jonah seemed pleased to see me as he is a bit lonely I think, his wife and family being in England. Mr. Ajayi is here of course, of International House and sends his greetings. Yesterday morning he took me round some of the village schools and I took the odd photo of the children at play to the sound of their drums. I had at one school to make a short impromptu speech which was warmly cheered though I don't expect they understood very much, though of course they all learn and are taught in English.

In the afternoon I rested and then in the evening Jonah said he would show me some native shrines where folk offer their sacrifices. So in the dimness of the evening we drove to a point in the road and then went into the bush to the shrine.

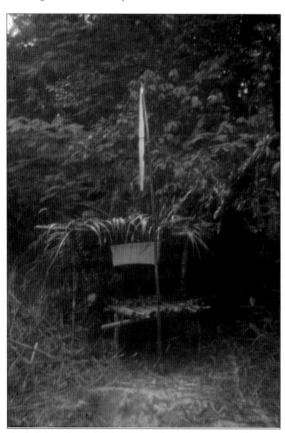

Juju Shrine

In the sort of little house there is a sacrificial slab large enough to take a human body carved with little gutters to let the blood run away and so forth. A most eerie experience especially as Jonah remarked that we should not be left long, and sure enough about three minutes later the keepers of the shrine turned up to see what we were doing. So we decided it was time we went back! We then went to the chief of the village and ask permission to go to the most important shrine in the village which is near his house. He showed it to us himself and the large speaking drums with which the villages communicate with each other. They stand about four and a half feet high and about fifteen inches in diameter. In the shrine is the holy of holies wherein no man can enter except the priests and juju men. Afterwards the chief's wives danced for us in order to get a dash (tip) which Jonah brought forth. A most interesting evening, though a trifle hard on the nerves!

This morning I set out to take a photo of the place and took Jonah's steward though he was rather reluctant. However he took me to two more in another village which again I photographed in colour so there should be some interesting exposures on this film. At one of them I found some women who were worshipping which made it all very real. There is a vast amount of this sort of thing under the surface if only we could see it, far more than we could ever imagine and when there are times of stress they go back to their own shrines. No farmer would think of using a new hoe without first offering a sacrifice to the god of iron, and if there is a shortage of water they will go to the rainmaker who commands the whole village to shut itself up for 24 hours, and it will, not allow anyone in or out.

This afternoon is the college sports, which no doubt I shall watch and then tomorrow I wish to go and see some American Baptists near here who have asked me to call when up this way. The rest and the fresh milk which I am drinking are doing me the world of good, and this glimpse into the dark part of Africa is most interesting. I will finish this at the weekend when I return.

Now back at Ilesha having had a very restful four days, and a good trip back last evening. Found the folk here well, and that Andrew had had an easy week, which was good news. He looks better though he still has to put on some weight.

In my absence the house was being finished off and I am looking forward to seeing it this afternoon. The wiring has been done and the finishing touched to the paintwork are being completed. All that remains is the built in cupboard and some furniture which has to come up from Abeokuta. We shall be living there within three weeks I suppose, as the Wrights are in this country three weeks yesterday. Jonah has suggested that I purchase a .22 rifle against odd creatures which will abound on the new site and also to deter anyone of an acquiring nature. I shall make enquiries anyway.

I have also been persuaded to coming home by air, via Rome, Geneva, Zurich, Amsterdam and London, staying a week in Rome and the odd night in the other capitals. A most interesting trip, but we shall see!

Much love, David

Sunday, 3rd May 1953

Just now you will be having the Chairman of our District with you and he no doubt will have told you of the happenings here, and of all the personalities. I hope he has been gracious to us! I shall be most interested to hear what he had to say and just how the weekend has gone.

On Monday work went much as usual, but in the afternoon Andrew and Elsie went up to a Coronation committee in the town hall. We are going to have fireworks, native dancing, tree planting, ceremonies and so forth to mark the day, and of course a Bank holiday or two. We shall listen on the wireless and make a festive occasion of it.

On Tuesday I did the work which needed to be done and then went out shopping for curtain material. Jean came too, to get some ticking for the mattress covers so we went round the many cloth shops. I found some smashing curtain material in maroon, black and white, the maroon just matching the paintwork of the outside of the house. I am having twelve pairs made up out of it and some material left over for cushion covers so that will be a real scheme. As Elsie says though, they will have to be a trifle careful what they wear when we have the housewarming party! However they all think it is rather nice so I am quite pleased. The curtains cost one and three pence to make up and the material 3/6d a yard.

On my return on Tuesday morning I had a caesarean to do which went well. In the afternoon I had a lesson with Mr. Ajayi and then the results of our last midwives exam came through. Four have passed and three failed. Rather surprising really the ones who have come down we rather expected to get through. However after a rather trying scene when they were informed they seem to have settled down again.

On Wednesday we hurried through the work in order to receive the acting Inspector General of Nigeria. He is the most senior man in the medical service of the country and is a very nice chap, Dr. Menzies. His wife came too and is, we think a South American - she had much to say about Rio. He is a Scotsman and I should think most efficient. We looked around this place first and then after lunch went up to the new site and looked round there. He seemed quite impressed, though as he says, two of the nurses lecture rooms will be rather stuffy as there is no through ventilation.

Thursday was theatre day as usual and we were busy most of the day.

My seeds that I had ordered from Suttons arrived and I got them put into seed boxes. I have paid for them by cheque, it means less trouble all round I think. I have just got beans, cabbage, cauliflower, lettuce, cucumber, radish, parsley, carrot with a few flower seeds which I am going to try, though I don't know if they will come to anything here.

Yesterday morning we had some theatre cases, but only two, so we got down to some office work and got out an order for equipment, beds trolleys and so forth, coming to about £600 but where the money is coming from I do not know. In the afternoon, Ken and I did the accounts and then went up to measure the kitchen and fit in the furniture we have. It should make quite a nice place for William to work in I think. On the 18th Ken and I are going to Lagos to meet the Wrights. We shall send the lorry down as well as they have 30 pieces of luggage! It will be some task getting it through the customs. However a trip to Lagos and the opportunity to shop will be welcome. On Wednesday this week I am off to Ikole and Andrew to Afon on Friday.

Much love, David

May 10th 1953

Another letter in longhand, this time because my left arm is sore due to TAB jab, which you will remember, makes the arm sore for a day. I had the injection last night, so by this evening it will be quite better, though at the moment it is difficult to type.

The missionary supper seems to have been a good do, certainly with good measure! Enid's sermons tend to be much the same and Mr. Angus has been known to go on for some little time! I rather think that he was distressed with John commencing the building scheme here and then retiring to work back in England.

Here the week has been a usual sort of week. The weather is a little cooler and we have had some rain, so it feels as though our winter is coming, better known as the wet season. Everything will start going mouldy again and clothes want watching carefully.

Last Sunday evening I went to service and heard Mr. Fashade, the Ilesha man who went to Travencore a most interesting sermon, it has done him the world of good to visit India. He is coming next Friday to show us some filmstrip of India and Britain.

Last Monday I cyclostyled the Pearson's Newsletter for them. They send two or three a year. I think it is too impersonal, however. Jean helped me with curtains, mending my mattress etc. so I felt it was some return I could make. On Monday evening I went to the evening class at the church and then am taking it next week.

On Tuesday we ordered some cushions for three chairs 2'x2'x5', six altogether. They have to be covered yet, but arrived yesterday. Later we bought four African mats for the floors, so gradually we are getting our furniture is accumulating. Andrew had to attend an exhumation at a village 14 miles away but the grave was filled with stones, the body had gone and possibly used for making native medicine I fear.

On Wednesday I went on trek to Ifaki but the brakes failed, all the fluid came out 15 miles from Ifaki. I drove very carefully in, with no brakes at all. I then borrowed a car to return. Ken then brought spares and fetched it back on Friday. Good old Ken! Otherwise, an uneventful trek! On Friday Andrew and family went on trek to Afon and are due back today. On Friday I had to do a post mortem, then during the night had two emergencies one a Caesarean and the other a *perforated typhoid ulcer, so I didn't get to bed till 4.30am.*

On Saturday I gave TAB to 60 of the staff in the hospital, as there are several cases of typhoid in the town. Yesterday evening, modified our beds, making them the divan type. Have done a round this morning and now about to have coffee - a great institution, though I would give a lot to have ground coffee with milk rather than Nescafe with a dash of made up milk! Am very fit except for one arm! Much love, David

Saturday, May 16th 1953

It is Saturday evening, and I have just been for a walk in the jungle close by to see if I could find any bush fowl, the African equivalent of grouse, and very good for eating. I haven't got a gun but I thought it would be fun to see if there were many about. Mr. Jobling saw some when he lived up here, but I did not see any this evening. As you may gather we are now settled in our new house though we shall move back to the compound when Andrew goes on leave in August, he, by the way is flying home as he will have such a short time.

How very fortunate you are to have the opportunity to buy seats for the Coronation. I do hope that it is fine for you, and as we listen here in Ilesha and hear the description as the procession moves down the Mall we shall all think of two Cannons sitting prominently there. I should get a camera set up for the occasion if you can. It might almost be worth putting in a colour film if possible to pick it all up. I am most impressed with colour photography. By the way I shall be acting superintendent when Andrew goes home, a solemn thought.

This week has been spent in moving all our belongings to our house on the new site it was a day later than scheduled because the stove was not fixed in. However we have been in since Wednesday and things are looking very nice. The cushion covers for the chairs were completed last night. They look very classy, toning in well with the curtains. Tonight, in about an hour's time we are having a house warming party, with the Sisters and Pearsons' in. It will be rather a squash but we shall manage. It will be interesting to see how they all like the scheme. Afterwards we are going to play Beetle if all is well, as Florence Cutler tends to frown on cards I think. Beetle will be a pleasant change anyway.

On Monday Ken and I set off for Lagos where we have a terrific amount of shopping to do, a colossal list from every member of the compound and a great number of things for the hospital. On Wednesday the Wrights come, and we are looking forward immensely to meeting them. They too, will have a lot of shopping to do as they have to equip a house.

Work has been much as usual this week. I have had two Caesareans to do, and all four main characters are well, though one has a very infected wound for some unknown cause. Our typhoid cases are decreasing fortunately. I had my second injection this afternoon and am well so far. Keeping very fit, and should have much news next week. Love David.

Saturday 24th May 1953

As you see we are now back in Ilesha having had a very good though busy week. I will answer your letter first and then deal with things in a chronological order.

Then on Monday, Ken and I set out for Lagos, with William and a nurse who we took to a hospital near Lagos for an opinion. We had a puncture a few miles out whilst Ken was driving, but we changed the wheel and when we reached Ibadan got a new tyre and inner tube. We went to the Day's at Wesley College for lunch and then I went to see the Public Works Department engineer about the Hospital plans, which he states have never been seen by the engineer at all! However he will get things put in order for us. We called in at Abeokuta at the Blaize Institute where we saw my furniture being made, and it will look lovely as it is in African walnut! It will soon be ready, and may be here at the end of next week.

We then went on to Lagos and arrived safely about 6.30 having found the nurses home in Ebute Metta on the way through the suburbs of Lagos. We stayed with Mr. and Mrs. Mann and had a good time. On Tuesday morning we went shopping and bought many things, such as scrubbing brushes, twelve boxes of soap (crates that is), baths, latrine buckets, cotton and lots of food for each household. In the afternoon we went fishing for five hours on the lagoon with Bill in his boat, a sailing boat eighteen feet overall. When we went over the bar I was sick unfortunately but soon recovered when we re-entered the lagoon. The largest fish Bill has caught in the lagoon is 168lbs. last year and he had his photo in the English papers. However we only had one bite on Ken's line. In the evening Ken and I went round to Gordon and Barbara Cooper's to chop and were two of a party of eight, and I must have been the second oldest there, being three graduated teachers, two engineers and two doctors!

On Wednesday morning we went shopping again and then in the afternoon went to meet John Wright and his family. I had a pass to get onto the boat and helped them down to the customs shed. Mrs.W and the children then went away in the car and I stayed with John and got his 33 pieces of luggage, mostly large crates, through customs and onto our lorry, which had come down. We arrived back safely at the Mission House about an hour after the others arrived, all the boxes travelled well.

In the evening I went with Bill to the Broadcasting station and watched him do the 'Lift up Your Hearts' broadcast. He wants me to take a broadcast service next month on Sunday evening for half an hour! I'm thinking about it. It means rather a task getting down to Lagos on a local lorry.

On Thursday we finished the shopping and bought again much food, went for a sail in the evening and then loaded the lorry.

Friday was a very wet day in Lagos and we debated whether to start but rang

Abeokuta, where it was fine and decided to go on. Sure enough we ran out of the rain and stopped at Abeokuta for coffee and a look round the factory. We then pressed on and stopped short of Ibadan for a picnic lunch by the roadside and then went on to Ilesha, arriving about 5.30, which was in very good time. John is a grand chap and I am sure will be an excellent colleague. Yesterday we unpacked, and then in the evening two doctors came from Yaba to look into our typhoid, but they will return today.

Am keeping very fit, much love, David

Sunday, May 31st 1953

At home there will be great excitement over the Coronation, and decorations everywhere no doubt. In Ilesha we have a Coronation committee, which sits periodically, but all boils down to Ken organising the putting up of decorations and lights!!

On Friday night Ken, Andrew and I put up some bunting by the entrance, which gives it quite a jolly appearance. Tomorrow the wards will be decorated with the decorations that we use at Christmas time with a few Union Jacks thrown in to make it Coronation Day. We are going to have two days holiday, though they are filled with events, such as ceremonial tree planting, some at the Town Hall and some at our new site, so next week I should have a lot of news for you.

Whilst you and Father are watching the procession we shall, all being well, be listening to the wireless, though I doubt whether the commentator will say that the procession is now passing the seats of the Revd. and Mrs. Cannon. Everyone here is most interested to hear that you have got tickets and are slightly envious I think, you must let us know exactly what it was like. I do hope it is a fine day for you.

Glad to hear that the garden looks well, I should love to see it. Here the rains have really come and things are beginning to grow again. We have seedlings of cabbage, cauliflower, lettuce, cucumber, beans of various kinds, in time they will come-we hope to fruition. I shall be down here when they are ready for eating and they will have gone.

On Monday we unpacked some of the instruments that John has brought out with him, mainly as gifts from friends. He has some marvellous laboratory equipment that we have spent the week preparing and standardising and we are now able to grow the bacteria that we get out of abscesses, and so see what the organism is. It is all very good and will raise the standard of the hospital no end. At the moment we are a bit short of room but when we move into the new hospital then we shall have much more and be able to get all the apparatus into action. John has done one or two operations and showed his proficiency.

They want me to deliver their infant, which is due on June 12th by my reckoning. A bit of an undertaking, but as it is the third, there should be no difficulty. I examined her the other morning and all is very normal.

On Tuesday afternoon we gave a series of TAB injections to the town folk, but it was a fantastic scrum and we got completely overwhelmed by the people who are coming for free injections. If we have to give any more we shall make a nominal charge in order to reduce numbers and try to create a spot of peace.

Wednesday was Fellowship in the evening, a very good time then afterwards we discussed the arrangements we should make for the Coronation celebrations.

Thursday I went with Margaret Ingham to the Ijeda dispensary to see the people there who want us to re-open it. We spent about an hour looking at the furniture they have made and then I returned to a language lesson. In the evening. I lectured to the four girls who are doing their midwifery exam next time, and then we had a Hospital Week Committee to welcome John and Sylvia. It was quite brief. Andrew gave a short report of the work of the hospital and then we promised to show our colour photos to them in ten days time, and then ask them to give money to the Stella Liony Memorial Chapel, which we are going to build on the new site. Andrew and John will be away at the time so it will fall on my shoulders.

Friday was busy and yesterday we had to pay the men and do the accounts, as well as a number of operations one of which was a cataract operation, which Andrew did. It went quite well, though we shall see what the result is when the bandages are taken off in a weeks time.

Am keeping very fit, much love, David

June 7th 1953

Your letter of the 24th arrived last Monday, and is the most recent I have received. It is very nice for Michael to have the privilege of playing at Lincoln College

Incidentally I have half promised to take the English service the last Sunday in July for Jean as she feels it too much for her.

Monday was a busy day of preparation. We had the usual routine work, and in addition had to put up bunting, which was provided by the District Officer. Andrew, Ken and I draped this round the front gate of the Hospital and one or two of the verandahs. In addition Ken draped the cars with Union Jacks so we looked quite festive. In addition he rigged up some lights on the Town Hall, which make it look almost pretty.

John and Sylvia came up to chop and we had a pleasant time. They thought that it was a very nice house, and were most interested as it is nearly the same as the one they will have except that theirs instead of a box room has a second children's room.

Tuesday was a great day, and it began with ward rounds as usual. John,

Florence and I went to the state service in the CMS church lead by the Archdeacon, with the lesson read by the District Officer, admission by ticket only. All the chiefs were there, including the Owa on a throne. After the service, our nurses representatives were taken to the service by Ken in the lorry, and then on to the tree planting ceremony at the Town Hall. Andrew went to represent the Hospital. The Owa and chiefs planted trees to commemorate the day.

It was quite a good do I believe. I was on duty so could not get up to it - though Ken took some photos with my camera. We had a sign for the new hospital painted for the occasion, which looks very well. Meanwhile we listened

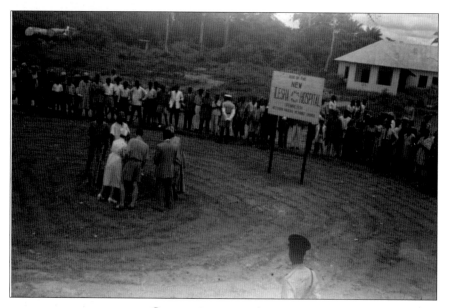

Coronation tree planting

to the radio and though reception was not good until 1.30 we heard snatches of the ceremony, including the moment she was crowned, which is after all the climax.

In the afternoon we went to sports organised by the District Officer for adults and children. There must have been thousands there. Some of our nurses won prizes.

At 6pm we all went to a cocktail party given by the District Officer. There were 57 of us altogether and it was a great opportunity to get to know the prominent men and women of the town. There were many more Nigerians than Europeans of course. After toasts and the National Anthem, sung with much fervour, we rushed back for chop, through pouring rain which cancelled the fireworks which were to have been held. However at nine in the evening we showed our colour slides to the nurses after which we had a few songs and games an? then extra food for them, quite a jolly evening though as you can imagine at the end of it we were absolutely exhausted.

On the Wednesday we did the routine work and then thought of going out for a picnic Unfortunately Elsie said she wanted one of us to stay in so I remained at home whilst the others went to Imesi. They had a good time but on the way back Andrew panicked when the brakes failed, though no-one was hurt. In the evening Ray and Daisy Rowland came from Afon as Daisy was going to a committee in Ibadan on Thursday. We had chop together at the Ps and then fellowship.

On Thursday I had a Caesarean to do, and then the list followed. In the afternoon I had a Yoruba lesson, and then lectured to some nurses. In the evening I had an abdominal laparotomy to do, followed by a lecture to the nurses, so you can see we are busy even with three doctors. Saturday was operating again and then in the evening we had the Pearsons' and Ray and Daisy to chop, playing Lexicon afterwards, a very pleasant evening. Sylvia felt as though the baby was coming about 8 o'clock so I went down to the compound and slept in the camp bed, which they had made up for me! As they say it is not often that you have the accoucheur sleeping in the house! I sincerely hope that all goes well with her.

On Tuesday we had some first day issue stamps with the Ilesha stamp and I am sending these by sea mail today. They should be quite valuable in time. About sixteen of them altogether, though I shall only send a few now.

Am very fit, much love, David

June 14th 1953

It was grand to get your letter describing the Coronation. I read most of it out to the other people, as I was the only one to have a first hand account of the procession, though John's parents saw it on television. From the account we heard on the wireless, it minimised the weather, but from your letter it seems to have been wettish but no doubt a very memorable day for you both.

We haven't received the Weekly Times for this week so we are a little out of touch. Incidentally, the Pearsons' will pay half this years sub. by cheque straight to you if you will let me know what half is, and then they will receive it when I am on furlough. The paper is greatly appreciated here.

Here the week has jogged along much as usual. Last Sunday evening Ken and I went down to church, and then to hymn singing, in the compound, the first we have had for many months. It was very pleasant, there being a good number of us there. Margaret Ingham was back after a week's holiday in Ibadan, looking better for the change as she had been quite unwell before going.

On Monday Ken and Ray went to rescue the latter's car, which was stuck in the bush 30 miles away. They had procured the right spare part and fitted it but unfortunately the last nut would not fit so they had to return and go down to

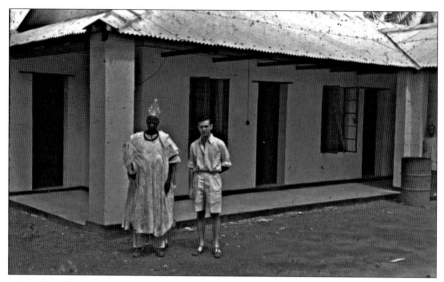

Owa at David's house

Ibadan in the afternoon for one nut, so on Tuesday morning they left at 6am went to the car, put the nut on and then drove back to pick up Daisy and the baby and set off for Afon. Andrew had a note yesterday to say they had arrived safely, which was good news. Ken and I had chop with Jean, and then the others came in for family prayers, which I led.

Thursday was a normal operating day. I assisted John with a prostatectomy, as all the clerks were away it being a public holiday for the Queens Birthday. In the evening we had a staff committee to discuss aspects of the dispensaries and matters to be arranged at Jos. It was a long drawn out session. It was agreed however that I go to the Joint Advisory Medical committee in Ibadan next week to represent the Protestant missions there. It should be interesting.

On Friday morning Andrew took John to be introduced to the Owa, again a most interesting experience. The rest of the day was routine, I lectured to one year of nurses in the evening.

Saturday however was an interesting day. Out of Andrew's visit to the Owa, the latter expressed a wish to go to the new site, so at ten am we called at the Palace for him and he came out in his superb car and followed us to the new site. Despite his age and his dropsy he walked all the way round and did me the honour of sitting down in my sitting room and admiring the house. Sam brought out some squash which we all imbibed, saluting each other meanwhile. He was very friendly. Afterwards Andrew took a colour photo of the Owa and me outside the house which ought to be amusing if it comes out. A memorable morning, the Owa was wearing his crown throughout and all the workmen on the site fell on their faces when they saw him coming.

The visit lasted about an hour and then he returned to the palace once again. In the later morning, the Rev. Geoffrey Parrinder, lecturer at the University of Ibadan, his wife and son brought up a physicist, Dr. Duncanson, of University College, London, who is examining at Ibadan this week, but is a keen Methodist - wanted to see Wesley Guild Hospital. He knows Uncle K very well and Derek Morris works in the next room to him.

They had lunch but could not stay to tea. In the evening Andrew and Jean came up to chop and we played Oh Hell, a very pleasant evening.

That I think ends the news for this week, except to say that I am very fit. Andrew is off to Jos tomorrow for two weeks, which again leaves me in charge.

Much love, David

June 21st 1953

You will notice that this is a strange typewriter, it is in fact one of the office ones as mine is on the new site and I am here on duty this morning. At the moment the whole compound is organised in giving Sylvia a medical induction of labour. We all hope that this will start it off, but if not then I shall doing a surgical induction tomorrow, when I return from a committee in Ibadan.

Ken returned from Abeokuta yesterday afternoon, and seemed in good blow. However as we were talking with Jean in the house after tea he mentioned that he had involuntarily regained bachelor status, and had been jilted. The time was not propitious to open a heart to heart talk but after chop last night (Jean and Margaret came up) I had a few moments with Ken, and he is very cut up about it and does not really understand what has happened. Anyhow most of us on the compound know, Ken having let us know, and we have each, in our own way, given our support.

Last Sunday I went to service in the evening and heard Sister Florence preach then returned to take up my week of night duty.

On Monday Mr. and Mrs. Mann from Lagos came abut 11am and had an early lunch with Andrew and then they all set off for Jos in the car.It is a three day journey by car from here the first day being 250 miles, and they did not start until after mid day as the boot locked and would not unlock despite much effort on Ken's part so they had to enter the boot through the back seat. However just as they were going off again, Bill Mann found another key which fitted and so it was opened. Since Monday John and I have been on our own and I think John has found the work harder than he expected when there were three

On Wednesday we had chop with Jean and I led the Fellowship afterwards, which was kept on a high plane of thought. It was most interesting, and we are all gradually bringing along odd commentaries that we have in order to be able to contribute something to the evening. Both Sylvia and John place a lot of emphasis on the intellectual approach and the need for keeping ones 'interest' alive in all kinds of things. They feel rather the lack of cultural pursuits but I have no doubt that when they have had a year of temperatures in the 80s and 90s and occasionally over 100 they will relax too. By the way the highest temperature this year was 117F in the sun in January. Margaret has a thermometer that records the maximum and minimum during the day.

I must go and change as I have the children to take to chapel. At the moment I am compound father to four children, Andrew being away and John looking after Sylvia. Now it is the afternoon and I am on the new site. Jean reminds me to let you know that her mother will be at the garden party at Methodist House, London, and that it would be interesting for our mothers to meet. Tomorrow I have to go to a Regional Advisory Committee in the Secretariat Ibadan.

Much love, David

Sunday, June 28th 1953

The main items of news is that the Wright babe arrived safely on Thursday morning at 1.25am and that the travellers arrived from Jos last night, 24 hours late as Enid's plane was delayed. She brought my watch however which has gone well during the twelve hours that I have worn it. It looks as though the second hand was catching because a fraction of an inch has been sawn off it, the glass also seems lighter and it has been cleaned. It is a very good job I think.

On Monday I set off at 7.30 for Ibadan but got stuck in some floods just outside Ilesha, the water getting into the engine. However the heat dried out the various parts and it started again. The committee was most interesting with some important people on it, though I learned that we shall not be getting the money on our Philipson grant that we had hoped for. This means that we shall have to think seriously about increases of salaries, which has been expected by the nurses. I returned in the afternoon and then had to help John with a D&C which he had not done before! Then in the evening I had to do a Caesarean, which meant a late night and the ending of a very heavy day.

On Wednesday Elsie went to the nursing equivalent of the committee I had been to on Monday in Ibadan. Elsie quite enjoyed the change I think, though she felt not much had been done. In the evening we had a conference about the Wright babe I said that I would do a surgical induction. So with much palaver at 8pm I ruptured the membrane under an anaesthetic administered by John. She went into labour shortly after and delivered at 1.25am the next morning. It was a perfectly normal delivery, but the baby weighed only 6lb 6oz which is not very big for a third baby. It is a lively baby though, but does not feed very well as yet. It is a little girl, but the name not fully decided. Needless to say they are very pleased.

Thursday was a theatre day with the usual run of surgery. John has been very tied to the house, managing the two children, and Jean finds four of them a bit of a handful. Today I received a letter from Ilford Church asking me to speak at their annual missionary meeting next January. I don't really think I shall be home quite by then though the Mission House had put my name forward. Anyway I don't want to do any speaking until I have had a months holiday after landing, so please don't let me in for any until I know more when I shall be sailing.

Friday was a heavy day, as John was looking after Sylvia. We expected the travellers home but they did not arrive. Jean was a bit worried, but there were many things which might have delayed them, and in fact they had a good journey down. Whilst they were there, Bill Mann had all his clothes, keys, files, cheque book stolen from their chalet, during a meal time. On the key ring were the District safe keys, so they are in a bit of a mess.

It is now the end of the day, 11 o'clock in our house on the site. Andrew preached this evening, very well, and then we had a singsong, to welcome Enid and to say farewell to Elsie who leaves on Friday for furlough. She is coming back about December for the move too.

This week we have several hospital committees to try and get things settled before Elsie goes on leave, so the nights are pretty well booked, though I am not on night duty thank goodness. Incidentally I shall be having a weeks holiday soon, before Andrew goes, which will be very nice.

Am keeping very well, much love to all, David.

Sunday 5th July 1953

As I write this I have two letters before me, one from Mother and one from Michael, and it was very pleasant to receive these last Thursday.

Incidentally, I am going on trek to Ifaki and Ikole and then on Saturday am going for a few days holiday to Afon, also on trek so my next week's letter and perhaps the one after could be late, so don't worry if they don't arrive in under ten days as Afon is very much out of the way.

Here the weather has been wonderfully cool for a week or two and it is necessary to have two blankets up here, but only one on the other site. Nevertheless we still wear shorts and open shirts with no socks. It will be difficult to get used to longs all the time but no doubt the weather in the early part of the year will encourage me to get used to it quickly. Glad to hear the garden is looking trim. Outside this house we are trying to get some semblance of order in it but when one thinks that four months ago it was jungle it is not at all bad, as in my enclosed garden there are cucumbers, beans, lettuce, radish, ground nuts growing. I have not put in any of the longer term things as cabbage and cauliflower as they would not grow before we move down at the end of the month. Andrew and family fly on the 29th July and then I take over as superintendent of the place, some headache with Elsie away.

They are hoping to look you up at some time in the early part of their furlough but will ring you up first, and would like to come over for the day, if possible as it is a long way from Gillingham, about one and a half hours on the train.

This week has been very hectic. I went to chapel last Sunday and Andrew preached very well.

On Monday we had the usual work and then in the evening the Missionary Staff Committee at which Enid Blake asked for a transfer to the United Training Hospital, Umuahia. This is a terrific blow to Ilesha, and to Elsie in particular as we made it possible for her to take her Sister Tutor course one furlough and Elsie had been depending on her to build up our training school, which has taken so long to develop and which is now just getting on its feet. It looks as if she took the Tutors course with the aim of getting into this new and bigger hospital now being built. She says there is more scope for her talents. We all think she is giving Elsie a raw deal, but don't want her if her heart is elsewhere. This means we must look out for another Sister Tutor. In addition this is Florence Cutler's last tour for family reasons, her mother is still alive and must, we think, be approaching 90.

On Tuesday afternoon we had a compound workers meeting and then on Wednesday evening we had another staff committee and drew up a constitution for the new hospital, which took me hours to type up, however it is now done and we have sent copies off to various folk for their comments.

On Thursday evening we had a farewell party for Elsie, eleven of us and played beetle afterwards. It was a very pleasant evening.

On Friday I had to take the nurses class and after it Ken and I and the sisters went over and had chop with Florence Cutler, again a very pleasant evening. Yesterday was Roger Pearson's birthday and all the European children in the town were invited, seven altogether. The 'Uncles' rallied round and played ball afterwards. In the evening Margaret, Jean and Andrew came up to chop and a game. Once again a very pleasant evening with an early night, as we are all ready to drop. Nevertheless it is nice to change into well pressed trousers and clean collars and to see the ladies in evening dress It bucks up ones morale Am very fit and am looking forward to my break. Love David

Saturday evening, 11.7.53

My heartiest congratulations to Michael, well done brother mine B.A. A.R.C.O. Your comparison between the dreaming spires of Oxford and the tall chimney of Billingham is a natural one, but you will get just as fond of the factory. Whitechapel is not exactly salubrious, yet I think of the place with affection. Brother! do not worry, mental adjustments have to be made sometimes and these adjustments, if we manage them, then our character is molded in a better way, - here endeth the sermon.

This week has been one of variety, as on Wednesday I went to Ifaki and stayed with Jonah for the night, and went on to Ikole the next day where I found Margaret G. in good form. There was not a lot to do at either place, but the roads were atrocious. They are as you know made of a sort of mud, and after heavy rain it is treacherous. Other parts where the rain runs down in a stream, there is a gully perhaps one and a half feet deep, very difficult to get out of, and hard on the springs!

It is now Sunday afternoon. On Friday I did the routine work of Outpatients, Operations in the theatre, antenatal clinic in the afternoon, lecture in the evening, and then later on I was invited round to the Sisters' for chop. After chop they got out the gramophone and we listened to the new records that Enid brought back with her. Then on Saturday I began my holiday packed my case and briefcase, two lots of drugs, and enough instruments to do most operations, anaesthetic both general and spinal, put in my camera and it's accessories, gun and ammunition and set off! In addition to the above approved list of equipment for those going on leave, I had a cat in one box and four kittens in another!

The drive took 3¾ hours, again over very bad roads. The cat was not very good, but the kittens did not turn a hair. I stopped on the road to shoot two grouse sitting there but missed both! I arrived in time for lunch, and found Ray, Daisy and the baby well, though Daisy has since got a bad cold and is in bed today. I rested yesterday afternoon and we talked in the evening. This morning I went with Ray to the little chapel, which has got no walls, where he preached. We then went on to the village chief and saluted him, and then on to the rest house where a District Officer from Ilorin was staying. They are coming to chop tonight. I have just had a further two hours sleep and look forward to another nine tonight. It is grand to get away. In a short while we are going down to hold an open air meeting in the market, which should be most interesting.

Trust all are well at home, am very fit and in good form.

Much love to all, David

Sunday, July 19th 1953

After a breakfast of grapefruit, porridge, two boiled eggs, toast and marmalade, and a new ribbon for my typewriter I feel that I am in a fair state to write a letter, and think it is unlikely that I shall have to stop for want of food.

I arrived back yesterday from Afon after a good and uneventful journey about tea time, and looked through the mail which had accumulated. The New Testament had arrived from Grandma to whom I will respond today, and I had a letter from the Cattersons, but none from home

I have had a grand rest at Afon with Ray and Daisy Rowlands. The terrain is quite different from that of Ilesha, as we are in the forest belt here, and they are above it with the distant views over low scrub inhabited by antelope and similar small wild game, though it is not easy to see them unless you go out specially with some of the local hunters to find them.

In the evening Ray and I entertained a District Officer and his wife to chop as they were staying in the rest house, being there for a change and to get to know the feeling of the people about self government in 1956. They were a nice couple whose son is soon to go to Sedbergh and was flying out to them this week for the long summer holidays and they were looking forward to it immensely, though they were afeared lest he get bored there being few white children of his age in Ilorin. Daisy was in bed with a shocking cold which I fear may be catching as I had a thick head last night and a runny nose. However we hope for the best.

On Tuesday morning we went into Ilorin as Ray had business in the District Office and looked round the town - what there is of it. The most imposing building is the palace of the Emir, which is a large white structure with domes and so forth. We called at his palace and asked him by letter if he could come to tea on

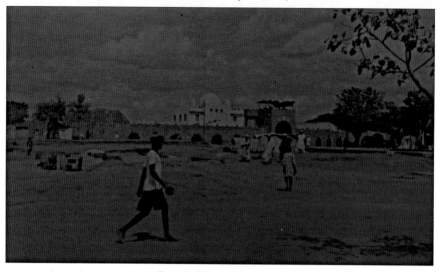

Emirs Palace at Ilorin

Thursday and to our delight he consented to do so. It would be his third visit to the mission at Afon.

On Tuesday evening we again went out with the gun and this time I shot a bush fowl which is much the same as a grouse in England, with similar markings and habits. There was great rejoicing and my reputation was saved.

On Wednesday I spent the morning in the dispensary seeing patients who had come specially to see the doctor, and then in the afternoon Ray suggested that I went with him to one of the small villages nearby on a routine visit. He hired a bike for me and with the catechist we set off. At first it was a normal mud path about 18' wide but it deteriorated into the bed of a stream where we had to walk, and incidentally got soaked three times by falling off whilst crossing streams! Eventually we had to push the bikes the last few hundred yards as it was through loose sand. Some ride!

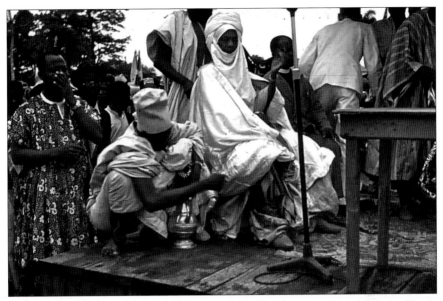

White robed chiefs

The village has about 40 people in it, and we heard some of the boys read, they are being taught by the only man in the village who can read and who is a Christian. All the others are either those who worship many local gods, or Muslims. After we had heard them read we had an open-air meeting in Yoruba with a simple story. In the evening I took the class meeting at Afon and we had quite a good time I hope.

On Thursday morning I cleaned out the little car and gave it a thorough overhaul, and then in the afternoon the Emir came to tea. Half an hour before, all the village chiefs began coming in on their horses dressed in their white robes and white gowns they looked like something out of Arabian Nights. Then at 4.30pm promptly the Emir's car swept round the drive - a modern Austin 'Princess' with a large mace in one corner, and as the doors opened we could hear the radio working! a most interesting contrast! After saluting us, he turned to the 60 chiefs who immediately went do on their knees and touched the ground with their foreheads. I hope that my photo of that comes out, a real example of the feudal system which pertains in this part of Nigeria. These are the people who realise that they are not ready for self - government yet. We had tea and then he looked round the place and he asked me to take his photo with the Rowlands and some of his chiefs. I shall try and finish this spool as soon as I can and get it home as he wants a print and it will not do to keep him waiting. He has absolute power in his Emirate which is about the size of Derbyshire. On Friday evening we went to the night market in Ilorin a most interesting sight, all the sellers have one small bush lamp but thousands of these lights make it quite bright.

The radiator tube burst on the way home so we had to go slowly. Last night Andrew, Jean and Margaret came to chop, Ken is in Ifaki.
 Much love, David

July 26th 1953

I am envious of your visit to the Strand Theatre. It is one thing we miss out here, at least I do, and look forward to the odd visit when furlough comes round.

We are huddled up in jackets and thinking of getting into longs. Jean had had a frightful job getting clothes aired by the sun before packing them away as sun has been notable by its absence and the humidity has been great.

John is worried about his son Andrew, who is nearly two has had fever for ten days and been in bed, John almost rang up a pediatrician in Ibadan but Andrew looked at him and said there was nothing special to worry about. In addition John himself has been laid up with an ulcer on his foot which has not healed and which is giving him trouble. This should be a warning sign I feel that he should take things easily which is rather a blow to me.

On Friday evening we had a staff committee which went on till after midnight, quite a big part concerned the Stella Liony Chapel. We have now launched a fund for this chapel and hoping to raise £2000. Anyway we are thinking of designs and plans and Andrew, whilst on leave is going to approach the Rank Trust and see if they can give us any help. They might as it is part of the evangelistic effort of the hospital rather than concerned primarily with the medical aspect. I understand that the Rank Trust does not give anything to Missions as such, so we shall have to see.

Yesterday was the Christening of Christine Sylvia Mary Wright. Jonah came over from Ifaki and we had the service in the hospital chapel, followed by tea afterwards. It was a very nice ceremony, especially the part where she was given her Yoruba name - Ayodele, which Jonah gave in Yoruba. There were a number of nurses there, the senior of whom were invited to tea afterwards. The District Officer and his wife, and Miss Dibble were also there, a very happy gathering. Jonah was very thrilled to be asked and really enjoyed his visit I think. He paid his first visit to the new site and was most interested.. He was amazed at the size of it and the amount of work completed, and I suppose to look at it with fresh eyes it is a big scheme, and one that would cost three times as much at home with the material available

This week has been a bit hectic with the packing of the Pearsons' as they are flying their luggage is limited so they are having to pack all their other things in trunks. On Wednesday I am going with them to Ibadan to see them off at 9am so we shall have to be up very early. On Wednesday John is going down to examine for the Nursing exam of Nigeria, in Ibadan. I am taking the evening service tonight in Otapete, and shall be glad when it is over. Much love David,

August 2nd 1953

It was good to get both your and Michael's letters this week and to hear all that is going on there, especially that Michael has got the job with the ICI.

Here we have had a busy week. Last Sunday evening I preached in the circuit chapel here. The service seemed to go quite well as far as I could tell. There were no major calamities, and it lasted about an hour.

Monday was pretty busy, as I had now taken over as Superintendent from Andrew in order that he might have time for clearing up. In the evening we had a party in the Wrights house to wish them bon voyage and had some very nice food indeed - quite different from the usual run of things that we have out here. Afterwards we listened to a piano concerto on their record player, very restful. I was on duty so pressed on with night round and so to bed.

We tried unsuccessfully to get to bed in good time ready for an early start. Ken had gone to Lagos with the lorry to bring back the 32 beds we have bought for the new hospital, and also to take six nurses to Lagos to have their eyes examined.

On Wednesday morning the alarm woke us at 4am and we rose had breakfast, packed the car and I drove down to Ibadan in just two hours we arrived about 7.30am. We had no difficulty in finding the aerodrome, but it is a very amateurish affair with wooden buildings, and only one runway. The baggage was weighed and we found that they could have taken another 30 pounds of clothes, which was a bit galling. The plane arrived at 9.00 from Lagos and three business

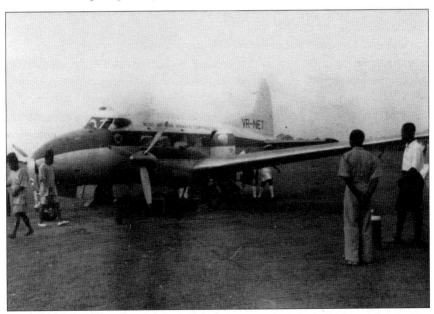

Ibadan aeroplane

men got out. It was an eight seater with two engines and they were the only passengers so it would be rather fun. This plane is to take them to Kano where they pick up the BOAC plane which would bring them to London at 8am the next morning, less than 24 hours after leaving Ibadan. I then drove home, calling at an agricultural farm to buy the fruit trees we had ordered, and the ones we have bought are in fact, Lisbon lemons, grafted onto sour oranges. It was a most interesting two hours. I then pressed on to Ilesha arriving soon after one. In the afternoon I settled down here and then supervised the planting of these trees, on the new site.

On Thursday John went to Ibadan to examine for the General Nursing Council of Nigeria, and had a good day meeting one or two people that he knew. He left at seven am and returned at eight in the evening. I had one or two things to do in theatre and then some office work Ken returned from Lagos at five having had a good trip, though he was ill in Bill Mann's boat whilst fishing. He brought up the 36 beds and the six nurses safely.

Friday was very hectic. Outpatients was busy and then we had a caesarean. John had never done one so he asked if he could do it, so I gave him a hand. Then he had arranged two hernias, but his leg was bad so he went to put his foot up and I did a hernia for him and he postponed the other one to the afternoon when he should have helped pay the men. However, Ken gave me a hand and it went quite smoothly. In the evening Ken and I went out to chop with Mr. and Mrs. Gear, and had a nice time. However when I returned Enid told me that the first year nurses had refused their salary because they were not satisfied with their rise, and Enid had said that if they did not come for their money they could leave the hospital. This I felt was a most unwise move because they might easily do so and then we should be in a difficult position and ultimately I am responsible at the moment to Synod medical committee and then to Mission House in London. I fully expected them to walk out the next morning but they have continued to work quite happily despite the fact that they have not come to collect their salary. Yesterday was fairly busy again, I had four operations in the morning, but John went to the new site to see about the new hedges round his house. In the afternoon I had a deputation from the church asking me to give a lecture on 'Alcohol and the Body' at Otapete in connection with the temperance and social welfare department. and could I let them have the theme so that it could be printed on the handbills and posters!

Recently I have been realising what a likable, companionable, capable sort of person Margaret Ingham is and wondering whether she might be a future Mrs. C. She comes from a Methodist, Derbyshire family, though her mother died last furlough and father now lives in Liverpool. She has one married sister, a niece of Dr. Craddock of China, a well known missionary, and she has just turned 29.

I am aware of the danger of isolation and am not overlooking it. Anyway we *will see. John has just looked in to say there is a swab coming! out of an operation wound of one of his patients!*

All well here, and don't worry, much love, David.

Sunday, August 9th 1953

I have done well for letters this week, receiving yours, and a brief one from Michael, one from Dr. Bolton and one from Andrew. Andrew told me of their journey home, which was uneventful and most enjoyable, though Michael was sick once or twice, and Jean felt unwell on the small plane. He says that the planes are luxuriously furnished and there is a powder room for the ladies containing every known preparation and a similar room for men, containing aftershave lotion and so forth which are all 'on the house. He seemed very pleased to be home, and was on his way to Liverpool to see his people. Immediately after they arrived in London they had lunch with Dr. Bolton. The following day Dr. Bolton wrote to me a most encouraging letter, for the additional burdens, which I now have to carry. A very nice letter indeed. He is going on leave during August so I shall write for his return.

On Tuesday we learnt that at the Women's Training College are having the British Council film unit showing a film and Miss Dibble invited us up to it. We all went except Enid and John who were on duty. We saw the Coronation film and Henry Fifth in colour. I had seen the latter before but as it was the first film I had seen for fourteen months if not more, it was most enjoyable.

On Tuesday also I received a letter from the Director of Medical Services asking me to examine for the Nursing Council of Nigeria Grade 1 and Grade 2 Midwifery examinations at the end of this month. I shall be in Ibadan for three days staying there for three nights. It is quite an honour and I am looking forward to it as a new experience. John went down for one day in place of Andrew who was asked to go for the preliminary exams which are the first that they have had to take. That is on the 26-28th of this month. I went to see John who should have gone on trek, but as we had a note from Jonah to say the bridges were down in places he felt it would be unwise to take the family and did not yet want to leave them, so I had to go again, which I wasn't keen to do. However it all went without trouble and as I wanted to speak to Jonah I had to cycle up to the compound having taken the bike across a stream over a narrow plank, the bridge being under reconstruction.

On Thursday I got back without trouble having stayed in Ikole where I was well looked after by Margaret Gregory. She had unfortunately, prepared cots and so forth for the Wright family and was most disappointed when I turned up. that made the situation just a bit awkward. All was well on my return, and I found Bill Mann and family here, just pausing on their way through to Owo for some discussions.

Friday was a busy day and then yesterday was the opening of the new hospital at Ado Ekiti. It is a CMS Maternity Hospital with about 30 beds. We were all invited but it was agreed that Florence, Margaret and two nurses, and two of our male staff should go. We set off at 7.30 and got there just at ten when the ceremony started. Despite the fact however that we had official invitations which we had answered, Florence who is pretty deaf and I could neither see nor hear. Miss Dibble from the WTC who is an ex CMS missionary and quite senior, though has not the 28 years in the country that Florence has, didn't have a seat either. In the afternoon too, there was a long gap between the opening of the hospital at ten and the dedication of the chapel at five and there was no provision made for tea so we all had a picnic under one of the trees in the compound. The whole situation was made more complex by Miss Dibble's driver who had taken her car away without permission so left her stranded all afternoon. However I took the whole party up to the Christ's School there, which has a marvellous view, and a lovely cool breeze. Our party did not stay for the dedication, as I wanted to get home in the daylight, as the roads are shocking. On the way we passed through one of the nurse's village and she insisted that we all went inside her house which, compared with some, is good. I was presented with a cock and five eggs which I brought back. On the way back we were involved in an accident- a large lorry hitting the side of our car. It scratched off the paint but did not stop. When I saw it sweeping round the corner on its wrong side I pulled over to the edge of the ditch and stopped otherwise it might have been much worse. John's leg ulcer is very bad so he is stopping in bed this week. Once again solo for me!! Otherwise all well. Much love, David

Sunday, 16th August 1953

John has been in bed for 1 week and looks as though he will be there for some time yet. He had an insect bite on his ankle over a patch of varicose eczema, which developed into an ulcer. This has meant that I have had a lot of work this week, and have been on duty all the time.

Difficulties may arise this week as I have to attend court three times Unfortunately I don't know which mornings it will be. The following week I am examining in Ibadan and have been invited to stay with the Director of Medical Services, so I shall have to mind my Ps and Qs. I have met them on several occasions, it is the spot where Jean and Andrew were ill!

On Friday we had a Staff committee. This was the first full committee in which I was in the chair, but it seemed to go quite well. Many interesting points were brought up including the suggestion from John that we had another Sister appointed to do Health Visiting in the town. We all agree that it would be a good thing, and John thinks that he could get the money from the Nuffield Trust. However there is some doubt whether the Mission House would appoint another sister even if the money were found. There is considerable doubt if they will replace Florence who is retiring at the end of this tour. If they do not we shall be in a very bad way. Our hope will be to try to find an Nigerian Sister and consequently we are looking out for one. Primarily we should like one who would look after theatre and are advertising for one in the Daily Times

Yesterday afternoon Sylvia asked me to go to the District Officer's to take her and the children to a party for their youngest child's birthday. It was quite interesting to see the mix of dark skinned and white children, the former doing very well considering the way the table was laid and the type of food being quite different to that which they are used

The weather has been very cool lately, down to 60, I believe so we are all wearing woollen clothes, long trousers etc. It hardly gets warmer at mid-day which is most unusual. The garden flourishes and we are having cauliflowers almost every day, as well as carrots, runner beans, butter beans, lettuce etc. These vegetables with the drop in price of potatoes makes living a bit cheaper than when we have to rely on tins of vegetables, as they are most expensive. I don't know whether you have heard but all the missionaries in Western Nigeria district have had an increase in their salaries It varies a bit as to whether one is single or married and the size of family but Ken's and mine is £30 p.a. Nevertheless I have decided against flying home as it would cost an extra £40 unless I could find any reason to persuade the Mission House to let me come at their expense. Looking forward to hearing from you, and also to hear of the Pearson's visit when it comes off. All well here although I shall be glad when John is back again.

Much love to all, David.

Sunday, 23rd August 1953

I was so glad to receive your letter of the 11th and to know that Margaret is well thought of and that you like her, because I am quite sure that I love her and she loves me, and we should like to get married.

It has been a bit difficult the last year because when two people such as us are put in the same situation, our names are likely to be coupled and the inevitable occurs. We both knew this and were quite determined to take no notice until we were sure that it was right and part of Gods' plan for us.

Margaret's father is a schoolmaster. He retired ten years ago after being senior science master at Chesterfield Grammar School, but since then has been teaching in Liverpool to keep himself occupied. He was treasurer of the Methodist Conference the last time but one, when it was in Sheffield, and is a foundation member of the Esperanto Society. Margaret's mothers' sister is Mrs. Craddock, and they have three children one of whom is a doctor and the other I knew slightly at Kingswood School. Dr. Craddock was of course in China as were two relatives, one on each side. One of her uncles is a director of a stone quarry in Derbyshire.

Her sister is married to a telephone engineer working for a private firm in Liverpool, and they have recently had a baby. In addition the third child of the Craddocks has recently married a doctor, the son of a Methodist minister and they have one young baby too. Most of these people live near the sea south of Liverpool where Dr. Craddock is in practice and close to where Margaret's father and sister live.

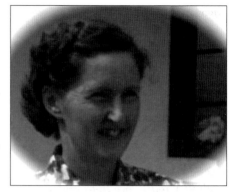

Margaret

That exhausts my information at the moment, but I could fill the page with eulogies of Margaret, but in the fullness of time they will be apparent to you. Our furloughs should come together and we hope we may be on the same boat, perhaps in February, though it depends when we open the new hospital.

Otherwise the week has not been outstanding. John has not been up at all, so I have had considerable work to do. Operating has been very heavy and tiring though the weather has been delightfully cool 60-70 degrees most of the time, though Friday afternoon was very hot. In addition we have had two Muslim holidays to mark the end of Ramadan, the period of fast and it is celebrated by much slaughtering of rams, dancing, drumming and merry making which has added somewhat to the confusion.

This morning Margaret and I went to church chaperoned by Florence, bless her, who suspects something may be in the wind and shows that she thinks it would be a good idea. The service was longish so we, and all the nurses came out after an hour and 50 minutes as we were singing the hymn before the sermon, the spirit might have been willing but the flesh was distinctly sore where it met the bench.

On our return I had the most difficult case in maternity I have yet had, a breech delivery in a woman with a very small pelvis, and everything stuck that could stick. The babe was dead sometime before I got it out but the mother will recover. Maternity has been pretty busy recently, and we are expecting that we shall have had a record number of deliveries.

By the way Margaret saw my photo the other day, the passport one but a bit larger you remember, I brought one out just in case! Anyway she said I looked older and a bit thinner, but it really is no wonder taking into consideration the weather here and the responsibility one has to carry, especially now Andrew is away. However, a fortnight on the boat given good weather will get the roses back to our cheeks.

Eileen Searle, our new sister arrives next week. She will be coming up from

Lagos by train as Bill Mann says we must save money. Then either Ken or John will meet her at Oshogbo 20 miles from here and bring her back. I shall, of course be examining in Ibadan if all is well, when she arrives. I expect to go Tuesday evening and return on Saturday afternoon, a welcome break though the time will be pretty full.

In September there is a possibility I may have to go to Shagamu to speak on Medical Missions? I have never been, but it is a well known station in Nigeria where we have a secondary school and a layman's training institute. My address would be to the Wesley Guild of the Methodist Church. Incidentally, I have received an invitation to be a member of a Missionary team for a week in March. With very much love from your very happy and affectionate son, David.

August 30th 1953

Here the week has been one of routine largely except for my trip to Ibadan. John, I am pleased to say got up on Monday and began work so on the whole it has been lighter and I have been off duty at night for five nights, which has been most welcome. His leg is healed but he still has a limp. But it does not interfere with his work at all.

Monday and Tuesday were much as usual but early on Wednesday morning at 5.30 I set out for Ibadan, taking the four girls who are sitting their exam, three for the second time. We had a good run down but I had a frightful job to find the house where the Bury's lived. By the time I found it he had left for the Secretariat and his wife had gone to England. However I went on down to the Adeoyo Hospital and met the other three examiners, a doctor from Abeokuta and two sisters, one from Lagos and one from the East. We examined the grade I midwives first, 15 minutes with the doctor first and then 20 minutes with a sister examining a patient and so forth. It was really most interesting to be on the other side of the table in the examination and to ask the questions and not have to answer them. We worked from nine to 2.30 with break for tea and then I went back to my co-examiner's house for lunch (all government people have lunch at 2.30 and do nothing else for the rest of the day.) He welcomed me warmly and we had chop, an hours rest and then tea. After tea I went down to Wesley College and saluted the Days and then returned for bath and chop. After chop we discussed many things and had a most interesting evening. He has travelled quite extensively in Africa and in the Middle East and of course has the medical situation of the Western Region of Nigeria at his finger tips. I had a wonderful night, my room had its own bathroom and proper toilet, drinking water was ice cold in a thermos jug and the bed wonderfully comfortable. At 6.30 next morning, the boy came in, un-tucked the mosquito net without disturbing me and left a tray of tea by the bedside, not just a cup but teapot, hot water etc. — marvellous. At 7am the shaving water was brought and breakfast at 7.30 and examining at 8.15. Again we worked through and managed to finish at 2.45. Unfortunately two of ours failed, I did not really expect them to pass, actually. The other examiner examined them, so I had nothing to do with it, but I can foresee trouble when the results come out.

In the afternoon after lunch I went to the shops and bought a film and chocolates, returned and had tea and then got back to Ilesha at 7.15 having had a most interesting and comfortable time. On my return I found that I was going to be arrested for contempt of Court as I had been wanted on the Thursday, However I rang up the Assistant Superintendent of Police who is a friend of mine and apologised to the magistrate the next day and all is well. I had three cases in court on Friday, two of which have been referred to the Supreme Court which is a bit of a bind. It means it will be judged by a full Court, after Christmas and it may be that I shall come home before the move.

Yesterday evening Ken and I went round to the Sisters to chop, a pleasant evening except for the main dish which was palm oil stew and neither Ken nor I liked it and I don't think Eileen did either, very odd indeed. We played Chinese Chequers afterwards, which I won oddly enough. This morning Eileen has been welcomed in church. I had to go up and introduce her to the members but all went well. Next week John is going to a retreat in Ibadan for two days, and the following week on trek. Then on the 23rd of next month I am going to Shagamu to speak to their Wesley Guild on Medical Missions. It should be most interesting as I have never been and all expenses paid!

The weather has been delightfully cool for about a month now but is beginning to warm up in the afternoons again. I rather gather that you have had it hot at home recently with your 93 in the shade.

I enclose some stamps including a sheet of Coronation ones, they will be off the market soon. I should keep it as a whole sheet and one day it may be valuable. In addition the high value British ones will also be valuable

I hope all is well at home and that you are fit for the new Methodist year. I am very fit indeed again, and the work is easier.

Much love, David

September 5th 1953

It has been again a rather busy week, but over all a very happy one, in fact almost unbelievably happy, and the future looks absolutely wonderful. Despite the fact that I have been out here for sixteen months, almost, I feel on top of the world and full of energy - love is a very wonderful thing.

I am very pleased to hear that you are happy at acquiring a daughter at last! Of one thing I am sure and that is that Margaret will fit into our family life in a very real way.

I have been thinking about Michael a great deal in the last week and wondering how he is getting on in 'Industry'. I am quite sure that given a little time he will settle down very well, and make a number of friends in the church and at the works. I wrote to him last night in reply to his letter.

I wonder if you could send out an AA handbook if not too expensive, by airmail, but if it would be prohibitive, by sea mail, as it would reach here in a month or two. I have asked all the Europeans here but they have all left them at home!

Our plans for the future are necessarily a bit vague, but if all is well we hope to come home on the same boat. I don't know whether you were thinking of coming up to meet us, that is both of you, but if so you could stay with the Craddocks overnight if you wished, and meet Mr. Ingham, and then come to meet us at the dock next morning.

Then during the first month Margaret would like to stay with us for some time in London to get to know you, and then perhaps we might go through Derbyshire to see her folks and then to Yorkshire to see ours. After the first month I shall have to do deputation for at least three months, based around London I expect, and Margaret will gather unto herself those things which brides do at that time.

Perhaps then we should get married about a month before we are due to return, a fortnights honeymoon, two weeks in which to pack and then a further fortnight on the boat before we arrive.

It all sounds extraordinarily inviting, but of course it is all very much in the air and we should be very glad to hear any suggestions from your experience.

The week has gone very quickly despite the fact that John was away at the retreat for three days. The work has not been especially heavy, until the last three days when John has done his full share, and some very big operations, for which I have had to give some long anaesthetics. However all has gone well and on looking back it has been a week of achievement. Next week is the trek week and John and family are going at last. As the family is going they will take an extra day otherwise it is hardly worth setting out.

Mr. Mellanby has arrived to put our electrical installation up at the new site. He is staying with us and looks as if he will be here for a number of weeks. He had intended to be back today but he has not arrived so it must have been more serious trouble than he first thought. Jonah was through the other day and was delighted at our news. He does not think there will be any difficulty about getting married despite the fact that I am not out of probation yet. However I have written to Bill Mann who as Committee representative, is the man who knows.

I don't know whether I mentioned it but Margaret is a trained hospital dispenser, having obtained the Society of Apothecaries certificate before she took up nursing.

Time is moving on and I am becoming more and more sleepy so I must close. The weather here is warming up considerably, I fear our cool spell is nearly over.

Eileen is settling down quite well, though tired as she is not sleeping well yet, no doubt due to the heat and the strangeness of it all.

I hope all is well with you and I look forward to your next letter. I am in the best of spirits.

Very much love, David

September 19th '53

Dear Mrs. Cannon,

It was very nice to receive your letter. I had been looking forward to it since David told me you would be writing.

Of course I remember meeting you at City Road - that was a very happy day. It will be an even happier day, when we can meet again and know that I am really one of the family, although do already feel the assurance of your welcome.

David may have told you that I lost my own mother 18 months ago, just a few days after I arrived home on furlough. Now I can look forward to the day I may be allowed to call you 'Mother' and to share in the home which has made David so happy.

These last few weeks have been very wonderful. We are sorry that distance has made it impossible for our families to keep pace with developments, but it has not been difficult for us to come to decisions because we have both felt so sure that this is the right thing; that God has guided us in this as He has throughout our lives.

I was very sorry to hear of the death of David's Great Aunt. He had spoken of her very often and told me what a fine Christian she was.

We are looking forward to our visit to Lagos this next week. Our primary concern will be an engagement ring but the shopping list is already assuming gigantic proportions.

We shall do a certain amount of window gazing too and shall probably return feeling thankful that we live so far from the shops and their temptations.

You will perhaps have heard that Jean and Andrew have a baby daughter, it is very good news. I am so glad you were able to meet the family. We are fortunate to have excellent colleagues here. I have always found life here very happy but now it is just wonderful.

With love, Margaret.

September 20th 1953

This week I have done well for letters, receiving two from you and one from Michael, as well as odd ones from folk in the District here who have sent congrat-ulations.

It is very fortunate that Gladys has been with you for the last week or two as you seem to have had an exceptional number of visitors. I have had a note from Andrew and he enjoyed his night very much. Incidentally Jean has had a baby girl, 8lbs12oz on September 11th. I don't know if you have already heard, but no doubt they are all thrilled. The nurses here made a wild noise when they heard, they are most interested of course in all the happenings of the European staff. Also most interested in the prospect of a new car. It has been a very hectic for you, but without doubt you rose to the occasion as always.

Margaret was very thrilled with the letter you wrote her and is I believe writing today. I am awaiting a reply from my prospective father-in-law, a rather anxious time!

I had a letter this week from Ralph Bolton containing his congratulations but he also put in the words 'engagements in the field inevitably lead to certain changes in appointments'. This has obviously put a query in our minds as to whether we shall be moved from Ilesha next tour or whether he means that Margaret will be moved for the rest of this tour. Both are a trifle disturbing so I have written to him to explain the sentence and so put us out of our misery. However if it is decreed that we move then no doubt we shall settle down in a new situation, but we should both be exceptionally sorry to leave Ilesha now we have got settled in. Still we shall see. The week has progressed as much as usual as far as the work of the hospital is goes. It has been quietly busy. One of the more interesting things was a visit of John and myself to the District Officer's office to meet the Medical Officer and nursing sister from Oshogbo hospital in order to discuss the rural health work of this division. It was quite interesting, though I rather feel that the District Officer's move now to give the smaller villages dispensaries and maternity homes, is more or less a political move. At the moment he is having to tell the villagers that they have to pay much more tax, and in order to get them to agree he is having to promise them better health services, but it will be a long time before anything concrete can be done.

Later on Friday evening I went to see the Hon. J. O. Fadahunsi who is one of the leading men in the District, a Methodist and a member of the House of Assembly under the old system. I took to him the proposed constitution of the hospital and asked him to look it over and let me know his reactions and suggestions.

We had quite a pleasant half hour discussing the new hospital and I am hoping to see him after the service this evening when he will let me have it back again. In addition this week I have been thinking about the November Committee and the agenda and so forth for that. There is quite a lot of work to be done there.

I don't know if I mentioned that I have been asked to lecture to the Shagamu Wesley Guild on Medical Missions, next Wednesday evening, all expenses paid. Enid Blake said that they could do without Margaret if she would like to go. We had actually thought of it but didn't like to suggest it as it is hard work with only two sisters, but as it came from her all is well. We wrote to Jonah to ask *permission for her to leave which he has granted so if all is well we motor down to Shagamu on Wednesday, and I lecture in the evening, then on Thursday we go into Lagos to shop, if all is well for a RING, and return to Shagumu in the evening and then home next morning. Space gone. Am very fit except for a small ulcer on my tongue, but that will heal soon. Very much love, David.*

Sept. 26th 1953

Margaret and I have had a wonderful time, three days away and the most important fact is that Bill Mann has booked up passages on the boat sailing on the 2nd of February so we should be home on the 15th.

The time will soon pass now and already we are quite excited about it and on our way back from Shagamu we made plans as to what we should do next furlough and how we should spend the time.

The boat gets in on a Monday and we wondered if it would be possible for Father to have the Sunday off so that you could both travel up to Liverpool on the Saturday, stay with the Craddocks and then meet us on the boat on Monday morning. It would be rather fun if some local preachers could be prevailed upon to take the odd spot of preaching on that day. Anyway think it over. Margaret says her father can get passes onto the boat for two, one for himself and one for one of you, so we could entertain you to coffee in the ships' dining room that morning, and show you round the boat. Then we could supervise the luggage through the customs and get it onto the train for London and we could return later in the day, to No.1 Then I should like Margaret to come and stay in London with us after about a week, for ten days or so, and then we might go visiting the Aunts, some of M's in Derbyshire, then to Yorkshire and finally Liverpool, where M remains and then I come to London. During the next few months I shall have a lot of deputation to do and Margaret will have to gather the odds and ends together she requires. We are thinking tentatively of getting married early in June followed by a fortnights honeymoon, and then two weeks to pack our things ready for sailing about the middle of July as we should be due back out here at the beginning of August. However it is all in the air at the moment, though we shall have to get things fixed soon in order to arrange deputation, as I am getting several invitations to speak.

This week has been a very happy one. The early part had nothing very marked about it, but on Wednesday, Margaret and I set out at 9.15 and drove to Ibadan where we had lunch with the Days at Wesley College. Charles has been in hospital about ten days and did not look at all well. Margaret, his wife seemed in good form however. We met Jonah there who was up on business in Ibadan and also John and Mary Boshier, whose mother you met in Guildford. They have been out there a fortnight now and are settling down in their little house at the college. They are very happy and full of energy. In the afternoon we drove down to Shagamu where we were warmly welcomed and congratulated by the staff at the Girls High School there. After tea and a bath we went to the church, where I lectured to a audience of 300 on the Medical Missions. I then showed some coloured slides which I have just received from Kodaks which went down very well. Then followed questions and a District donation to the hospital. The most embarrassing part of the do was their introduction of Margaret who 'loves Dr. Cannon so much that she could not let him come alone and you would be right to think that she is his girl friend'. All frightfully difficult for us but well intended by the secretary. After this confusing start all went well however.

On the Thursday Margaret and I drove to Lagos along a road through the swamps, most picturesque, but a place where brigands have held up vehicles recently at night. However we travelled both ways in daylight so had no trouble. In Lagos we saw the Manns and he fixed up the passages. We did some shopping, had some coffee in the store there but could not find an engagement ring, so we shall have to wait until we get home for that. Disappointing, but it is better to wait than to enter in on a postal scheme, which one shop runs. Learnt that Harry Jobling may not return and that the government have no money to buy the place - rather worrying.

Very much love, David

October 4th 1953

Have been very fortunate this week receiving two letters from you and one from Michael. Your letter of the 19th took eleven days to come, hence the delay.

I have had a letter from Ralph Bolton in which he says that nothing is further from his mind than to move us from Ilesha, so we shall be returning to our small house on the new site.

It is not going to be easy this Xmas, as Ken and I will be living on the new site and I don't think we will be able to have any guests. However we shall see nearer the time.

Here the week has been one of routine work chiefly. On Tuesday John had a big operating list so on both these days I did the whole of Outpatients over 90 of them on the Monday.

On Thursday afternoon Margaret and I went up to the new site to our enclosed garden to be where the men were working and started our nursery garden. Yesterday we went up again and putting about a hundred cuttings of one sort or the other and many seeds from a certain tree, which bears pink flowers. Our vegetable garden (enclosed) is coming on too It is larger than any we have at the moment, but if all is well Margaret will have more time to see that it is in order, and ensure rotation of crops. During the war Margaret and her father ran a large allotment on highly scientific lines with very good results, She has ideas about compost and so forth which I shall have to implement when we return, in the shape of a large wooden frame to hold it all and then allow it to rot, whilst filling the second frame.

On Friday I had one of the European teachers to see me and she is suffering from sinusitis. Yesterday Margaret and I went up to give her an injection of penicillin, and this morning I hear that Miss Dibble the principal is also suffering from the same disease and would also like to see me so I seem to be developing quite a general practice there.

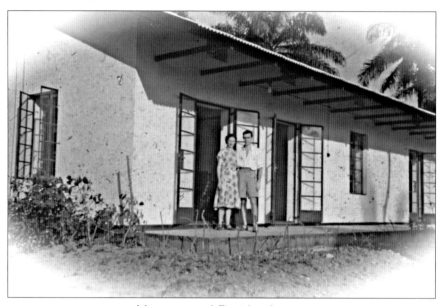

Margaret and David at house

Yesterday afternoon a children's party was held over in the Wrights house in aid of their Birthdays which they had some time ago. The District Officer's children came and also Billy Gear with four Nigerian children. It was a very happy time altogether. M and I were also invited and assisted in the amusement of the children. One very good thing they had was a fishing pond into which they put lines with cup hooks on the end. John was out of sight behind a travelling rug over a clothes-horse and he hooked on presents for each of the children. The children were completely mystified!!

The District Officer and his wife were in good form and have invited Margaret and me round to chop next Thursday evening.

Am keeping very fit and happy, much love, David

Sunday, October 18th 1953

This had been a hectically busy week, as I have had to prepare for the November Medical Committee of Synod which is due in about three weeks time. In addition there is a committee with the government in Ibadan shortly to which I shall have to go, so the future is going to be a trifle busy. However despite it all I am keeping well and remarkably cheerful! John has gone to Afon on trek and is staying a while, a spot of local leave. It is not very convenient just now but Sylvia is needing a change badly so I agreed.

I am sorry to say that Margaret is not very well. She has a cough, cold with some fever and vomiting and has been in bed for a day and a half, but is much better this morning and will be getting up this afternoon for a while and perhaps will be on duty tomorrow again

I rather envied you walking round the London parks. One of the things one misses most are the parks with the green grass and fields etc. Out here it is just forest with massive trees in unending succession and very rarely any view, and even if there is it is only of trees in unending succession. The only change is up towards the north where there are wide vistas but then only of short bush without any real pasture.

This week has passed very quickly without anything untoward. John and family left on Friday morning and get back sometime this week. I am not sure just when. On Friday evening I had to take the nurses class which I quite enjoyed and then had chop with the Sisters but as M was not very well I did not stay long afterwards. Most evenings however I have spent in the office duplicating the constitution, and minutes and so forth for the committee, and have cut ten

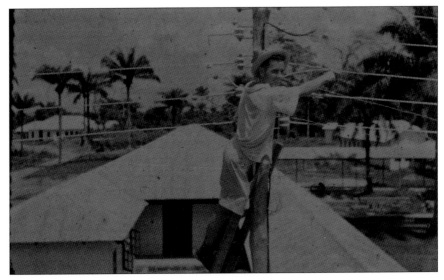

Ken with electric wires

stencils and rolled off up to 45 copies of each which is quite a task single handed. In addition I have to write to the Chairman and other folk to see if there is anything they want putting on the agenda.

The new hospital is going on steadily. The wiring of the buildings is progressing and the overhead wire poles are going in. The plumbing is being organised and we are considering the generators.

However there are still certain problems, which have to be solved of which water is the biggest. The water engineer, who has been in charge of the job has been transferred and we don't know when we shall get someone else to finish it. This means that once again we are faced with the problem of digging some wells, again to fill the large tank, which I hear is now on the way. The site is being cleared and grassed and is beginning to look quite trim.

In addition the seeds of trees which we have put in have also sprouted so we have about 40 small trees on their way which we can put round the compound next year. Our grapefruit and orange seedlings are very slow, and don't seem to make much progress. Perhaps next year when we thin them out they will do better. The banana trees which were put in almost three months ago have all sprouted and most of the lemon trees too are growing, though there again not many leaves have appeared. When I am at home I must get a book on fruit trees growing in the tropics for there must be some available I am sure. Ken has had a bad cold but he is improving, and Mr. Mellanby has had stomach trouble again, but he too is on the mend.

Incidentally the notice of our engagement should appear in the Methodist Recorder any time now. Airmail out the cutting when it comes can you please! Much love, David.

October 25th 1953

Your letter of the 17th arrived on Thursday and I was very pleased to get it. Here the week has gone quite quickly. John and family returned on Wednesday which has eased the situation quite a lot, though I still have a great deal to do with the November Committee which I learn has been fixed for the 11th at 2.30pm which should be quite convenient.

Last Monday I had a very difficult decision to make over a boy from a secondary school in Ado who had a fracture of his leg set and plastered in the new hospital there. Two weeks later he complained of pain and then the plaster was changed. However unbeknown he developed an abscess in his leg which constricted the circulation under the plaster and he developed gangrene of his lower keg. Thus on Monday morning I had to amputate his limb below the knee. He was very ill before but since his temperature has come down and he is very much better. I have written off to see if we can get an artificial limb fitted so that he can return to school.

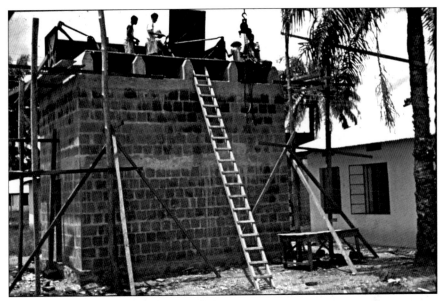

Building of the water tower

On Friday evening I received a phone call from Lagos to say that Dr. and Mrs. Cundall plus children were motoring through with Mrs. Haigh and her boy on Saturday and would like lunch. However yesterday we had another phone call to say that they would be late and would like to stay the night. As it so happened Ken has gone to Ikole with Louie Trott who came through on Thursday so I had his bed and they had my room and Margaret put up Mrs. Haig and her boy (2 and a half years) in their house in Enid's room as she is in Ogbomosho for the weekend inspecting Guide Troops, so it all worked in rather well.

They arrived about 7.15 after a longish journey, late in starting because the car wouldn't start. The children were fed and put to bed and then after baths we all had a meal together, a merry party with me at one end and of the table and Margaret at the other.

After chop I showed Bob round the hospital and he was most impressed with the work that had to be done outside the routine medical work. We were rather late to bed and up early this morning for they left at about 7.30 having had breakfast and packed up and so forth. It was very nice indeed to see Bob and Monica again and to talk of mutual friends They are very excited about the prospect of work out here and looking forward to it immensely.

Louie Trott was through on Friday, stayed the night and then went on with Ken to Ikole. She seemed in very good form and looked very well and said how well you looked when she saw you in London. She too was anxious to get to Ikole, back to her home. Ken should return today if all is well.

The new site is progressing and we found that the vast majority of the cuttings we made have taken and are showing signs of life. Ordinary wooden cuttings from plants have sprouted and seeds of trees we have planted have grown. It is really most marvellous the quick way in which plants spring up here.

I heard this week that our large tank is on its way, and in addition we have found a well digger who starts tomorrow, so that we shall be independent of the town water supply which once again seems very doubtful. They have only tested three miles out of 23 miles from the intake to the reservoir, but they have found many faults and leaks so that it may be many months before they get the water through to us.

The electrical work is proceeding, the buildings wired and the poles up ready for pulling up the overhead wires. It should all be finished within the month.

The plumbing is underway but this will take quite a bit longer but should be finished by Christmas if all goes well. The decoration is ready to start and one ward is finished. Furniture is being built. On the whole things are not too bad, but it is quite a strain keeping an eye on things and people.

Tonight we are having hymn singing.

Am keeping very fit except for a cold. Much love, David

November 1st 1953

I haven't a letter to answer this week for you have been busy with the Hull weekend I expect. I am wondering how you enjoyed the service at St. Martins. Andrew heard it on the wireless and Dr. Bolton said how impressive Father was.

I am also wondering how the new car is going? and how Father is getting used to the steering column gear change. I am sure that the secret of these gear changes is to be very gentle and slow in doing it especially from first to second. Second to first is usually satisfactory or are there four forward gears?

The week here has been one of routine, without anything very spectacular. One outstanding thing though was an operation we did last Thursday. A man had come in with dislocated and fractured hip which he had had for three weeks. After X-raying it and attempting to reduce it with traction we decided on an open operation, but this required blood. We put up two notices and before long had six volunteers. We took samples of blood and cross matched them against the blood of the patient. The first three were suitable so we took a pint of blood from each and stored it in the fridge. Then before the operation we put up a drip and gave him the three pints during the two and a half hour operation performed by John, with anaesthetic (open ether) which I administered. The whole operation went quite well and the patient is remarkably well.

I have had, unfortunately, a maternal deaths in the midwifery department yesterday quite unexpected and for which I have no answer. I had to do, a caesarean section for an accidental haemorrhage and she was much better when I did the round in the morning and then died suddenly about mid-day.

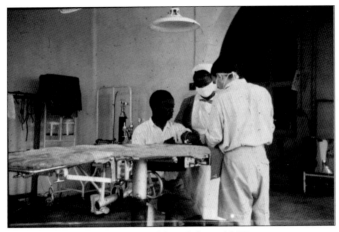

DSHC taking blood from William

This month promises to be a very busy one with several committees and then December is always busy with the end of our financial year and numerical year. Then Christmas comes into view with its jollity then the move (perhaps) though I feel it is a bit doubtful really. I have also heard from Dr. Bolton and Andrew and Margaret has heard from Jean. They are now up in Chasetown with his people I think and the baby, Alison Margaret is doing quite well and feeding a little better.

On Wednesday this week I am going to Ibadan for a Government committee and then on to Oyo where the Rev. Longley is opening a new maternity home and he has asked for a representative from here. I have never been and I am quite looking forward to it. Tomorrow we are expecting a visit from the Western Region Minister of Public Works who is going to inspect the place and see if it is suitable for an Educational Training Centre. We are hoping for a fine day so that the buildings are light. Both M and I are very well and happy.

Love from us both, David

Saturday, November 7th 1953

We have had a most interesting week here. On Monday I had a visit from The Minister of Works and the Minister of Health who came to visit the old hospital and see if it is suitable for an Educational Training Centre. They are reporting back to the education committee on the 11th and will let me know the result on the 25th or so of this month. They had several secretaries and advisors and the District Officer also came. The visit went off quite well and we parted with mutual good wishes. The Minister of Health is a barrister, though his law is in abeyance at the moment. The Minister of Works has no special qualifications and I believe, was at one time principal of the Christian School Ado Ekiti and had to leave rather hurriedly! They were both quite affable, looked into every room including the staff houses and left with mutual good wishes.

The District Officer thinks on the whole that it is quite hopeful and that they will purchase the place. I shall be very pleased to get it in writing anyhow!

On Wednesday I left early in the morning for Ibadan to attend the Medical Advisory Board. I got there in good time but the committee itself was most disappointing. The Minister of Health has been so involved with the changing constitution of the country that he has not been available to discuss the various proposals made at the last committee five months ago. However I got in a further suggestion which would give us a further £6,000 per annum if it went through which I don't think it will.

I left Ibadan at mid-day and drove to Oyo, 30 miles away to the north, where Frank Longley was opening his new four-bedded maternity home. There is much trouble in Oyo just now between two rival chiefs, and the police are having to stand-by armed with tear gas and so forth in case of trouble. This being so, neither of the two chiefs were permitted to attend the opening on account of trouble developing so there were not the great crowds which were expected. When I arrived I found that I was expected to make a speech and found that I was the Guest of Honour, after the Resident and his wife. The Resident is responsible to the Lieutenant Governor. The three of us sat in the middle of the front row and got on quite well. I spoke after Frank and after me the Resident's wife opened the doors with a key. Then local folk opened every door and window which took rather a long time which distressed the Resident a little as he had an appointment for 5.30pm and didn't get away until nearly six. I returned to Ibadan and called in on the Days for coffee. I arrived here at twenty to two having had a good run through.

Our well digger is a flop so we shall have to see if we can find another. Much love from us both, David

Sunday, 15th November 1953

Before Andrew returns there are the numerical returns to cope with, and the financial account to prepare for the auditors. In addition there is a report of the medical work of the district to prepare and this year it has to include the work of Ikole, Afon and Oyo as well as our own, so it will be some task. However I have written to the other centres for their individual reports

The new site work proceeds. The wiring both internal and external is finished and we wait for the engines from England. The plumbing is under way, though it is only just started and there is a great deal to do. However we got the pipe yesterday which we have been waiting for so it should go ahead more quickly. Decoration also is a big job, and the mortuary and nurses wash-houses are yet to be built, so whether we shall actually move in or not at the time expected is a bit doubtful. However move or not Margaret and I are coming home on the Feb. 2nd boat for there will be sufficient folk to get the move over.

We are so short of room here that our new intake nurses will have to go straight up to the site, and Miss Cutler will live up there with them and be the first into the sisters house to live. A lot of organisation is required to fit all that in though.

Here the weather is getting warmer and warmer we have not had any rain this week and think that we may have had the last. There is a lot of work entailed in drawing water from wells and tank for the whole hospital, a most expensive item. Our well digger is a bit of a flop but has borrowed some apparatus which should help. We hope for the best?

Love from us both, David

Sunday, 22nd November 1953

We have heard that Ken's photo is a bit aggressive (in Kingdom Overseas). I do not think he will stay with the Mission unless something else crops up, for we shall not be able to keep him, and I do not think he would care to stay once the hospital is built. He is not keen on accounts and so forth. Incidentally he has asked Bill Mann to book him on a mid March boat, six weeks after M and I sail.

This last week has been a heavy one with night duty as we have had a number of difficult cases which have necessitated several night visits. Yesterday was a bad day, John had a difficult skin graft first and found that the knife had not been sharpened as requested which caused a little disturbance, then I had a case which I had hoped to be a simple one, but it turned out that the woman had cancer and it necessitated a most involved operation lasting two and a half hours. Then I was called to maternity to do an obstetric operation, and then had to return to remove a piece of dead bone from a girl's leg. I had my lunch at 3.45!! After this I had hoped to rest but the Sisters wanted to look round the new site to see about cupboards for the wards. This was an exhausting procedure, though it was cooler being evening time and there was the compensation of a very lovely sunset, which we can see to advantage from the higher vantage point.

In the evening Margaret and Margaret Grant, the latter being the new WTC teacher who is a Methodist, came in to chop and we had a very pleasant evening. Unfortunately I had to give an anaesthetic for John just as we should have started, but I was not very late. After chop we played 'Oh Hell', and it is some time since we did, about three months I should think. During the game the phone rang and it was Bill Mann who rang to say that he had just heard from the Mission House that the loan which they promised us for rebuilding of £3500 had lapsed and Dr. Bolton had said that we should not need it. Bill Mann and Mr. Angus met last night and decided that if there was not a cable from the Mission House by Wednesday saying they would in fact lend us the money then we should have to stop work on Thursday. This is a serious situation as you can see and we hope that it is just a misunderstanding which will in fact be straightened out. It looks as if Andrew has been too sanguine about the financial situation and given the wrong impression. I am quite sure that it is nothing that I have said or written for I know how every penny is going to be needed.

Last evening I had a subpoena for a case in the Supreme Court for next Wednesday in Akure, a town 60 miles from here. This thrust me down into the depths of depression, for it is an unpleasant task. However when I got back from chapel this morning a telegram awaited me to say they would take my evidence in Ilesha on December 3rd which is I suppose, in private before the judge and so save me the journey to Akure. It would have been an interesting experience in retrospection no doubt, but one which I am quite happy do without.

On Friday we had a staff committee that did not go too well. The Sisters wanting two more buildings, which have not been budgeted for. However if the £3500 does not arrive there is no question of it and we shall just have to make do with what we have.

Andrew will have had his operation now (last Wednesday) and be getting better. I feel that Jean will have a lot of work to do with packing for the family but will no doubt get through it. It will be very nice to see them all back with us again. We are all well here, with much love from us both, David.

November 29th 1953

Your letter arrived on Tuesday of this week, and I was very pleased to receive it. Deputation requests continue to come in, another five this week.

I have accepted one for March 29th in London SW11 - Beechwood Road Church for a Guild evening, and I am about to accept the Overseas Mission Anniversary services for the Rev. Tom Baird in Surbiton on May 9th. Thus the time is getting filled up. I am not very happy about accepting preaching appointments, but feel that it is expected of me.

The week has been a very busy one here. We have had a great number of patients in and it has meant a considerable amount of night work. John has actually been on duty, but I seem to have been disturbed most nights too, for some reason or other, either to give an anaesthetic, or for my keys because John has lost all his keys including the office, store and laboratory keys, which are rather important. In addition we have had a nurses concert. This has been produced by the nurses themselves, in aid of the Stella Liony Memorial Chapel fund. All I did was to see to the printing and send round to all the Europeans in the town with a complimentary programme and arrange for the seats and screens for the stage. It was held out doors, on the lawn outside the Sisters house, part of which is raised up and makes a very suitable stage. We had footlights which were adequate illumination on the stage and hung 20 hurricane lamps in the trees and bushes around the auditorium and make it look like a *piece of fairyland. It was most attractive. The District Officer and about ten other Europeans came though some went in the interval as the whole thing - in true Yoruba fashion- lasted about three hours. There would be about 300 people there and on the evening from selling programmes (admission by programme) and from the collection we made £19 odd so we feel to have done quite well. There were several prominent Nigerians there who have much money, but I don't think they gave any very great donations, which was disappointing. However some gifts may come in later.*

It was a great success, and due I am sure to the fact that we did not interfere in any way but let them go ahead. We saw the dress rehearsal on Thursday evening and suggested that two items might be cut out to shorten it to which they readily agreed.

We are very busy just now with our numerical returns and reaching a balance with our accounts. Our turnover has been about £35,000, so there is some work to do. We hope to get the books within striking distance of a balance and then Ken will take then down to Bill Mann to have them audited. It will mean quite a bit of work this afternoon. We seem however to have a balance on the right side and will be able to give the building fund a further £1000 and still have £500 in hand with which to start the new financial year.

Love from both of us, David

Sunday, December 6th 1953

Very pleased indeed to hear that you have fixed up to go to Liverpool for the weekend of the 14th February so that you will be on the quay to greet us and perhaps come onto the boat itself. I will let you know which cabin I am in so that you can come down and meet me there.

However I think I shall have to buy a tin trunk myself to bring out again, because they are absolutely essential to pack linen and blankets in when on furlough.

Andrew and family should be on their way now and I heard on Friday evening that Harry and Nellie are sailing on the 8th from Dover, so we should all be here in January. I am looking forward to seeing them all again and then only a few weeks and we shall be sailing ourselves from Lagos. On Wednesday this week I heard through the District Officer that the two Government ministers who looked round here a month ago failed to make their report to the Executive Committee of the Ministry of Education and that it is not likely to be prepared in time for the December meeting. This means even more delay in the sale of these premises and the arrival of the £10,000. This is a most disappointing blow and I am sorry that Andrew will return to it, I should have liked to have had everything fixed before he arrived, but evidently it is not to be so. The District Officer is very disappointed and advised me to sell to some of the private individuals who are pressing for it, and are interested. However I have written to the Chairman and he, as it happens, will be staying here a week tomorrow for a few days as he has a committee in Ilesha. We can discuss it then. I had hoped to meet Andrew but John has to examine that day in Ibadan which means I cannot get away. However the car will go down with a driver and Bill Mann will go to the boat, as he usually does.

On Thursday I had to give evidence in the Supreme Court of Nigeria, complete with High Court Judge and Counsel for the Crown and for the defence all in wigs and gowns and all Nigerians. It was most interesting, though a rather harrowing experience. I was of course an 'expert witness' and so my cross examination was not as severe as it might have been, though I was in the box for half an hour. The Crown lawyer met Andrew's father at Swanwick last year and was most interested in the affairs of the hospital. I had quite along chat with him before the court started.

Then on Friday afternoon I went to the Agricultural Show with John after we had finished our clinic in the afternoon. It is the first time that they have had one in Ilesha, and it is an attempt to stir up interest in new methods of farming. As we went round we met the President who remembered me from our meeting in Oyo and said 'Ah! Hello Cannon', so I was very bucked that he had remembered my name, and I was like a dog with two tails. He wished to show his wife the new site, as she had not seen it, so at ten yesterday I met them on the site. I rather feared there might be a large retinue of followers but just he and his wife came up in their own small car. We walked round for half an hour or so and they asked some very pertinent questions about the place and were apparently most interested. He used to be District Officer many years ago at Ife 20 miles from here and at that time stayed with the Ludlows who were at the Mission House here then. They also knew Dr. Hunter. A most interesting and friendly time. I think it is well worthwhile to be on good terms with these people, for they can help or hinder so much.

I had a letter from Shepherds Bush Road this week asking me to speak at their Guild on March 25th and enclosed a booklet that had been printed at least three months. It looks as though I shall have to accept, although it falls within the six weeks I am supposed to have rest before starting deputation. Not very tactful of them. Looking to February 15th! We are all well here, work is as ever.

Love from us both, David

Sunday, December 13th 1953

Another Sunday is here, and I have just finished a round and so down to the letters. I have had a letter from Auntie Ruth asking me to speak at a garden party sometime in June or early July. As arrangements are at the moment it would seem that June 1st would be most suitable. I told the Mission House that

I would not accept any deputations after June 1st but I think that private ones should be accepted. Auntie Ruth wants a Tuesday and I believe has asked you to take the chair. If June 1st suits you therefore, would you let Auntie Ruth know that we shall be happy to go.

Earlier this week I heard from the Mission House that I have been chosen to go to the Channel Islands for my deputation from April 1st to 15th, and thus get it all over at once. I am very sorry to be away for a fortnight together, but rather pleased to think that I shall see the Channel Isles. I have had a letter from the Circuit minister there and I am in the Guernsey, Victoria and Sark Circuit and the other deputation is a minister from India.

Last night Margaret and I were looking at the diary and really the time is filled in remarkably, what with the trip round the relations, the Channel Islands, a week at Swanwick and then a Honeymoon.

The week has again been a full one one, with progress all round. I completed the numerical returns earlier in the week so they are finished with for the year, and a nice piece of news with which to welcome Andrew.

Mr. Mellor of Badagry arrives this mid-day to take a service here this evening and Mr. and Mrs. Angus arrive tomorrow, and will be staying with me. We shall be having a constitution committee tomorrow morning which may be a bit stormy. On Tuesday Ken and Mrs. Angus go down to meet the boat. I had hoped to go but John is going to examine in Ibadan on Wednesday, the day they dock. John's going away is making it very difficult indeed, as I shall have to move house at the same time. Ken is moving his things today, so there will not be his to worry about. Friday I shall be here to welcome them. By this time next week we shall all be settled down, with Ken and myself on the new site again. During the week I had a letter from the Gills in Lagos, asking if they could stay for Christmas so I wrote and said yes. They will be here for three days only and we will put them in the Sisters house on the new site which will be ready. Very fit, love from us both, David

Sunday, 20th December 1953

My love and best wishes to you all for Christmas, though I fear that this may be a bit late. I know you will all have a lovely time, with no doubt some of the men from the hostel in too.

Here we are beginning to think of things, though work has kept us busy most of the time. The big news is of course that Andrew and family are here although he has not taken over. They all had a very good journey though the children picked up some infection from the other children on the boat and arrived with fever and spots, but on the whole they have settled in very well indeed, Michael saying that he has reached home at last, which is most interesting. It is very good indeed to see them.

Your letter arrived during the week, and was read eagerly. In addition I had one from Dick West asking me to speak in Hull, the date to be left to me. It seems a frightful way to go to speak, but I think that I ought to fit it in some time if at all possible.

This week has been a very busy one. Monday and Tuesday were very busy ones in the hospital and we had one or two very big operations. Early Wednesday morning John and Enid went to Ibadan to examine for the Nursing Council and did not return until late on Friday evening.

The Chairman of the District arrived on Monday morning with Mrs. Angus. Mr. Mellor having arrived the evening before. I entertained the chairman. We had a Constitution committee of which I was secretary and it went quite well. In the afternoon I showed Mrs. Angus round the new site whilst Mr. Angus had a committee with the local church leaders. In the evening they went to Florence's for chop. The next morning Ken and Mrs. Angus drove down to Lagos to met the boat, leaving the Chairman and myself to amuse ourselves. We had a quiet time and he spent most of he morning writing letters. In the afternoon I showed Mr. Angus around the site and though he did not say much I think he was quite impressed with the progress. He left on Wednesday morning for Ifaki for a valedictory service for the boys. Wednesday and Thursday were both busy days as I was quite alone and at the same time had to pack up my things from the Pearson house and have the house cleaned for their arrival.. On Friday again I was very busy but at four o'clock went to the office where I could watch the drive and at the same time get on with some work. Promptly at five the car from Lagos drew in and I was the first to welcome them back to Ilesha, and I was indeed very glad to see them. That evening we had chop with the Wrights and then Ken came up to sleep whilst I had a shake down as I was on duty. I had a bad night operating on a woman who had attempted to commit suicide, so last night I came up here to sleep and had a wonderful night, sleeping for nearly ten hours without any disturbance. Today, here on the site is wonderful, my cares rolling away one by one, Christmas coming and above all Margaret.

Tonight we are having hymn singing and there should be a good number at it. Guests arrive during next week and our two will be on the new site here. Unfortunately I learn they will arrive about 8.00 pm so that I shall not be able to go carol singing. However it will be very nice to see them.

Andrew came up yesterday afternoon for a look round the site and seemed quite pleased with the progress. The Chairman too said that I done well when he was up which was praise indeed from him.

When Christmas is over we must think of the annual report and Synod matters so that they are ready in good time. In fact we ought to get them done during the next few days. Margaret is going to her dispensary at Imesi tomorrow and as I have never been to it I hope to go as the driver. We are taking a picnic lunch.

Best wishes for a happy Christmas, love from us both, David

Sunday, Dec. 27th 1953

Dear Mrs. Cannon,

This has been a wonderful Christmas. It would seem strange to me to spend Christmas at home after sharing in so many 'hospital Christmases', where generally speaking the activities take the same form year after year. The carol singing on the wards, the nativity play the nurses concert and presents to staff and patients are received as eagerly here as anywhere in England. But this Christmas has been for me a very special one.

As usual we felt a few days before the festivities began that we should never have everything ready in time, but everyone enjoyed sharing in the preparations and when the time came I was too happy and too busy even to feel tired. To be able to share things with David made such a difference.

I expect David has told you about our joint giving and receiving of presents. Did he tell of the piles of sandwiches which we helped to prepare for the nurses party yesterday evening and the squeezing of oranges to produce three large jugs of juice?

I want to thank you very much indeed for my Christmas present a delightful foretaste of furlough. I couldn't wait six whole weeks until we shall be in a climate where such apparel will be a necessity so I wore them at our Christmas party and they added much to my enjoyment of the evening.

It is in some ways a relief to have Christmas over, now that Elsie is back we can give more time to hospital work which could occupy more time than we ever have to give to it. But during these next five weeks I hope to have time to clear out cupboards so that everything is in order both for going home and returning to 'our home' again.

I am so pleased that you will be able to stay with my aunt in Waterloo when we arrive. What a wonderful day that will be! I'm sorry that we could not entertain you at my own home, but apart from friends in the flat upstairs my father is on his own so I am sure you will understand the difficulties.

With love from, Margaret

Sunday, December 27th 1953

Christmas is nearly over. We have had a wonderful time, and Margaret and I feel that it has been the most or one of the most wonderful Christmases we have known. Being in love certainly adds to everything! And what is more, there are only five weeks before we sail, in fact in five weeks time we shall be in Lagos if all is well waiting for the boat.

Thank you very much for the pen which I opened on Christmas Day it is lovely one.. My old one had been on its last legs for a long time Margaret was very thrilled with her nylons, and wore a pair on Christmas evening for joy. It was a most thoughtful gift. I gave Margaret a nylon slip that Jean got for me in England

and brought out. She was very pleased with that too.

In addition we received some very nice gifts from the compound. We gave gifts together and we received them together so that it was easier. Jean and Andrew gave us two glass bowl things for table decorations I find it difficult to describe, sort of semicircular gutter things of glass. Elsie Ludlow and Florence gave us a Pyrex casserole the sort which you can use the lid for something too. Enid Blake gave us a towel and two tea towels all of which we have put in our 'bottom drawer' with the tea towel and pillowslips we have been given already.

We have indeed been very lucky in our gifts and have a very good start to our housekeeping. Next week Margaret is going to start packing, and we will make an inventory of all the things we have so that we know where we are. We shall be well off for towels, sheets and pillowcases I think. All those sorts of things we shall pack in one of Margaret's airtight trunks and leave it in the store here.

Yesterday I helped make hundreds of sandwiches for our nurses party last evening so I can appreciate something of the task. In addition I had a letter from Auntie Sarah. I shall try and write though I fear that life will be very busy these last few weeks and I hope to see them in early March if all is well.

Here we have had a very busy time indeed as you will remember we did last Christmas. Guests arrived on Christmas Eve, Charles and Margaret Day to the Pearson's, Mr. and Mrs. Gill to us on the new site and a Miss Jean Packet to the Wrights. Both the Sisters guests could not come unfortunately. Carol singing round the town was good fun, and we enjoyed a drink of Coca-Cola and chocolate biscuits at Mr. Fadahunsi's. We had early Communion on Xmas morning at 6.30, some job for those of us up here. However we arrived on time but Charles Day was late as he couldn't find his cuff links!

Afterwards we had breakfast in the Sisters house then gave presents to the labourers in the compound who came for their gifts, five shillings each. Then we opened our presents, and a very happy time it was. Services in the wards followed. I took the Gills to the leprosy village where we took the service and gave them their Christmas presents. Then we gave presents to the patients in the wards followed by coffee and Christmas cake. At one o'clock went to lunch of cold turkey and so forth at the Wrights - 20 adults and six children. In the afternoon most of us retired to our beds to rest and then at four by our time listened to the queen, though reception was not good. Then tea in the Pearsons' house followed by the nurses Nativity play for the patients in the male ward. During the play we had a conference to discuss the programme for the nurses party last night and we all trooped to the theatre where we made masks of each others faces with plaster of Paris.

Ken who was the first to undergo the procedure practically passed out so the rest of us had a breathing tube incorporated. They were most realistic when they had been coloured. On Christmas Day evening we had our Christmas Dinner proper in the Sisters house Andrew carved the turkey and I carved the ham, John was not well unfortunately and spent yesterday in bed and has fever. Yesterday, Boxing Day, we rose late and then did the odd spot of medical work as was required. At lunchtime we had a duck, Margaret and the girls and Florence being our guests. It was very nice indeed though not as nice as many I have had. In the afternoon we had the preparation for the nurses party and in the evening the party itself a great success.

With very much love to you all from both Margaret and me, David

Sunday, January 3rd 1954

Another Sunday is here and as usual the sun is high in the heavens and the temperature high. Ken is not too well, just having had a booster dose of TAB and is lying on his bed. I have just woken after a post-prandial snooze having had a full morning without opportunity to write this letter. William the cook is ill so it looks as though a little later I shall have to rustle round and get some chop. Margaret is very well. She has been on duty this morning and no doubt at this moment is having tea in the Sisters' house on the other compound and will shortly be getting down to writing letters.

I haven't received any letters this week, though we got a parcel from Gladys, containing a tie for me and a hand embroidered tea tray cloth for Margaret which was very nice indeed of her, and I hope to drop her a line when I have finished this.

The week has been a busy one. Monday and Tuesday were work days, with routine things to do. On Wednesday I went on trek and as Margaret and Charles Day are still with us they wished to come also, and drove back Louie Trott's car, which was down here.

I set off first and got to Ijeda where I did the dispensary and gave such injections as were necessary. They then joined me and after taking sundry photographs we set off in procession with me following. The roads are incredibly dusty and before long the car was thick with dust, my eyes sore and my hair filled with it. The steering too was a bit faulty with half a turn play on the steering wheel so I felt like a tram driver! We stopped at the Effon intake (water) and they took further photos, and I took one of them on the dam looking at the water. It was shaded and delightfully cool at this place. Unfortunately as we had our elevenses we left a thermos in the middle of the road which had to be rescued in the nick of time, but otherwise a very pleasant break. We then set off for Ifaki and travelled very slowly due to the ailments of the two cars but arrived safely at 1.30 where Jonah was very glad indeed to see us. He hadn't expected the Days so chop was a bit late but as there were very few at the dispensary it being just before the New Year, I caught up with the work. On my return we were having a chinwag when a boy came in to say that a heron was on the compound. We

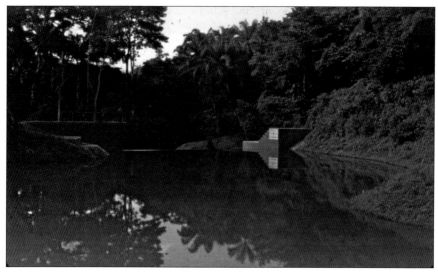

Dam at Effon

went down to look and I stalked it about two miles into the bush.

In the evening the Days went on to Ikole to stay with Louie and I stayed with Jonah as there would be four at Ikole with David Head who was staying there already and not room for me. Jonah and I had a look at the car and he said that his man would fix it. We had a quiet evening talking and retired at ten when the lights are turned out. The next morning I set out in good time for Ikole and arrived about 9.15 and found them having breakfast. Louie and I got on with the work and then we listened to some records and talked until lunch time. After this we set off back home. The steering now in addition to there being a lot of play on the wheel began to get stiff and you will hardly credit it when I say that at the end if we had to go round a sharp corner Charles had to get out of the car and push the wheels round with his hands as if it was too stiff to turn from inside. However we came home very slowly and without incident though we were later than I am usually and found Margaret rather anxious, though she tried not to show it. Next time I go that way she will be with me if all is well, and treks will be something to look forward to.

That evening we all had chop in the Sisters' house and we had a most hilarious time. We all enjoyed it very much indeed.

Friday was New Year's Day, and we all spent it quietly, Margaret came up here for tea in the afternoon and we planted out 73 small seedlings of orange, grapefruit and tangerines which we have grown from pips in a seed box. It was a back breaking task but is now complete except for the second box. We have put them outside the bathroom window so that the water from the bath and basin runs onto them and waters them automatically. They should be ready for planting in the orchard next season if they do well.

Yesterday we did the accounts and so forth and in the evening had chop with the Pearsons' after which had a game called 'I commit' a most interesting game of crime. After this several had their TAB injection and are not too well today. This morning I went to the other Methodist Church in the town and this evening we have a compound Covenant Service. Much love, David.

Sunday, January 10th 1954

Another Sunday is here, making one less until we reach home. Despite valiant attempts to remain calm and unruffled I find myself getting very excited.

Two of your letters arrived this week and I was very pleased to get them and to hear how the Christmas celebrations had gone at home. I was glad to learn that Michael had been able to get home for the week, it would make a very nice change.

Rather disappointed that the car will not take the luggage however as you say the important thing is that I shall be home. We dock early in the morning, having anchored outside during the night. If all goes well Margaret tells me we should be away from the docks by mid-day. If we are going south by train it would be as well to go down on the boat train, sending the luggage straight to the station. The docks will know all the ins and outs having met many boats and entertained many parents meeting their missionary children, so I leave it with you to fix up with them the arrangements of the day.

It was very nice of Gladys to suggest an electric toaster, we were thinking of getting one, and we could use it in the mornings and evenings when the generators were on so it would be very useful I think.

You seem to have had a wonderful time at the theatre, a galaxy of stars! Interested to hear of Michael's bookcase. I don't know whether I mentioned it but I am hoping to buy a selection of tools, both carpentry and engineering so I can do a little of the work that Ken has done. It would be most useful on trek where one has to be self-sufficient.

The thought of a week abroad is a very nice one and I should love to do it, but it is not easy to find a week in which I have not got an appointment of some sort. The only week is the one before I get married. On the back of the letter I will give the dates of my present engagements so that you can enter them in a diary. I really think I have as much as I can manage in the way of deputation especially with my other commitments this leave! Abroad would be very nice, but a week would be reduced by travelling to four or five days, and if we are going to pay travelling fares it would be more economical to have longer. What about Lands End or flying to the Channel Isles which I should know a little.?

The week has been a busy one with patients and the Doctors took a record amount of cash in outpatients that will be a mite in helping to offset the loss which we shall sustain while moving. In addition too we have had a good number of operations and this morning there was a lorry accident from which we got nine casualties, five of which have had an operation so it was a busy time.

Yesterday the Dr. and Mrs. Haigh came up from Shagamu, you remember that I stayed with them one night when I went to speak there, and they brought his Mother and Father who have come out to stay with them for a few weeks. It was nice to see them again and they were most interested to see both the present and the new hospitals. They went after tea and soon after they went Mr. and Mrs. Evans and their boy aged five came up at our invitation. He is a water engineer and this morning we have been discussing our problems here. It is complicated but we hope to have found a solution.

On Thursday Andrew and I go down to synod for the Medical committee. After it I return and John goes down. With them both away it will be rather a heavy load, but the thought of next month will no doubt buoy me up. Below I will append my diary so far as it goes.

Feb 15th - Home, Feb. 22nd Margaret to London. March 1st to Adwick? Brig.? Hull Liverpool? 9th, 13th London. 14th-21st Deputation preparation - i.e. making sermons and talks, March 23rd Pinner Youth Club, 25th Shepherds Bush Guild, 29th Broomswood Guild. April 1st-15th Channel Isles, 16th home for Easter? Margaret to come down and both go to Matlock for next weekend to see her aunt and uncle. May 4th Rivercourt, May 9th Surbiton M&E 15th and 16th-Norbury M&E, 24th-31st Missionary Swanwick, June 12th Wedding, You see what I mean about deputation!!

When will Michael be on holiday? Is it feasible whilst we are at Brighouse, say, to go up to Middleborough and see him? During this last week we have had a new intake of nurses and as there was not enough room on the old site they are living up here which makes quite a community of us. I fear that it will be for quite a time as the water palaver will delay us still longer, I think. We are counting the days now!! Much love from us both David

Wesley Guild Hospital

Dear Mr. and Mrs. Cannon

I should just like to take this opportunity of thanking you very much for your Christmas present. It's always been my ambition to own a pair of nylon socks.

We had a very pleasant time at Christmas, as I am sure David will have informed you, and now we are pushing ahead with the work. This weekend Mr. Dan Evans, a PWD water engineer has been staying with the Pearsons' and has advised us on a number of matters. Tomorrow I shall start getting a supply of water from our stream by means of a small ditch. This water will be conveyed into a well via a sand filter. In this way we hope to be able to have our own water supply and be independent of the town water. I am afraid that our lack of water may delay our moving, and I want to stay here until we move, so I may not be home for some time. I am looking forward to seeing all my Rivercourt friends again, the time seems to have passed very quickly and I am sure that it will not be long before I am knocking at the door of number I Rivercourt Road!

I must close now and will do so by thanking you once again and remaining Yours sincerely, Ken.

Sunday, January 17th 1954

I have just returned from the pre-Synod Committee with a sharp bout of fever, which is however on the wane now and by tomorrow I shall be fighting fit again. However I am in the Pearsons' spare room, with adequate attention from John, Margaret and Jean, but the light is fast fading and the engines are not yet on. Thus I write this reclining in the gloom.

It has been an eventful week on the whole. We have heard that the £10,000 for the premises is assured, which is good news and in fact Jonah has said that the cheque for £5,000 is en route, which is good news, we shall be happy to see it arrive.

The early part of the week was very busy with a large number of operations, and then on Thursday, Andrew, Enid Blake, Kathleen Wood (who has been staying here for a holiday) and I set off in the Standard for Lagos. We had lunch at Dan Evans the PWD water engineer who was up here last weekend and discussed further with him, the sanitation of the new hospital. After leaving there we pressed on to Abeokuta to see Miss Skeats and to learn that Harry and Nellie Jobling are on the way! In fact they should be here by next Thursday. This is very good news.

In Lagos, Andrew and I stayed with the Manns, and on Friday a.m. went to Igbobi Artopo Hospital to see about septic tanks. In the afternoon we had the Medical committee, which passed off without incident. Afterwards Andrew and I watched a cricket match and then returned to the Manns for chop. After chop eight of us went out to the pictures, open air, interesting but a very poor film. The next morning I woke feeling sick and shortly after attempting breakfast, was sick. By 3pm my temperature was very high, but folk rallied round with the necessary and today I am much better, having had a good run up this morning (a driver drove me) I shall be back at work tomorrow if all is well, and Ken and John go down to Synod.

In two weeks time should be in Lagos waiting for the boat! Thank you for your letter. You will have had my letter with itinerary. Thrilled to think Michael will be down the weekend after I arrive. Much love from us both, David

21, Marina, Lagos, 31.1.54

Well here we are in Lagos, very, very thrilled, having said goodbye to Ilesha and its inhabitants for six months.

Your letter arrived on Thursday and we were very glad to receive it and very pleased indeed to hear that you are better. We have had a very hectic week packing, and getting all the linen aired and washed so that we could pack it into the two airtight trunks of Margaret's that we have left behind.

On Wednesday they gave us a farewell cum Birthday party which was very enjoyable. On Friday we had a good run down and received a very warm welcome from Mr. and Mrs. Angus. Lagos was very hot and sticky. Yesterday we shopped in the morning, and then in the afternoon all went down to the beach and swam, magnificent!

The Ashley's with two infants are also staying here - they are on our boat. The Prescotts from Dahomey are at the Coopers and Mr. and Mrs. Hodgetts from Umuahia are at Bill Manns, so there are eight and two children we know on the boat so far.

Now for a fly in the ointment - last night thieves made two attempts on my room and on the first managed to steal the travelling rug. However it is covered by insurance so we should get the money back out of it. I am claiming £5. It was a most disturbing experience as twice I got out of bed to chase them away! without being able to catch them. A broken night! They cannot get in but managed to hook the rug with a long stick and pull it under the steel guard and out of the window.

Yesterday Margaret had to purchase a new case- a rather nice one, which will do for the honeymoon also. Tomorrow we shall pack the suitcases and get our tickets etc. and I believe we sail about midday on Tuesday. Could you bring some money to customs in case I need it please, should there be duty on anything in customs?

Incidentally, yesterday we bought a supply of anti-sickness tabs in hope of staving off any untoward happenings! Also bought some very fine swimming trousers so that I can sunbathe and try to get some colour! It seems unbelievable that we are almost on our way. Looking forward to two weeks tomorrow.

Love from both to you all. David.

On board mv AUREOL
Feb. 2nd 1954

A scribbled note to say that we are safely aboard. Margaret has a cabin to herself and I think I am sharing with a R.C. priest but I have not met him yet.

It is a lovely day, though very humid, and the sea looks calm - long may it remain so! The cabin class on the Aureol is very well equipped, everything much smaller though than on the Apapa 1st class.

Our companions seem very nice folk and we are looking forward to a very happy trip - weather permitting. One glorious relaxation, deck quoits, table tennis, swimming and eating (weather permitting). Mr. Angus thanked me this morning as we left for the work done in the tour - very nice of him.

We have had another wedding present of a damask tablecloth - very beautiful, from the folk who were up for Christmas you remember.

Well not long now, in two hours we shall be casting off (it is now 10am). Tomorrow Gold Coast, end of the week Sierra Leone then Gambia. Next week Canary Islands and then a fortnight yesterday - home.

I noticed on the news last night you had the coldest night for six years. Pray hard for warm weather!

Much love from us both,   David

SECOND TOUR, 1954-56

M.V. Aureol
Aug. 12th 1954

Here we are safely on board and have just had our lunch with our other Methodist colleagues including Margaret and Charles Day. They both look well especially the former.

Yesterday we had a good journey, with the taxi waiting at Waterloo when we arrived. We went round to Thea's for a meal. She is very well, as is Roger. Ernest is still in Lisbon, but will be back on Saturday I think.

This morning Auntie Florence called in and Thea has come down to the boat with us. We had a bit of a wait till the customs opened but thereafter did not have any trouble.

The weather is poor, foggy this morning, but it looks now as if it is going to clear - the sun is just peeping through.

I should like again to say how very much I appreciate our home and how very much I love you.

Love and affection from us both, David

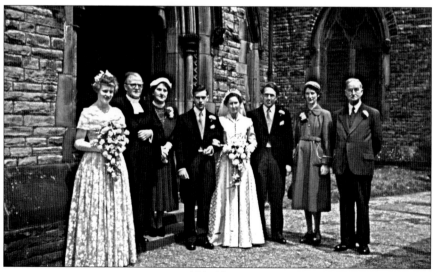

Wedding

160

On Board
August 18th 1954

A week has gone by since we left, and as I write this you will be on your way to North Yorkshire I expect. I do hope all is going well and that you have a very happy and restful time.

As I said in my letter on board we got here safely, though rather fear that one holdall got lost between customs and the boat. It contained three of Margaret's dresses, two pairs of my trousers and other odds and ends. It is just possible that it may turn up when we unload, but we are not over hopeful about it.

It was a dull and rather foggy day as we sailed down the Mersey, but it cleared towards evening, and as we went to bed it was beautifully calm. Friday was rather rough and Saturday very choppy indeed. None of us felt very well. Margaret and I missed one meal each only, though Charles Day and several others spent all day on their bunks. On Sunday however our uneasiness left us and we have had a remarkably good trip so far, even though they say there is an abnormal amount of swell for this time of year and the boat rolls most alarmingly at times.

There are over 80 of us in the Cabin Class, with a large proportion of Africans. There are a large number of Americans on board belonging to the Sudan Interior Mission chiefly. There is an African Bishop, and English SPG brother who has not taken off his dog collar yet despite the heat, and a strange young man - ex Cliff College who is going out under the London United mission as an engineer. So you can see we have all shades of religious beliefs! as we have in colour of skin.

The food is good, though not as good as it has been, we have margarine instead of butter all the time for instance! But it is a real joy to wade through the menu with unabated zeal.

The weather has gradually got hotter and hotter, and to varying degrees we are all sunburnt - one or two really quite seriously, but it is pleasant to feel the warmth of the sun upon one.

We have not seen land now for six days but yesterday we had a bit of an excitement when two stowaways were transferred to us to take back to Africa. They had stowed away on a cargo vessel. Tomorrow we reach Bathhurst where I hope to post this and purchase some stamps of the country.

We are both very fit indeed and hope you are having a good holiday with fine weather. Love to you all from us both, David

Lagos, Thursday, 26th August 1954

Here we are safely in Lagos with all our goods intact, and what is more the missing hold-all has turned up again!

It was grand to receive your letters when we arrived at the Mission House. I am sorry the weather has been so poor. Everyday I looked at the news sheet for the cricket and every day it said 'rain general' - but we hoped that perhaps North

Yorkshire was being spared.

We landed at Takoradi, the acting Chairman came on board and took us all off in his car for a cup of coffee at his house - Rev. and Mrs. Kenward - brother of the Kenward in Guernsey.

We had a full day in the harbour and sailed in the evening, arriving in Lagos in fine and cool weather at 2pm yesterday afternoon. The immigration and customs authorities came on board and I paid £1.3.0d in duty. Mr. Angus then hove into view - we all had tea together and then went into battle in the customs shed. All our baggage turned up and I asked one of the customs men to come. He asked me what I had got and seemed a bit sceptical but I didn't have to open anything - nor have to pay any more! Then came the problem of loading seven lots of luggage (MMs & CMS) but Mr. Angus had brought a lorry, a kit car and a saloon car! He took the ladies, I supervised the loads onto the lorry and came with that.

We received a warm welcome from Mrs. Angus, though we are staying next door. Today has been very busy. We left at 8.00 am and went shopping - and bought a sewing machine £23.5.0, a modern Singer portable a very nice model. The fridge we will buy through UCH Ibadan. A watering can, a hoe, and rake were amongst our purchases and food including fruit for cakes and mincemeat for Christmas. The hospital car turned up last night with notes from Andrew and Jean. They seem well and are looking forward to seeing us. They asked us to buy one or two things, which we have purchased but we shall have a car full!

In addition we have to arrange for our heavy loads (-1/2 ton) to be taken up by lorry and we are fortunate in that they are going up over night and should be there before we are.

We are setting off in good time tomorrow morning and hope to get there before dark - we shall not bother to call anywhere en route except to enquire about chickens! We have bought a small book about keeping hens in the tropics - should be very useful.

I do hope that the latter half of your holiday was better than the first. We are both very fit   Love from us both , David

Sunday, August 29th 1954

Here the tale is continued from our own house and home in the compound, having arrived safely with all our luggage intact.

We had a good night on Thursday evening having had chop with the Angus family and we set out on Friday for Ilesha. The Vanguard car is not too good at the moment so we set out in good time after making one or two calls in Lagos to get printing paper and a hat for me.

It was a very wet journey and 40 miles out of Lagos we stopped to have a banana. When we tried to start the car it wouldn't and there we stuck for one

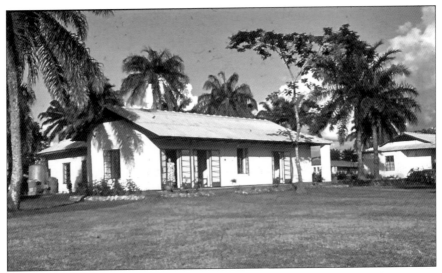

Cannon House

and a half hours. Several cars stopped to help but without avail. However we said that we would give it one more good push before sending for help and it started. We were very pleased, needless to say and carried on right through to Ilesha, without a further stop except for petrol. Just outside Ilesha we stopped briefly to change my shirt as it was wet and dirty with car repairs, and also tied a piece of white ribbon to the car. In this way we drove through the new gatehouse and received a rousing welcome from the staff, and since then we have had many individuals up to salute us and welcome us back. Andrew, Jean and the Sisters were very glad to see us and seem in good form except for tiredness.

When we arrived we found our loads intact and after dinner with the Pearsons' we retired.

Yesterday we began to unpack and what a job it was! but we had Joseph the carpenter in and as soon as I unpacked the bathroom cupboard and so on he fixed them in, so really we are almost straight. All the boxes, trunks and cases are empty and put away and homes found for most of our things, despite the fact that six drawers are stuck due to the dampness. All has arrived safely except that two cups of the picnic case are broken and the mirror of my microscope cracked, which isn't too bad considering.

Our house has been painted up in honour of our arrival and really looks very nice and with the tray Michael gave us and the Patterson bowl everything looks extraordinarily nice in the living room. Our bedroom too is almost straight but the spare room has many things on the bed that will have to be put away in time.

I do wish you could see the house, but perhaps one day you will. Last night we were really tired. This morning we have been to service 1 hour 50 minutes and then we crept out! Coffee in the Pearsons' house and lunch will be ready very soon. William is in good form and is going to stay and make good we think.

John returned last night in very good form and we have several visitors this weekend. The grounds look very nice! but we have not even been to our garden yet, so will tell about it next week. Nor have I been up to the Hospital! We are going to get quite straight first and then tackle other jobs

We have thought of you a great deal and look forward to hearing how you fared. We are both very fit and happy. Love from us both, David

Sept 5th 1954

It was grand to get your letter on Tuesday and to hear how you all are - though I fear your holiday will have been completely washed out from what you say. Here the weather has been very cool for this time of year and consequently we have more energy for getting things done.

On Monday and Tuesday we spent the time in getting the house in order, putting up pelmet rails, putting in the fittings and so on and really the house now looks most attractive - it is much the nicest house on the compound. There are still many jobs to be done - especially in the garden but they will have to be tackled one by one in due time.

There has been a great deal of work put in on our garden - but the vegetables are not growing as well as they might. I think the ground needs some compost and other treatment to get it quite right. The compost pit is now started and a little is added to it each day, and Margaret says it is getting warm at the bottom, which is a good sign.

Our chicken run is ready - but no chicken house- so we have got to start thinking about that. We are asking John Powell who is definitely coming out to bring some day old chicks - by air- and we are hoping that we may be able to rear them.

On Wednesday I started work in the wards and it is almost like starting in a new hospital - I didn't know where things are kept and so on, but I am learning now. The wards look so much cleaner and more attractive and it is more possible to work them efficiently. We get much the same number of patients and the work will be much the same, though easier when we get the official opening over.

On Wednesday evening the compound gave us a party, held in the Wrights. We were met by the whole staff, each playing an instrument - the Wedding March. John as Best Man and Eileen as Bridesmaid and were led to the Wedding feast. We had a lovely meal, finishing with the top tier of the Wedding cake and speeches! Then we played games and then showed the colour photos - it was a most enjoyable and successful evening.

On Thursday Margaret and I held a reception for the Nurses in the Out Patient Department in the evening. We welcomed them all at the door and then showed the photographs, which were greeted with loud cheers. After this we cut the cake into 70 pieces and gave each one a piece, and then they gave us three cheers and we closed with the benediction - a most successful time.

On Friday Margaret made pelmets for the living room, having made curtains for a screen earlier in the week. The cotton broke many times, but we think this is due to the poor quality cotton bought in the local market. Last night Andrew and Jean came in to chop.

This morning it was our turn for coffee. We had everyone in and will go to the service this evening. On Tuesday we are having dinner with Elsie and then on Wednesday we are going on trek to Ikole and Afon. We shall be away for three nights.

We are busy writing invitations for the New Hospital opening ceremony at the moment - a gigantic task - will send a copy off by slow mail.

We are both very well indeed and settling down in our new home. Much love from us both, David

10.9.54

At the moment it is Friday night and we are on trek at Afon. William is just finishing in the kitchen. There is a brilliant moon and a clear sky after a very wet day. Tonight - at this moment, Michael will be in his train travelling up to London for his vacuum course and will no doubt be a trifle late at Kings Cross!

Last Sunday we spent quietly at home after entertaining to coffee in the morning and in the evening we went to the Hospital Service, which is held in the Outpatient Hall. It was taken by Enid Blake who spoke at some length on humility. Monday was a usual sort of day with outpatients, and one or two minor operations, and again addressing of envelopes. In the two days we got over 400 ready for the post, many containing a stamped addressed envelope for the return gifts which we hope will pour in.

I did my first op. in the new theatre - not a very big one - about half an hour. All went well and it seems a very satisfactory place to work.

Incidentally the plate is fitted to the Rivercourt Table and looks very well. The table is getting a good deal of use in the Outpatient theatre and I have used it half a dozen times already.

On Tuesday evening we went out to Elsie's to dinner, with two of the Apostolic Missionaries Mr. and Mrs. Wood - Americans. She has got her house looking very nice indeed and we had a very pleasant evening.

On Wednesday we set off on trek for Ifaki and Ikoli. At Ifaki (Jonah is still on leave) we camped in the house for lunch and then went down to the dispensary where there were very few patients, as they had not been told of our coming. After this we pushed on to Ikole where we received a warm welcome from Louie Trott who seems very fit.

On Thursday we saw the in-patients and some very interesting ones too, and

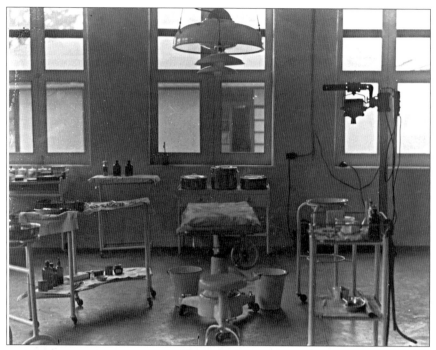

New theatre

then about 30 out patients. After a rest we went for a short ride in the car to distribute a letter of invitation. In the evening Margaret made some curtains with the material we brought out. It was raining so hard that we could not hear each other speak, so I just read and Louie sewed,

Today it has been rather wet and the roads appaling in places. We left Ikole in the driving rain about 11.30 and set out for Afon along a road I have not been on before. We stuck fast in the mud at one place for half an hour until we had seven men, and together we lifted first the front and then the back of the Morris Minor out of the rut and out to a hillock of mud and then with many pushes we were through but covered with thick brown mud!

We had a picnic lunch from our case, which does very well indeed. On arriving here I took the gun out of the car and shot a bush fowl which we have had roasted for supper tonight- delicious! We are sitting around two pressure paraffin lamps with absolute silence except for many crickets outside.

Tomorrow we return to Ilesha after seeing the patients in the morning.

(PS shot another bush fowl for tonight!)

Now Sunday. We returned safely after good journey to find all well. Your two letters received with great pleasure. Thea has had a baby daughter - Brenda. Glad to hear all is well with you all.

There are two books I should like please as my Christmas present but could I have them at once? - The New Bible handbook edited by GT Manley - 12/6 and

Search the Scriptures- one volume three years Bible Study course 12/6 both published by the IVF at 39, Bedford Square, London. I should be pleased if these could be sent as soon as possible as they will be invaluable for Nurses Prayers and study groups.

The hospital is very busy today, John and I and Andrew operating. Just used our pressure cooker for the first time - most successful. Mr. Mellanby turned up on Friday night! We are both very fit.

With much love from us both, David

19.9.54

Another very full week has passed. It is now Sunday morning and we are awaiting the staff, who are coming here for coffee. Andrew, John and four boys are down at Otapete, so we shall not be starting for a few minutes.

We were very pleased to receive your first letter and to learn of the activities (many at No.1). By now Glanville and Jean will be on their way- having a calm voyage I hope or else the sea will earn Glanville eternal disfavour! Glad you met Ray and Daisy Rowland - they are a very nice couple.

Your second letter arrived on Thursday with the news of Henry's waistcoat! It sounds a most beautiful creation and a pity a close up colour photo could not be taken and sent out, - or perhaps the present day colour film could hardly do it justice!! Yes Margaret wore her Wedding dress and I wore my going away suit for the staff party.

Dr. Craddock will have come and gone by this time - I hope you had a happy time together.

Here we are up to the eyes in the arrangements for the Opening Day next Saturday. The plans seem to have to cover every detail and it is taking most of our time and thoughts. Despite this the hospital has been very busy and to cap it all the lights failed one night and I had to do a strangulated hernia by the light of two 40 watt bulbs and a torch, which wasn't very easy. The patient is fine! In addition we have been busy in theatre and maternity has had one or two odd things. Last evening I had to do a forceps delivery on a girl of fourteen years who was having fits. Not very easy everything considered!

On Tuesday this week we had the Wrights, Elsie and Donald Mann, a visitor from Ado Ekiti in for dinner a most interesting evening, which went very well. Last night we had Eileen, Enid and the Pearsons' in and played Pitt afterwards which, was enjoyed by all except Enid who knitted and did not play

In the morning yesterday I had to go out to the post office and Margaret came to buy some curtain material and stuff for mattress covers. We got the latter at UAC then went to the Syrian shop for curtain material. The shop we went into belonged, as it happened to a Syrian lady who is a private maternity patient I am looking after and after we had chosen 7 yards of material we liked and tried to pay for it - she gave it to us!

This time next week we shall be tired in body and spirit. I am processing from the old site to the New, a two hour march in the sun. In addition I am treasurer of the Opening Day Appeal, which has now reached just over £60 - we are hoping for £2,000, but I fear we may not reach that figure.

This afternoon will be an office afternoon, as I have a great deal do and the Procession committee minutes to prepare for duplication. The Angus's arrive on Wednesday, Ken and the Gills on Thursday, so we shall then be up to the eyes in work. The weather is still comparatively cool 75-85 and down to 70 at night but still a lot of rain. We are both very fit and happy. Love from us both, David

26.9.54

Of course the great item this week was the opening. On Wednesday the Anguses arrived in good order and Mrs. Angus took our devotions that evening. Unfortunately the town water supply failed so Andrew and I went down to the pump by the stream - it was most eerie. Pitch black, raining and strange rustling all round. We started the engine and the pump but the latter would pump for about six minutes and then loose its suck and we would have to prime it again. This we did four times but could not find the leak so gave up, but fortunately the town supply came next morning.

On Thursday, Ken (who is now working in Eastern Nigeria) arrived with the Bennets of the Salvation Army. Ken very fit and in excellent form. John Powell also came, very fit and most thrilled to be back. He is staying with Elsie, and Ken

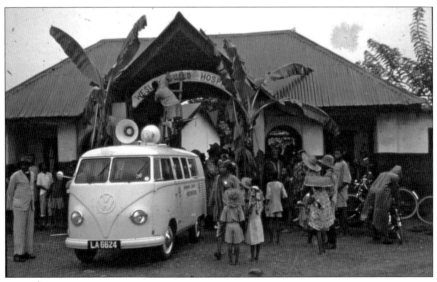

Removing the hospital sign

with us, though Ken left this morning and returned to the East. On Friday the Gills arrived from Lagos - bringing me a cream shirt which cost 57s.6d! It is almost too good to wear!

Mr. and Mrs. Inazelle the film producer also arrived as well as Margaret Swann from Lagos and Louie Trott from Ikole That night we had a discussion about last minute details. Incidentally I am in charge of the fund, now £760 which is reasonable, though we hope to get £2,000 at least.'

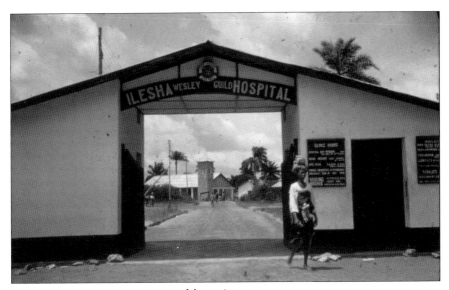

New site gate

On Saturday it poured with rain and it was so dark that we couldn't have a film taken - most disappointing! I dressed up in a cream shirt and suit with maroon tie and was told looked smart. I went down to the Old Site to organise the procession. It rained steadily. Then as we left the Old Site it began to clear and remained fine the rest of the day.

The procession headed by nurses with flag and shield and Drs. Powell and Cannon, stretched a quarter of a mile with Schools and banners and drums, colleges, societies, churches. Many photos were taken by the PRO of Ibadan and there was a loudspeaker van giving a Christian testimony throughout, given by the Rev. Adigbola. As we arrived at the site most had arrived. The badge and shield were received and put by the platform and the flag run up but not unfurled.

The Minister of Health arrived and the Owa and mounted the platform at the roundabout outside the hospital gate, with the guests of honour sitting all round.

There was a large crowd but not as vast as it would have been if it hadn't rained, I couldn't hear the speakers very well but Rev. Salako opened with prayer and a hymn and then Mr. Angus, Andrew, John Powell, Rev. Adegbola, the minster and the Owa.

The Minister, escorted by Andrew, unlocked the vast padlock and chain and opened the gates where a Guard of Honour was in position, consisting of nurses and compound boys and the rest of the staff, and the wives of the Staff.

Charles Day came and also Dr. Lawson the Consultant Gynaecologist from Ibadan. After the gates had been opened the official party looked round, then the folk who had give £2.2.0 opened windows, which had been allotted to them and people who had given £5.5.0 opened doors.

This passed off remarkably smoothly but the food afterwards was chaotic. By 5pm most folk had left, peace restored, the compound remarkably unspoiled. In the evening the Angus's came in to chop and we had a restful time, a most successful and happy day. The one disappointment was the film, which could not be shot in such poor light. We are both very fit and enjoying ourselves immensely.

Love from us both, David

3.10.54

Your tour of Cudley Hall seems to have been most interesting - but 23 miles of Swiss Roll per day seems fantastic doesn't it?

The piston rings arrived safely and intact thank you very much and have given great pleasure to Mr. Lanyon. I had 2/- customs to pay on them. Thank you too for the books and look forward to their arrival.

Glad to hear that Grandma is well, how is the weather with you? We have had quite a lot of rain, which makes the ground very difficult to walk on and white clothes do not stay white very long!

It has been remarkably cool in the mornings and evenings too, though is getting much hotter in the mid-day. Good gardening weather though and Margaret is putting in a lot of work, planting out seedlings - cabbages, lettuces, carrots and so on. Flowers too are flourishing but the white ants are depressing. They eat through the stems of the flowers overnight and next morning it is lying flat, just as if cut with an axe. The rain is causing the weeds to grow so that it is a full time task to keep the lawn weeded.

Last Sunday we went to Otapete and heard Mr. Angus preach, and the rest of the day had an easy time with the happy thought that the opening was over.

On Monday we were back to normal routine again and able to give our minds to the patients. On Tuesday afternoon we took the Gills to Imesi Ile where there is a very nice rest house where we had a picnic tea and then went to look at the road that is being made there by the people themselves in an attempt to increase the business of the village.

John Gill and I, whilst returning saw a large scorpion about seven inches long, blue/black in colour with large pincer claws in front. It looked like miniature lobster with a wicked looking tail, which comes up and over the body. A ferocious looking animal, but the guide who was with us said that the smaller ones are more dangerous. The sting of a scorpion can kill a man sometimes.

On Wednesday the four of us went to the Pearson's for dinner and then John Gill led the fellowship afterwards. Thursday was much as usual, except that in the evening I had to do a Caesarean section with a happy result and a very nice baby boy and both are doing well. Margaret Day has had a son and both are well. Everyone very thrilled about it.

On Friday the Gills went off to Ikole where John is going to install a pump for Louie, so that she has water laid on to all the buildings. John and Nancy will be returning on Friday. Also on Friday we had our nurses class - twelve or so of them - We had an introductory session and are going to study Marks Gospel. Yesterday we had a long committee in the afternoon and in the evening, amidst many other duties completed one end of our chicken house! We haven't any chickens yet!

This afternoon I am taking the leprosy patients service and this evening Sylvia is taking the service in the chapel here. To date the Opening Day appeal has reached £930. Andrew is going on trek this week.

Love to you all from us both, David

10th Oct 1954

We have received two letters this week the first concerned mostly with the London Committee and the latter with family affairs.

Here we have had a busy week. Eileen came into clinic on Monday, and on Tuesday Andrew and I paid £1600 in to the bank, whilst Margaret obtained cold store (food) for the compound. In the afternoon Margaret prepared to go to Lagos and on Wednesday about 7.00am left to go to meet Joyce Tompkins, the new nursing Sister.

Margaret picked up Major Roberts the Salvation Army man who hasn't been well and took him to the hospital for observation, and then went down to Lagos. Margaret did not actually go to the boat but did shopping and was at the Mission House when Joyce arrived from the docks.

On the Thursday they set off after more shopping which kept them rather late. But Joyce wasn't well on the journey so they stopped with the Days in Ibadan for two hours for Joyce to rest and sleep. Margaret had bought small gifts for the Days and Boshiers babies - both lovely children but the Days haven't a name for him yet.

Last night (Sat.) we had a party in the Sisters house - a very happy affair with the nine of us - most enjoyable.

Friday was work as usual but on Saturday I did a new operation which went quite well at the time though we shall have to wait many months to check the end result.

On the way up Margaret called at the Poultry Farm at Agage and collected ten eggs for sitting (1/- each) Jean has a broody hen and she is now sitting on them to our delight. The hen house is making slow progress, but should be ready by the time they are ready for a proper run! I have got the two ends made - one with a hole for them to pop in and out and the back is almost complete except for the nesting boxes on which I am working at the moment! The tools I have are excellent and it will not be for poor tools that the job is not expertly completed.

This morning we have been to Otapete where the notices lasted for 30 minutes, including a list of subscriptions in all the classes! Joyce was welcomed at the end of it. She is settling down quite well I think and is going on duty this afternoon for the first time. After chapel we drove round the old site and picked 20 grapefruit from one of the trees, by Yoruba custom as we planted the trees we can continue to pick the fruit. The weather is remarkably cool.

We are both remarkably well and very happy.

Love from us both, David.

17.10.54

We were glad indeed to receive your letter on Friday and to hear that all is well at home. Talking of the Methodist Recorder, I was sorry to read of the wrong date in connection with the opening of the new hospital, but Dr. Bolton says there is a good photograph within. If all is well we should be sending home a series of photographs of the opening but at the moment they have not come.

Very glad to hear that Jonah and Mrs. Jones looked in and that you liked them. Jonah is a very fine man and well liked by the local people.

We have had a quiet week here so far as it can be quiet - no anniversaries or things of that sort. Last Sunday morning we sat through the service and then in the evening had another service in the Out Patients department here for the nurses taken by a school master

This week John and Sylvia have had a week off to do language study and took their first exam last night and they will certainly have passed. It has meant though that Andrew and I have had all the hospital work to do. However despite it all I have managed to get the hen house built. It is made of wood, sides and floor back and part of front three nesting boxes which stick out behind and have a lid whereby the eggs (if any) can be removed. The front is covered with wire netting and also lifts up for ease of cleaning. On the side not seen is a small door with a little ladder affair for the hens to walk up!

The roof and top of sides remain to be completed and the whole painted with salignum to deter the white ants from having it for lunch one day. The hen is still sitting on nine eggs so we are hopeful but mustn't count our chickens!

The next item in the carpentry agenda is a shelter for the seed boxes. Unfortunately the torrential tropical torrents have washed the last batch of seeds into oblivion. However to compensate the compost pit and stack are both working very well and there is a nice lot of compost in the making. The lettuce has done very well but beans and carrots are disappointing. On Monday we went to the old site and brought up a stone of grapefruit and 30 pineapple plants, which we divided out. At the moment no-one is getting the fruit there so we sally forth occasionally and bring some back.

The trees are unfortunately covered in ants which eat the fruit so it is a somewhat painful pastime. The pineapples will not bear fruit for 2 - 3 years as they are all young plants.

Last night Andrew and Jean came in to chop - a lovely meal, pork and apple sauce and we played 'Oh Hell' which for a change I won decisively!

We are both very well with a lot of work. Love from us both, David

Sunday, Oct 23rd 1954

It is a really hot day today and one has to make a real effort to get anything done especially if it means going out in the sun!

A lady doctor (from Germany) has just gone. She arrived at 3.30 and for an hour and a quarter she, Elsie and I and two nurses have been round the hospital with teutonic thoroughness and I feel as if I shall never be cool again!

The news of Ted's death came as a great surprise naturally, and we have been remembering Henry and his family a great deal in the last days.

This week has been an uneventful one for us. The main item of news is that Andrew and family have gone on local leave. They have gone down to a beach near Lagos, very quiet, you have to go by canoe to get to it. It will be quite a job to get the children and luggage across and then one has to have bearers to carry the loads to the bungalow. The house belongs to a businessman in Lagos who uses it for weekends. They are going this evening and return next Saturday and the rest of the time they are staying with friends in Lagos. Thus I have the problems of the hospital to solve at the moment.

The maternity ward has been incredibly busy. At one time we had 25 mothers in and 21 babies - the other four being undelivered and today we have already had another three babies though some of the 25 have already gone home. Why they should suddenly all come at once I do not know, anyway it has been very thrilling to see our new ward absolutely full.

On Friday evening Margaret and I had our Nurses fellowship group. We are going through St. Marks' Gospel and have got to the baptism of Jesus - we had a most interesting discussion on it.

Our kitten Scales, seems to have come to stay at last. His mother seems to have cast him out so he is content to remain with us. He seems a most intelligent and friendly animal.

The hen is still sitting on the eggs and we hope to have some good news by the end of the week! The chicken house is progressing! It is now a question of completing the painting it with anti termite stuff and putting on its roof.

Have just taken a few photos in the evening sun of the chicken house, cat, Margaret and self. We must finish off the film quite soon, develop it and then send the negatives home to you.

We are all keeping well with rather a lot of work at the moment. The garden is thriving under Margaret's hands and from the books we are having many new recipes that are quite exciting.

Although it is 6pm it is still very warm and close. Went to Otapete this am. - one and three quarter hours and tonight the Salvation Army couple are taking our service here. Much love from us both, David

October 30th 1954

With sundry rude remarks about my writing I resort again to the typewriter in the attempt to restore legibility to my letters, though I fear that it will be necessary to spell more accurately as the doubtful letters cannot be hidden.

We were very glad indeed to receive your two letters this week or rather two from you and one from Stanley! The latter is a hoot, beginning with an original spelling of 'Margaret' and ending with some Greek.

The nature of the new operation was a salpingostomy - new for me - though I believe the operation was devised by Mr. Bonney in 1921, though I am open to correction on that point.

The big piece of news this week is that the eggs have hatched. Ten were set and of these eight hatched, but unfortunately one chick got smothered, I think after 24 hours, which leaves us with seven of the loveliest little chicks that you ever saw. Some are light Sussex crossed with Rhode Island Reds and some have the odd spot of Leghorn in them I believe. Margaret is feeding at the moment, though William seems to know what sort of food they like. The chicken house now waits only for its roof and given an hour or so that should go on without trouble. The painting with anti termite stuff is now complete.

The green sheets are very nice indeed, and both wear and wash very well, retaining the green colour and not apparently gaining any of the rather reddish earthy colour that white things do. They have caused a considerable amount of interest amongst the staff both European and kitchens in the compound! The apples have been a great success and the gooseberries have done very well. We had pork on two occasions, when we have had folk in and we have had apple sauce, absolutely marvellous and we have had one lot of gooseberry pie.

Another break whilst we dispensed coffee to the staff as it is our week. Margaret weighed the coffee yesterday and we find that we have only used one and a half pounds since we came and considering the amount we drink it seems most reasonable. The pressure cooker is a great boon also. This week on

Thursday night and Friday we had a Mr. Driscoll, a Methodist from Croydon, who is a representative from the firm Allen and Hanburys staying with us and as a special meal we had chicken. Normally, though cooked for a long time it would have been very tough, but half an hour in the pressure cooker made it beautifully tender, and then a short while in the oven to roast it made it look very nice too. It was delicious.

Mr. Driscoll was most interested in the Hospital and the work and stuck to my tail for 24 hours to see how things worked. He is flying home in about ten days time.

This week has been very busy one with Andrew away, with all the correspondence to cope with and all the palavers to settle. However only three days more and he will be back. We had a note from him to say that he had reached the bungalow safely, a wooden, two roomed place, with a patio for sitting out on in the heat, 20 yards from the shore, a fridge in going order and a two burner paraffin stove which boiled a kettle in fifteen minutes. There is a caretaker who tends to it and does the washing up but Jean would have to cook for the family, no small task. We shall be most interested to see how they look and feel after it.

I have been on night duty this week, and up every night, two nights getting less than four hours sleep in each! One was a very difficult maternity case (impacted breach) with marked disproportion and a long labour prior to being brought in, and last night an intestinal obstruction of four days standing. The first night - last Sunday- there was a whole run of calls starting soon after evening service. I shall be very glad to have a good rest at nights.

Last Wednesday was Eileen's Birthday and after chop all came round here and we played Pitt, which was greatly appreciated. David Head of the Student Christian Mission was here also, staying with John.

Last evening we had Eileen and Joyce in to dinner and afterwards we played 'Oh Hell' which seemed to be appreciated so we shall have someone to play with when the Pearsons' are away. Yesterday was payday, but passed off relatively smoothly considering the unrest in the Western Region over recent legislature ordering 5/- minimum wage (ours get 2/-).

We are both very well indeed, much love, David

November 5th 1954

It is now bonfire night and with many happy memories of parties on this night we wonder just what is happening at home and at Priors Court?

We, rather unexpectedly, are at Afon and I am trying to write this by the light of a pressure lantern but every time Margaret moves her pencil shadow falls across the page and my pen is in darkness, however I will try to keep it legible.

We have had a pretty full week here. Last Sunday John preached a very well thought out sermon but a bit above the heads of his congregation. On Monday Eileen went out in the truck to Imesi and to our concern failed to return at the expected time. A search party was organised but just as it was leaving she and the driver arrived tired and worn out. Their car (the new Morris) had trouble with the petrol pump. The next day I got the engine in the lorry and sent them off and some four hours later returned with the small car running well.

On the Monday night we were going out to chop with the Salvation Army folk, but sent a note to say we couldn't go as we had no transport. However an Apostolic couple were also invited and they called for us and brought us back, a very happy evening - with a rather over elaborate meal. Soup, beef, potatoes, beans, peas, cauliflower, onion sauce and mint sauce and gravy! Yorkshire pudding! and then sweet, coffee and cake.

On Wednesday John went on trek to Ikole and in the evening the Pearsons' arrived looking very fit after their holiday on the beach - it has been a marvellously quiet holiday for them. The only folk they saw were a few fishermen. When they wanted fish they went onto the beach and bought enough for them all for 1/-. At night, instead of a bath - a swim in the sea and so on. They are all nice and brown and very well.

On Thursday John returned having had a very tedious journey, so much so in fact that he stuck his heels in more or less about coming up to Afon.

On Wednesday Margaret was not well temperature 101, vomiting and generally below par. However a day in bed- and light diet have put her right and now she is quite better.

Yesterday we had a very heavy day in theatre. I had two caesarean sections, - which is most unusual - one for twins with abnormal presentation and the second a primigravida with a small pelvis. Mothers and babies are well.

This morning, I did the hospital work and we left about 11.30 and have come up through Oshogbo, Ogbomosho and Ilorin a much better route, though longer. Tomorrow we have to go back the old way - a very poor road. On the 11th we have the Federal elections there will be great excitement and Monday is a Muslim Holiday!

Now safely back in Ilesha. Books of Punches have arrived safely. Have written to Michael. We are both fit and well. Much love from us both, David

Nov. 14th 1954

Another week has gone and it is Sunday morning again our turn for coffee. Your letter arrived on Friday.

I noted from your letter the date of dispatch and registration number of the little parcel sent and wrote a note for the postmaster here. He had the parcel but it had been delayed in customs at Kano. The trouble being that on the declaration form you put films instead of photographs and their value at £1.5.0

instead of no commercial value. Films are dutiable photos - which they are not. The palaver has not been settled yet as I shall probably have to pay on them eventually. However the postman was very good and let me have them having signed for them. Most of the photos are excellent aren't they! especially the group on our doorstep and the photos of the hospital here.

Tonight is the last Sunday here for the Wrights before they go on furlough so we are having a little get together after the evening service and I am going to show them on the wall with the projector.

We were very interested to hear of you visit to Priors Court to see Stanley - days at PC do seem to be wet don't they? I don't think I have been on a dry one. Congratulations to Henry on passing his MB path., another step safely accomplished.

Interested to hear of taking up the dahlia roots. Our roots too will be taken up soon. We have not had any rain now for two weeks if we don't get any more this year the rains will have stopped very early with consequent distress to the gardening fraternity here. The ground is very dry indeed and the vegetables almost at a stand still. Soon the grass will be turning brown and the amount of dust will increase.

Last Sunday we went down to our Children's Harvest at Otapete. A vast crowd there - we only just got seats and that by some people being turned out to our embarrassment. The church was decorated with whole banana trees 12 - 20 feet high, sugar cane and paw paws. There was a native band, which beat out a rumba rhythm for the singing. Two weeks today it is the adult Harvest, which will be a real fashion parade.

The hospital has been very quiet as far as patients have gone and I have had a Yoruba week - had three days at Yoruba, which has been most useful. Now have a new teacher Mr. Ogunmokum.

On Thursday we had another public holiday for it was the Federal Elections, most exciting. The party in power in the West, the Action Group, looks like being defeated which will cause a bit of disturbance. At the moment it stands at NCNC 20 seats AG 18 with three to be declared so it is still in the balance. In Eastern Nigeria there has been a great NCNC majority. Whichever party is in power, I don't think it will affect us very much.

Our fridge is a great boon though it is a bit expensive to run about 11/- a day, which adds up in a year, but at the moment we are sharing it with the Pearsons' and that helps.

From now on we shall be incredibly busy, Missionary Boards in Ibadan, our annual accounts to make up and numerical returns to get out!

John and family go to Lagos on Friday or Saturday and sail next Tuesday.

Much love from us both, David

December 12th 1954

Another very full week has passed and a week of exceedingly hard work - and the week just starting looks as if it too will be pretty hectic. We had a letter from Michael too, which was very nice and heard again of the spectrometer, whatever it is supposed to do apparently it didn't! I remember meeting Dr. Bell at Pinner, unfortunately that is when the bulb of the projector broke so it was not a very successful evening.

Last Sunday Dr. and Mrs. Haigh of Ituk Mbang came through on their way to Lagos. Mrs. H is going home – Dr. Haigh is staying out a little longer. He said Ken was in very good form and, between ourselves, thinking of staying out longer. This would seem to be another of Ken's ideas - we shall see what comes of it when Keith the builder returns in January. Also Harry Haigh is not going to be Superintendent of the New United Mission Joint Training Hospital!! He says he cannot work for four masters three missions and the government. This is rather surprising but fits in with what we have heard of Harry H as an individualist. He says that John Gower (now on his first furlough) will be looking after it - another rather surprising fact. The Cundalls are well and fit and have settled down better now. They had a rather unfortunate beginning with ill health.

Last Sunday at service we had a thanksgiving for Elsie's 25th year but I think I mentioned that last week. On Monday we had a great deal of work and then in the evening, the nurses and staff and clerks gathered in Out Patients for games and then we presented Elsie with a new sewing machine to replace hers which the hospital has used for many years. I understand too that the Owa is going to hold a reception for her and she may be given an honourary title - in Ilesha town, which will be a well deserved honour.

On Sunday evening Margaret and I went out to the District Officer's for chop. We had a very nice meal and evening, but as usual it goes on rather late - dinner is not until 9pm. He his wife and family seem in very good spirits just now.

Wednesday evening was fellowship and Thursday we spent preparing for the hospital Transport Board, which met on Friday.

Most of this week I have spent doing the accounts. At first it was about £100 out - in £65,000. Gradually it came down to five shillings and then finally I found that. Great rejoicing so we were able to bring out a statement of the accounts for the committee.

On Friday, Margaret and Jean provided tea for the committee members - about eighteen - mostly local folk the Angus's and Jonah were with them. The committee sat two and a half hours but it was time quite well spent I think.

Yesterday after operating in the morning we spent time in the office, catching up with letters. In the evening we had many new patients, with several operations and then a difficult maternity case to finish with.

However I have put time aside to prepare for the service, which I have to take this evening in the hospital here.

The weather seems to get hotter every minute and it does not feel like Christmas at all! Incidentally will Jonah's son Alan be in the hostel soon?

We have hardly thought about Christmas yet but send our love and very best wishes to you all for a very Happy Christmas.

Much love from us both   David

26.12.54

Boxing Day - a day of rest we hope! Yesterday we had a very happy but exhausting day and we hope that you all at home had a very good and happy time. Your letter arrived on Friday with news of a parcel which we had not received but imagine our delight when late on Christmas Eve a parcel came from Afon - from Ray and Daisy containing your presents. Thank you very much indeed. Margaret is very thrilled with the broach and the tin of biscuits and the soap. The coffee is a wonderful idea too - we are so glad they arrived in time.

Here, as may be imagined, we have had a very hectic week. In addition to being Christmas week, the hospital has been very busy - maternity especially - and it has been my week on night duty, but tonight I am off thank goodness.

Last Monday Bill Mann came through Ilesha and called on his way to Ikole. He brought up our Lagos account, which showed we are still £63.3.0 out but on checking it through I found it, so at last I think the accounts are straight. He brought up our first guest -Marjorie Fawcett from Methodist Girls High School - a very quiet, retiring person.

Margaret has been out shopping once or twice to get presents for the staff here and food and one thing and another.

Last Sunday evening we had our Carol Service, which was very good - the outpatient waiting room full to the doors. On Wednesday we had our evening fellowship, which I took. On Thursday evening we had Marjorie Fawcett in to supper and spent the time making Christmas crackers but unfortunately the 'cracker' parts got wet and wouldn't crack but we put topical things into the crackers for each person, which folk seemed to enjoy.

On Christmas Eve the other guests - three teachers from W.T.C. came in to this compound to stay - Miss Dibble with the Pearsons' and the other two with Elsie. We have not had anybody - both our invitees already had engagements.

On Christmas Eve we went Carol singing round the hospital - very pretty - the nurses in a long crocodile with lanterns going round the wards. Margaret and I made our decorations with crepe paper and a sewing machine and decorated our living room - it looked lovely. I was up for nearly two hours on Christmas Eve with two abnormal maternity cases, which was not helpful as we had Holy Communion at 6am on Christmas morning. Margaret and I joined Elsie and Margaret for our breakfast after which we opened our parcels. How exciting it

179

was. We got towels, vases, dressing table mat, books, sweets and a large calabash with jam in it.

After breakfast we gave presents to the nurses and then it was the ward service and I took the one on the Female ward. Another maternity case and then I helped Margaret to prepare lunch for sixteen. We opened a tin of ham and a small tin of tongue, had Russian salad; potato salad, green salad, home made chutney, grapefruit, and ground nuts in our hors d'oeurve dish. It looked and tasted delicious. This was followed by flan. Margaret made three, one apricot, one gooseberry (bottled) and one strawberry (from a tin). They were all very much appreciated.

We all rested after lunch and then gathered in our house for the Queen's broadcast and thought of our folk at home who would be listening too. Reception was good but it seemed brief and vaguely disappointing we thought.

Tea-cakes of various types and mince pies in Jean's house. Andrew - assisted by me had made a wooden garage for the children for Christmas. They are thrilled and with their Dinky toys too!

Then the nurses Nativity play. I had to ferry patients in the lorry up to the out patients room where the stage is, but well worth while. Then there was Christmas dinner - thirteen of us in the Sisters' house. Grapefruit, soup, turkey and trimmings, Christmas pudding, coffee and sweets then games and to bed about 12.30 but fortunately a quiet night. It will soon be coffee time and in our house. It is Andrew's turn for chapel. Must do a round, and then return to the house. We have had a marvellous time, and are very happy

Much love to you all, David

PS Michael and Stanley's greetings also greatly appreciated.

Dec 28th 1954

It was wonderful to receive the parcel on Christmas Eve. Thank you very much for all the gifts. The brooch is beautiful and we are looking forward to making good use of the coffee, biscuits and soap. You must have remembered my favourite perfume!

We have thought of you all many times over Christmas, it would have been nice to be with you, but we have had a very happy time together here.

We were sorry not to have guests, but the Rev. Morton is coming on Thursday to stay over the weekend, and so we shall be having further celebrations while he is with us.

Yesterday evening was the Nurses Party. It was held on our lawn, with lights strung across between the palm trees. David and Andrew were responsible for the games, which went very well indeed. It was a lively two hours and we all felt rather exhausted at the end. The sardine sandwiches and orange juice went down as well as ever. They must have been ready for them as the party follows *immediately after the concert given by the nurses for the patients.*

The nativity play was most successful this year, in spite of the producer's despair after each rehearsal. This is the first year that I have not had a hand in it and I enjoyed being one of the audience. It was all in Yoruba and some scenes were rather unorthodox but it went over in a big way. It is so nice to see a real baby in the crib, this one was only a few days old and still quite pink. He played his part well waving his arms and legs and crying just a little. In the last scene a small patient from the children's ward came onto the stage with a nurse and placed a bunch of flowers by the crib.

David has just gone to the office after our afternoon rest to prepare for a statistics committee this evening. I am about to accompany our garden boy, Daniel, down into the bush to see if we can cut a way through to the coconut palms, which David planted last year. They became overgrown whilst we were away.

I have very much enjoyed my first Christmas cooking and hope that my beginners luck will continue. Tomorrow I am going to make some pineapple jam and Jean is experimenting with hers today.

With love from us both, Margaret

Jan 2nd 1955

A very Happy New Year to you all! Your letter arrived on Friday and we were thrilled to read of all your activities and to receive your sympathy in our recent loss of chickens.

Your Sunday evening suppers seem to be as popular as ever - I wish I could be present too, there is something about Sunday evening suppers isn't there?.

A trifle disturbed about the bottle of sherry! It will take a bit of explaining if any 'help with the rough' finds it! Freddie's explanation of a moat round the chickens house is a good one if we could keep water in it, but as we are in the midst of four months without rain and the earth dry and scorched he will have to think of something else.

Michael seems to have hit on something in his icing mixture which might revolutionise the building trade!! I hope the second attempt was more successful as far as the cake went.

Our food has been most sumptuous - the cake is most luscious and though quite large we have nearly finished it with folk who have dropped in. The mince pies have been the best on the compound! and there is quite a considerable competition over Christmas fare. The latest success has been pineapple jam. The District Officer gave us a beautiful pineapple - over 3lbs. in weight, but not quite ripe enough to eat. But as jam it is superb. Our chutney is finished, so that will have to be the next objective.

This week has been very full. Last Sunday evening we had a repeat performance of the nativity play - and a Bank Holiday on the Monday but it was filled with the Nurses concert for the patients in the afternoon and the party for the nurses, given by the staff in the evening. Andrew was out all morning, which made it rather a heavy day for me.

The party in the evening was quite successful but we missed the presence of visitors greatly.

On Wednesday Andrew went to Ikole on trek, just after an important Nigerian civil servant was brought in, very injured after a motor smash. He became worse during the day and in the evening I had to remove a ruptured spleen. He was better for a while but died early on Friday morning, and at the post mortem we found that the right lung was almost non-existent due to old disease. There was a paragraph in the paper about him yesterday. It was a very worrying and stressful two days.

On Wednesday the Rev. Francis Morton came to stay with us. He is chaplain at Wesley College and was at South Elmwall 1948-51 and knows Adwick and Hooton quite well though not the 'Smiths'. He has not actually preached there. It is rather nice to have someone to stay even though it is after Christmas.

On Friday evening we had a sort of Watch Night Service taken by Rev. Morton and this evening he is taking our Covenant service.

Yesterday was New Years Day and a Bank Holiday. I spent most of the day struggling with accounts but we had a good long rest in the afternoon. In the evening Elsie and the Pearsons' came in to dinner and we lit one pair of candles - they looked very nice indeed - a lovely meal.

A long quiet night and then this morning we have been to Otapete for service very many people there as they make more of New Year than Christmas. We had a 'Thanksgiving' when the nurses and us all, went to give thanks and some money, to give thanks for being preserved until 1955.

Margaret has a cold but otherwise we are both very fit and have had a lovely Christmas in our home. With much love and affection from us both, David

8.1.55

A swelteringly hot afternoon, quiet with just the birds calling to one another outside - peace after a hectic week and peace before a hectic fortnight.

Your letter arrived on Thursday, and we were most interested to hear of your Christmas activities - we should love to have been there to enjoy them also but also wished you were all here to enjoy ours.

Last Sunday night we had our Covenant service taken by Frank Morton. It went very well indeed with an extra ten Europeans mostly Apostolics to share with us. There were about 50 for Communion as not all our nurses are full members and so are not allowed to partake.

Tuesday evening we had a special treat for the compound staff and nurses.

We had written to the Public Relations Dept. in Ibadan and asked if they could run a film show for us here. They said they could so we had it in the outpatient department.

They showed four films, one a British Newsreel, a film on Northern Rhodesia and a cartoon abut malaria and finally a longer film about a Welsh farmers son, who graduates at Bangor and then comes back on the farm to work.

It made a very pleasant evening, though I had to go out at one point and missed one of the films, in order to give some methylated spirits to the hospital folk at Ife who are right out.

The latter part of the week has been overshadowed by the impending visit of the Auditors - so we had to straighten out our bills, receipts and so forth.

Friday began much as usual but about 11am a note came from a village 29 miles away to say that Mr. Mackenzie the District Officer had been taken ill and would a doctor go out. Andrew went to see him and found him with acute appendicitis and brought him back. He was not fit to send on to Ibadan - so we had to remove his appendix at 4pm that afternoon. I gave the anaesthetic and Andrew removed his appendix since then he has been in our spare room, with Margaret doing most of the nursing. We have been rather busy as you can imagine - with Mrs. Mackenzie coming up twice a day to see him. It was a perfectly straightforward operation and he is doing quite well, though it was a little worrying at the time.

Yesterday it was decided that I would have to go to Ibadan to examine, so I am off on Wednesday afternoon to examine on Thursday and Friday. I was going to stay with the Days but a phone call today from Wesley College informed us that Charles has been in hospital since Christmas and Margaret and the baby joined him a few days ago, but they were discharged this morning and could they come up here to convalesce and they are coming to the Pearsons'.

Next Sunday Andrew is off to Synod with Eileen for a week so we shall be pretty hectic. Certainly one cannot say that life here is dull! There is always something cropping up.

Hope you are all well and not overworking. We both very well indeed
Much love, from us both   David.

Jan 16th 1955

We have a slight lull during a very busy fortnight. It is Sunday morning and shortly before lunch time, and I have finished the mornings work, and hope that all remains quiet for the rest of the day.

We have had a very busy week here – Mr. Mackenzie has made good progress and is now getting up himself. Unfortunately his wound is a little infected, but will soon resolve I expect.

The early part of the week passed much as usual but on Wednesday

183

afternoon we had a committee and afterwards I went to Ibadan to examine. Margaret would have come if she had not had to stay to nurse the District Officer. I drove down to Ibadan in the late afternoon and stayed with the Bury's. They have a very nice house, beautifully run but although very nice folk they not the easiest of folk to converse with.

The next day, I began examining nurses in Anatomy and Physiology at 8.30 and went on solidly until 2pm when we had examined them all.

I returned to the Bury's for lunch and then went into the town to do some shopping but there were masses of people and it was very hot. There seemed to be very little in the shops so I returned for tea to the Bury's and then motored home.

Almost at Ilesha I passed a car broken down containing a Major Vivian, so I asked if I could help and he asked me to bring a message in for a Mr Gamra. Unfortunately I found he had gone to Lagos, so I had to find someone else to go out and help him get his car on the road, so it was 8.30 before I got in - a very long day.

I found all well on my return but we have been frantically busy the last few days getting everything ready for Synod and at last we have got our numerical returns complete.

Yesterday I struggled with accounts and in the evening we had an out of doors dinner party. The Pearsons' and we gave it, for the District Officer and his wife and in addition we had the Rev. David Head and an African who are up for the one day SCM Conference in Ilesha, a surveyor - Ted Palfreyman, and Eileen and Joyce - thirteen altogether. It was a very cool evening, down to 70 and we all felt it a bit damp, but most enjoyable. The District Officer managed to get out to the meal and then returned to the house where we played a rather good crossword game. A most enjoyable evening.

Early this morning Andrew went off to Lagos until the end of the week, which means a very heavy time for me until he is back again. Then the following week he may be going to a committee in the East - rather nice but leaves me alone again. There is far, far too much work here for one, now.

There is considerable subdued excitement in the town because one of the miners has found a rich seam of gold - richer than has been found before. This Major Vivien, whom I helped on the roadside is from the Mines Department and was coming up to investigate and the surveyor may well have to investigate the area before he goes. Anyway don't breathe a word about it as everyone here fears a 'gold rush.' It is rather thrilling isn't it? Last Sunday morning the bank manager showed us some of the gold - about £200 in a small bottle and a gold nugget in another. I fear that it will not benefit the hospital though.

Look forward to receiving your letter. We are both very fit and well and hope you both are not finding it too cold. Much love, David

23.1.55

It is Saturday night, just after seven. I have had my bath and Margaret is about to have hers. In a few minutes the Pearsons', Charles and Margaret Day are coming round for dinner and perhaps a game of Pitt.

You seem to be having rather poor weather. We are having a cold snap too down to 62F during last night - two blankets and long trousers this morning and most refreshing - one feels one can get much more work done.

We were very pleased to hear that Mary had passed her surgery and Pathology. - it won't be long now before both Henry and Mary are qualified.

Hope Father had a good time at Chapel Committee and with Auntie A. We had a letter from Auntie A in reply to one of mine earlier this week and also one from Mr. Cook of Kingswood School in reply to a Christmas card. His letter being absolutely illegible - mine is bad but his is infinitely worse!

Here we have had a very hectic week but Andrew returned last night so things are once more under control. The District Officer's wound was not too good so he was delayed returning home till Tuesday but as he left he presented Margaret with a one and three quarter pound box of Black Magic a marvellous sight!! We have just begun the top layer. Both he and his wife have been very grateful and through his stay here we have got to know them very well indeed and many other folk who came up to see them.

The hospital has kept us very busy the last week as you can imagine and there is the possibility that Andrew may be going to Umuahia next week which means another six days away! I hope he decides not to go!

This evening I had a few minutes to spare so finished off the soap rack for the bath, which has been under construction for some time! Now I must start Margaret's work box, which is to be a magnum opus. The preparation of the wood has been done by the hospital carpenters as it is very difficult to saw solid mahogany - but I am going to make the joints and so forth. I am looking forward to getting down to it.

The garden is still producing a few tomatoes we have had about seven pounds so far which have much more than paid the cost of the seed

Yesterday Margaret lifted our onions, They were put in a little late but have reached pickled onion size. One shilling's worth were put in individually and each onion has produced 6-8, so we have several pounds. We are hoping to pickle the onions. We have two recipes but lack some of the more exotic spices. However I am sure they will be jolly nice.

Tomorrow it is our turn for coffee and so we shall be going to chapel in the evening. In the morning I hope to get the Hospital accounts completed. Synod has been quite without problems. Mr. Angus is Chairman for another year 1956 - but the financial year to end in August so before long (and whilst Andrew is at home) I shall be doing the balance sheet again!

We are both very well and very happy,
Much love from us both, David

30.1.55

Your recent medical bulletin to hand! We were most distressed to hear of the illness at No 1, both yours and Stanley's but hope that by this time you are both well on the way to recovery, though it doesn't look as though Stanley will be back at school yet. His illness does seem to be rather surprising, probably some virus infection or other. What about infective mononucleosis (glandular fever).

Here we have kept very fit and except that I have had another bad crop of mouth ulcers – however, I hope they are going again now but eating and talking have been most painful, but this is a minor inconvenience compared with the Nursing Home at No. 1. Please congratulate Ernest and Vivienne for me - I am very glad. Thank you Henry, for your most welcome letter, which we appreciate very much indeed.

Incidentally last Saturday (eight days ago) I had to operate on a 4/12 old baby with a strangulated hernia (weight 8 lbs.), who is doing quite well and should be ready to go home soon. Monday and Tuesday were busy days with very many outpatients and a number of operations, then on Wednesday Andrew went off to a committee in Umuahia- he was deputising for the Secretary of the Christian Council of Nigeria Medical Board at the new hospital in the east (where Ken is). We all felt it was a bit unnecessary to go, but he decided to go, so there you are. It has meant rather a heavy week for me but he should be back tonight if all is well. My Birthday was very, very busy, but Margaret made a very nice Birthday cake, which we are still enjoying and we had roast chicken by candlelight in the evening!

I have begun work on Margaret's work box made possible because Margaret gave me a mortise chisel for my birthday. To make the framework there are 24 mortise and tenon joints - no small task - but it is fascinating task. So far I have made ten. Then there are the plywood sides to fit and the grooves to make in all the pieces of wood. It really is fun to have something to do, to take ones mind off all the problems of the hospital.

Charles Day has returned to Ibadan but Margaret, who is still not well, is still with us - the baby Christopher - is flourishing. There has been great excitement on Friday and Saturday. It has been the Ilesha - Ife Agricultural show. Margaret and Jean entered marmalade, jam, embroidery and biscuits. William entered bread. Margaret got a first and two seconds, William got a third and Jean got three firsts and a third so the compound has done quite well. Prizes consisted of alarm clock, material, enamel bowls - all quite useful.

There were 65 classes altogether, beasts, fowls, yams, etc., etc. Next year I am going to enter for the woodwork section!

186

Yesterday Margaret was pickling the onions - but to my distress I learn that they have to remain in the vinegar for three weeks before they can be or should be eaten.

At the moment I am chewing a chewing stick. The Yorubas, to clean their teeth, take a bit of a branch off the 'big tree found in the bush' and chew it for half an hour each morning and it keeps their teeth very white. I have bought one and am going to try it. At first it was very bitter but it was pointed out to me that I should first strip off the outer bark - now it is relatively tasteless!

Much love from us both David.

6.2.55

Another Sunday is here and so I sit at the desk in our living room looking out at the tropical scene, with the birds singing in the bush and the cock giving an occasional crow - it is very pleasant and peaceful. It is shortly before coffee time so I must try and complete this before the influx of people.

The past week seems to have been very busy without anything very special. The two gastronomic highlights are the biscuits which you sent us for Christmas which are really lovely and lasting a beautifully long time, and secondly the pickled onions. They looked so tempting we started one pot and they are really most refreshing! For lunch today we had cold beef and pickled onions (potatoes as well).

Last Monday was the first payday in the New Year. The labourers were not satisfied with their rates and went on strike – 35 of them. This rather dislocated the work of the hospital but the nurses turned to and cleaned and scrubbed very well indeed. I stoked the boiler for an hour or two so that we should have steam for the laundry, and Elsie did the laundry. The following day there were no signs of returning to work so we saw the men individually. They wanted a fixed daily rate, which we agreed. January worked out quite well for them but I doubt whether they have thought about February- with only 24 working days- so there may be more trouble then. However we are back to normal again now.

In the midst of the strike I had to go to Ife, 20 miles away to get the licenses for our vehicles - rather a thankless task which took a good long time. I found out that our Morris Minor is not insured! We have only got a cover note obtained by John so we must get that seen to at once.

Andrew returned last Sunday evening to our great relief so work has been a little easier. He brought half a dozen English eggs for sitting, we put them under a broody hen, which unfortunately died two days later, so we have had to put the eggs in our bacteriological incubator and have to be turned every four hours. The trouble is that the incubator is airtight and we fear there is not enough fresh air circulating. When they hatch, too we shall have to find a hen for them if we possibly can.

This morning it was our turn for coffee and this evening we are going down to Otapete for the service there. Margaret's work box is progressing but I am held up for a tool which I am going to buy with some of the Christmas present money paid in for me by you - a plough plane.

Much love to you all, and very pleased you are better, Mother.

Love from us both, David

13.2.55

Sunday morning, we have just returned from coffee in the Pearsons' house and just prior to going we went down to the morning service at Otapete. We took Michael Pearson and came out after one hour just before the sermon

This week has been relatively unexciting. Work has been a little easier as the folk are going out to their farms to prepare them for when the rains start in a months time. Still we have had enough to keep us busy. Elsie went down to a conference of Matrons and Sister Tutors from all of Nigeria (only 22!) which was held in Lagos. Helen Hooper flew over from the east but was not able to come up to Ilesha to see the hospital as Elsie did not have transport of her own having gone down with one of the Sister Tutors from Ibadan. She rang up on Wednesday to ask if she could be met on Thursday evening in Ibadan. At the last moment Andrew decided that the car needs attention and wondered if we could go with it.

So we packed a few sandwiches and set off - arriving in Ibadan just in time to get to the garage and then go to meet Elsie, who was two hours late! We sat in the house and talked to one of the sister tutors of the government nursing school there. At the moment I am making a sewing box on legs for Margaret out of wood, but wanted a plough plane as I mentioned last week. Elsie got one in Lagos! - it is marvellous , so I am able - when I have a moment - to press on with it, though there is still a good way to go.

I made a roller towel thing this week for the kitchen. It is made up of old box wood that we get from the sawmill for fuel, but the roller took a great deal of work as we haven't a lathe here.

Yesterday Andrew and I were giving injections to the nurses when the door opened and in walked Mr. Mellanby. He is staying at the sawmill in Ilesha having come up to mend their engines, which are defunct. He seemed in very good form and asked after Ken.

Also yesterday we asked a small boy to climb up a palm tree opposite our house to trim it so that we can see beyond. He climbed up with his rope cut one frond and came scuttling down - there are two snakes up there!

In a while I am getting out my rifle and try to get them out at a safe distance.

We are keeping very fit, very happy, looking forward to hearing from you, much love from us both, David

Sunday, Feb 13th 1955

Dear Henry,

Thank you very much indeed for your letter of Birthday greetings, which we were very pleased indeed to receive and to hear all your news. At the moment finals will be looming up and Margaret and I send you our best wishes for them and await the news in a few weeks time, that it is Henry Wyatt MB BS, that will be the day when your worries really start!

We were thrilled to hear of Mary's success in the recent exams and wish her a good time too in March/April.

Here we jog along from one thing to another, with always something unexpected happening. Last night I had to get up to see a patient who had fallen out of bed in his hip spica (fractured femur and compound fracture of tibia and fibula). Apparently he had got tired of it and cut the part around his middle and then tried to sit up! He is a French engineer who got entangled with a moving belt at our local sawmill He is rather a problem. His brother is in the House of Representatives here in Lagos (an MP).

The other day a woman came up with a story that at 9/12 she reached term, went into labour but nothing happened. Four months later a sinus developed in her left iliac fossa and foetal bones came out, followed a month later by a colostomy. She preserved the bones and I have seen and photographed them. On Thursday I closed the colostomy so far alright - but it is early yet to know how successful it will be. It is rather unusual and follows a Caesarean done elsewhere. I imagine the uterus ruptured, the foetus formed an abscess and discharged but bowel (small) was also involved to create the colostomy. I shall have to find time when I next go to Ibadan to look it up in the literature before putting pen to paper.

In what spare moments I can seize I am busying myself with woodwork and a fascinating pastime it is proving to be. Once one has the tools at ones finger tips there's no end to the things one can done, though as one goes on one requires more tools, before long we shall be requiring a lathe no doubt!

In the next four weeks Enid Blake, our Sister Tutor returns and Eileen Searle goes on leave, and well she deserves it and then the next arrivals will be the Wrights in May. When they arrive we shall go away for a fortnights break somewhere. Transport is our problem, as all the places we should like to go to are 500 miles away and to hire the hospital car a 6d a mile both ways is a heavy item to start with. We should like to borrow one if at all possible but there aren't many around to ask. We should like to go to the East of Nigeria and perhaps into the Cameroon, but we shall have to see.

Time has gone, a cool drink coming up (88F in the shade). Hope you are well, we are both very fit. Love from us both, David

27.2.55

We have had a busy week. Last Sunday evening we went down to a choral evening at Otapete, a most interesting evening, though Michael would have been distinctly upset I fear. The chorale 'Love Triumphant' was rather poor.

Monday was a very busy day and then on Tuesday I had to go to Ife (20 miles away) to give evidence in a police case, which wasted a couple of hours. In the evening we spent the time getting the car loaded up for our trek. Eileen took her language exam but had a very stiff time - the results are not out yet.

On Wednesday we set out for Ifaki and had a good run through. Jonah seemed in good form though a bit depressed about the state of Nigeria. He seems most grateful for his son Alan being in the hostel. I think it is this which has made it a financial possibility for him to become a solicitor.

We had a very heavy thunderstorm at Ifaki, which cooled the air marvellously for the time being. On Thursday morning we went on to Ikole and found Louie in good form. The great problem is to find a relief for her furlough, which is due in May. It looks as though part of the work will have to close down, as there is no-one to take charge of it and do the teaching. Whilst we were there we were rather unwell. Margaret was sick and my tummy was upset also - it was probably something we had eaten either at Jonah's or at Louie's. However we went on to Afon the next morning and were quite well by the evening. We had a restful time at Afon, Ray, Daisy and Stephen being very well. Unfortunately in the village they had a disastrous fire at least half of the houses in the village have been burned out - folk loosing all their possessions.

Saturday afternoon we had a good run home and in the evening went to the Pearsons' for chop and at 10.15 Enid arrived feeling fit and ready for work. It is very nice to have her back. We are both quite fit again now.

Much love to you all   David

6.3.55

Another Sunday morning and as I write I can hear Margaret grinding some coffee beans (ready for elevenses), which are in our house today. Andrew is at Chapel this morning - we shall go this evening, to our service up here when Rev. Salako is preaching.

You seem to be having a very cold spell just now, hardly the weather for climbing I should have thought. Henry no doubt will have had a most exciting time, with many adventures. I shouldn't be surprised if the Alps and Himalayas are the next item on his agenda - a pity Everest has been climbed - doesn't leave much scope for him!

Here we have had a busy week. Last Sunday evening we heard Pastor Elton preach on 'casting out devils'. Last week Andrew operated on a man with a hernia but did not think it wise to complete it. Last Thursday he completed the repair but yesterday morning the man lost his reason and ran out of the ward. After a 300 yard chase he was caught and returned to bed with sedation. During last night, whilst those watching him were doing other things, he jumped through the window and ran for the bush, being found in a nearby street eight hours later. Pastor Elton would claim he is demon possessed, so Andrew has gone out this morning to find Pastor Elton and to ask him to show us how he exorcises devils!

Yesterday we had another sod turning ceremony - A Mr. Lajide (pronounced Liede) who has been a private patient wishes to show his appreciation by building a private wing to the hospital (about £1100) and yesterday we started the foundations. He is a contractor and has already obtained stone and some sand and is starting the foundations proper next week. We hope that having put his hand to the plough, he doesn't look back, but sees it through. It is a most generous action. The only thing is we must make sure is that the hospital does not have to put any money towards it - our debt is enough as it is. The private block will, though, be a means of increasing our income, so that we are able to pay off more quickly.

We are still in the midst of a hot spell, surely our rains must come soon!- every thing is very dry.

We are both very fit and happy, with more work than we can manage. work box held up for lack of plywood and have started a clothes horse pro tem.

Much love from us both, David

3.3.55

We were most interested to hear of your appointments and visitors to be expected. It is a very long time since I have seen Anthony - I am sure I should not recognise him.

Miss Porter seems to be much the same as ever! Glad that all went well for your tea at International House. Should be glad to hear comments on Laymen's Missionary Dinner! We are looking forward greatly to hearing of Henry's mountaineering experiences.

We have had a busy week without anything startling happening. I forgot to mention in my last letter that on Tuesday of that week I acted as presiding officer in the Ilesha Urban District elections. I was in charge of one of the twelve polling stations, which was open from 9am until 4pm. I was given the ballot papers and was responsible for them and the discipline of the station. A total of 230 people could have voted. Of these 80 voted in the first hour and a half and after that only another fifteen voted, so you can tell it was rather a slow business. However for my efforts I received three guineas, which will go towards our holiday.

The District Officer has been so pushed with the election that Margaret and Jean have been checking the election lists - an exacting task for which one is paid 13/4d per hour! However they only had two lists each so they are now completed. The elections are taking place in the villages around about now, but should be over in another week. Mr. Mackenzie has been very, very busy with them, watching out for infringement of rules and so forth

On Wednesday we had a little dinner party to celebrate Enid's return and Eileen's departure. We had chicken, with peas, yam etc. but were mystified by large white masses covered with thin white sauce served in a tureen. We all thought that it was marrow until Margaret realised that it was white sauce!! - a trifle lumpy - in fact the bread underneath was in quarter slices. The meal was in the Sisters house and their cook thought he could go one better!

Yesterday morning, Eileen went down to Lagos prior to sailing on Tuesday. She asked for some woollies to be sent from home - but to her distress they have not arrived - she will find it a bit nippy I think.

Last evening we had the Pearsons' in for dinner - a most enjoyable time. We are all rather thrilled that the Governor is coming next Friday (Sir John Rankin) for a visit and coming here to look round and for tea. This week will be devoted to tidying the place up - cutting what is left of the grass and so on. We are hoping the District Officer will advise us to the procedure and so forth.

We are both very well indeed and hope you are also,

Much love from us both, David

March 19th 1955

It is Saturday evening after a very hectic day. We should have gone up to Margaret Grants for dinner tonight but as this epistle unfolds you will see why we are staying at home.

The main concern of the letter is Michael and we too have felt constrained to think and pray much for him in latter weeks. There seem to be a number of alternatives and I am sure he will be led into the right one. I have written recently - and am looking forward to hearing his thoughts later on.

You seem to have a great number of meetings to address still, and no doubt having a well established reputation they will continue after your term of Presidency is over.

We are looking forward to hearing of Henry's adventures - but trust by this time he has his books out again.

Poultry news. All Jean's hens, cock and turkey have died. Some disease got in the runs, and they all died within twelve hours, a most disastrous affair. Our bamboo hen run blew down in the first gale of this year, so this morning we have bought some wire netting and are making a more thorough job of it. There is just the possibility that Margaret may go down to Lagos on Monday with our lorry which has to fetch up a ton of milk (a free gift from Government) and on the way back purchase some three or six month old pullets, as our efforts at hatching and rearing seem to be abortive.

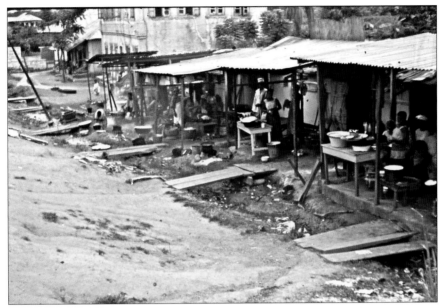

Ilesha town

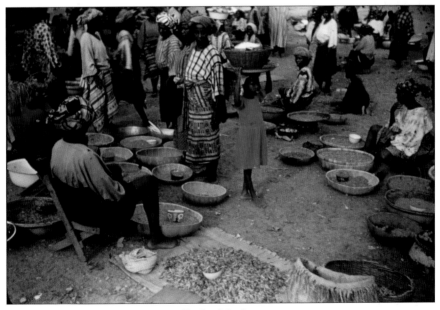

Ilesha Market

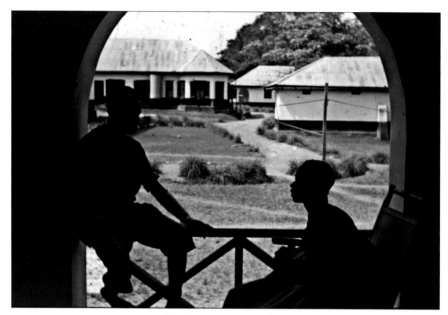

Patients on verander

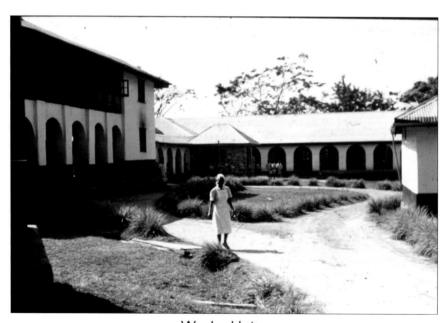

Wards old site

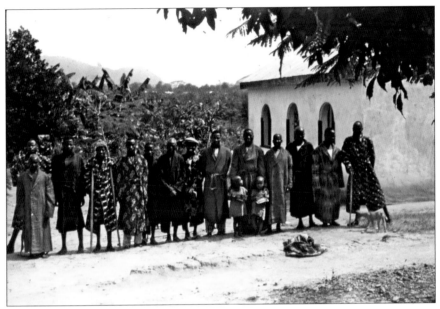

Leprosy patients in Christmas dressing gowns outside their chapel

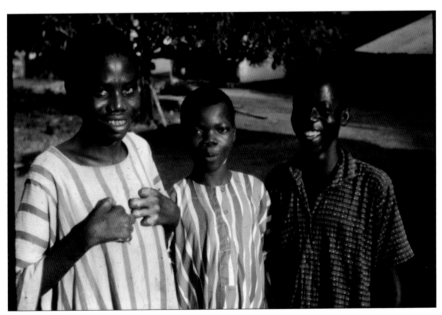

Three leprosy patients

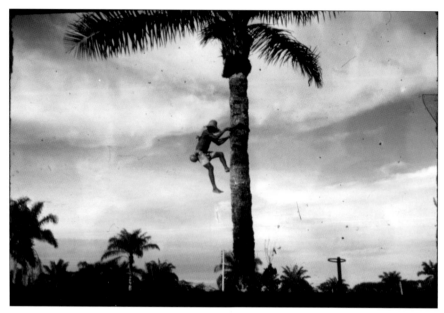

Collecting palm oil

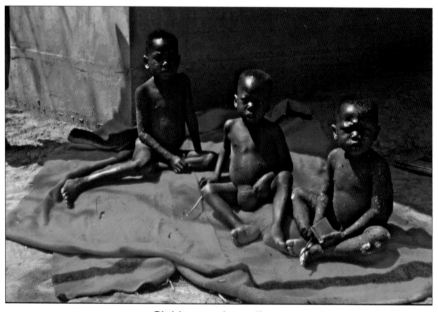

Children with smallpox

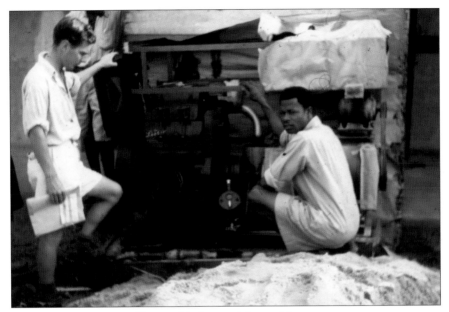

Ken and helper with machinery

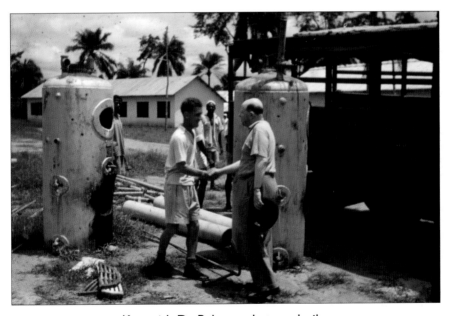

Ken with Dr Baker and steam boiler

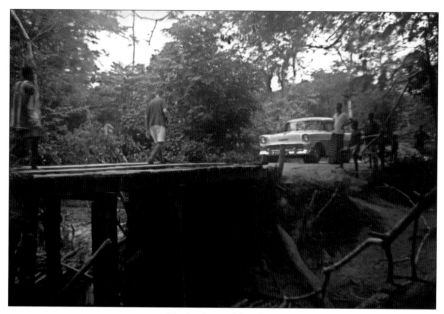

Typical road bridge

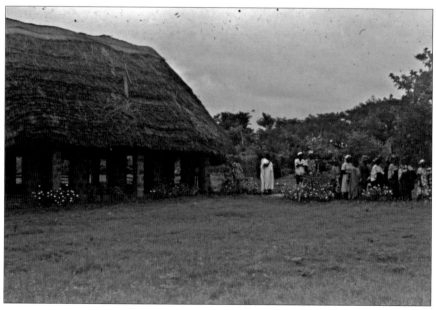

Afon Church

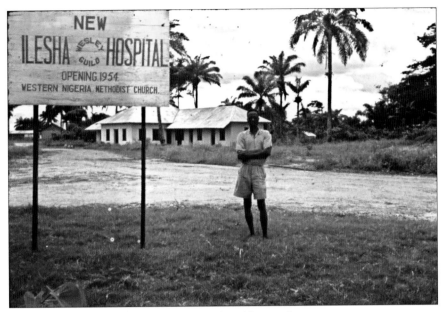

Early sign for New Hospital site

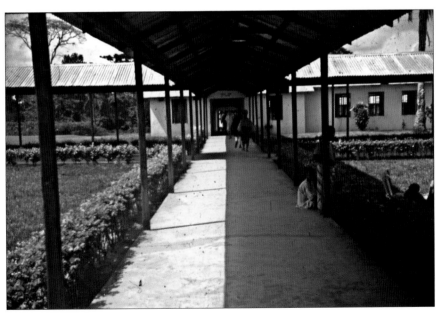

Covered way between wards

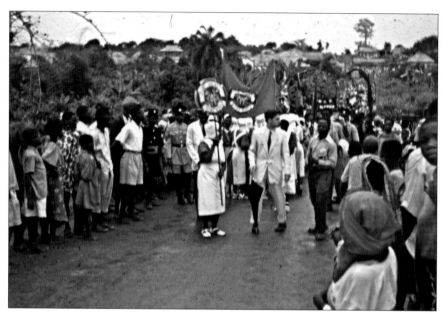

David leading the procession to the New Hospital

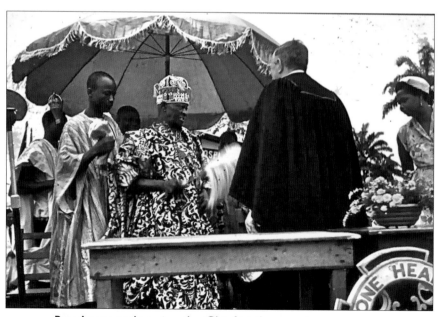

Rev. Angus welcoming the Chief at the opening ceremony

On Monday evening we went out to chop with the Woods, two American teachers in the Apostolic teachers training College here, They are a very pleasant couple indeed and we had a very nice meal. Afterwards we played Cluedo - a very good detective game.

The rest of the week we have been busy preparing for the visit of the Governor. Unfortunately, although Margaret had spent hours tidying up the compound, it was arranged he should come to the gate only. So we paraded there- and half an hour late he arrived, tall, quiet and statesmanlike. I was introduced, brief word and so on. In the evening there was a select cocktail party at the District Officer's, to which Andrew, Jean and Elsie were invited. Unfortunately Lady Rankin ate something, which disagreed with her and Andrew was called this morning. He saw her and suggested that, as Sir John had to go on to Ife today, that she came here to rest. So she is now in our guest room! That is almost unbelievable. Margaret is nursing her and they are getting on well together. Lady Rankin is improving rapidly and should be better by tomorrow evening when Sir John returns.

Needless to say we are rather thrilled! Now the governor has seen the compound - partly !

We are both very well indeed, Much love from us both to you all, David

22.3.55

A note to wish you 'Many Happy Returns of your Birthday from Margaret and me. I fear this may be a little late - depends on the planes, but it does bring our love to you.

Lady Rankin recovered swiftly, fortunately, and spent Sunday with us in the lounge. Sir John called for her in the evening and also had a cup of tea. When they departed they invited us to call and see them at Government House, Ibadan and seemed most grateful for all we had done.

On reflection it seems rather like a dream, but we have their signatures in our visitors book. Lady R remarked that we seemed to have a number of visitors!

In addition a friend of Margaret's arrived on Sunday to look round - she is a sister at Adegogo, and then, about 4pm Ken rolled up!

Ken has gone to Lagos to get some shopping done for United Mission Joint Hospital and for us but returns tomorrow for a day or two - it is good to see him again. He is going home in May I believe, so he says at the moment.

Time is going, Once again, our best wishes for your Birthday and love from us both, David.

27th March 1955

It is a very hot and dusty Sunday afternoon. Margaret is doing our accounts at the desk and Ken is reading Readers Digest, and Skates the cat is crying for a little attention which Margaret has now given him. A very domestic scene.

Your letter arrived on Friday by which time your trials will be over - we trust you will have strength to write to us and let us know just how you got on - though I have no doubt that all would go very well at the London Mission Rally.

Here we have had a very busy week. Last Sunday you will remember, we had her Ladyship plus two visitors from the University of Ibadan, one a nurse friend of Margaret's. On Monday, Ken went off to Lagos to do some shopping and was trying to get us some 3/12 old pullets. Whilst he was away Margaret and I put up the wire netting around our chicken run, just getting it finished in time. However, Ken did not manage to get the hens after all, but we heard later this week that Mr. and Mrs. Hands (he is a lecturer in ancient history at Ibadan) think they may be able to get us some so perhaps in time we may succeed.

On Wednesday Ken returned from Lagos and we went out to the Pearsons' to chop and Rowland Hughes, ex principal of Wesley College, now supervisor of schools was also there so we had quite a large party.

On Thursday we had a letter from Glanville and Jean and they are expecting a baby in July! We wrote inviting ourselves to French West Africa for our local leave - to stay with them. They will be very pleased to have us and it should be a most interesting visit! The one snag is the means of transport - we will try to hire the hospital car though Andrew may prove a bit sticky about it. However we shall see. It would leave the hospital a bit short. Friday was as usual a busy day and Saturday morning was a long busy one too. Ken has been busy with odd jobs around the compound, notably with the foundations of the new private ward which were not level!

Yesterday afternoon the BBC producer called Richardson - a West Indian-came to us with a letter of introduction from Dr. Lawson the obstetrician of University Hospital. A most interesting and charming man who came to look round and have a cup of tea. He is doing a programme on SCOA. Last evening we went to Margaret Grant's to dinner and today to Elsie's for lunch, so we have had a good time. This morning we went down to Otapete.

We are keeping very well and very happy. Hope you are all well despite your cold weather which continues. Ken back to Umuahia tomorrow

Much love from us both,   David

April 3rd 1955

This comes to wish you all a very Happy Easter from Margaret and me. You will be busy with Passion-tide services and Easter Communion in the morning but on Monday if it is a good day you will get out a bit.

Here I fear there will be little change except that there will be no outpatients on Friday and Monday, but many will turn up I expect.

Your letter arrived on Friday, as usual and we were very glad indeed to receive

it and to learn that you had survived sundry ordeals during the previous week. We look forward to seeing a report of it in the MR in due course. Very glad it went well.

You seem to have had a very good WW Council - glad to see that Mrs. Sangster has been made the next president. Glad too, to hear of the success with daffodils - considerably more success than with our poultry. However we have got our run up again, a small one of wire netting, and a large one of bamboo opening out of it. At the moment we have Sylvia's cock in the netting, and a turkey I have been given in the bamboo one. Our menagerie has increased this week by the gift of a rabbit (very wild). Quite why I have been given it I do not know! Anyway it is in a small chicken run at the back of the house. Feeding is rather a problem, as we have not enough lettuce to give it.

We are looking forward to seeing Edward Fields, Skelmanthorpe in the next issue of Good Housekeeping. We will look especially for it.

Ken left at 3.30am last Monday morning intending to get to Umuahia in the one day. We have not heard from him yet but presume he has arrived safely.

Last night we had the Pearsons' in to chop and a game. Jean is expecting another baby, which will arrive when they are on leave, sometime in October I believe.

The rains have not really started properly yet, though Margaret has many seedlings in doors almost ready for transplanting. There is still a great deal of digging over to do, but until the ground becomes softer it is too difficult for our garden boy who is not very strong - in fact whilst we were on leave he was very ill indeed and in the ward for a month.

A new lawn mower has been obtained, bought by the staff for themselves, very similar to the old one we had. It cuts well and easy to push so it should suit us all - if we have time to cut the grass.

Hope you are all well and gathered together. We are thinking of you this Easter time. Much love from us both, David

Easter Sunday, April 10th

Easter Sunday afternoon and as I sit here sweltering in the heat (3pm) and still half asleep from a heavy siesta, I can imagine you all at home in the sitting room or dining room, writing letters and thinking about the folk who will be coming in to tea.

Your letter came yesterday and we were very glad to receive it. We also had a letter from Ken who is going home at the end of this month, but is returning again to Umuahia- his plans do change. Very pleased indeed to hear that Henry and Alan Jones were received into membership of the Methodist Church!

Margaret has just cut our Easter cake - Simnel -very nice indeed - and this morning I had an Easter egg. Unfortunately as we went to church it was left on the table. Oliver (cat) came in, climbed up and ate it and returned to Jean covered in chocolate! The egg has been replaced with one of theirs but I am very sorry that Margaret's went astray!

This week has been quite a hectic one. Last Sunday afternoon about this time Mr. Cowan asked me to go and see his wife, whom I found to be in labour, I had been giving antenatal care but she was to have her baby in Ibadan. Mr. Cowan (a Canadian) was not very happy at taking her alone so Margaret went with them, after I had assured them that there was time to get there. Anyway they left at five, arrived at 6.45 and the baby was born at 7.25 a little girl to go with the boy they already have. Margaret stayed at Wesley College over night, and Mr. Cowan who has a very good position in a trading company arranged for a car to bring her back after doing some shopping. (He apologised because it was only a Vauxhall - his is a superb Chevrolet!) Mr. Cowan took Margaret on the Monday morning to the University where she saw the Hands, who had visited us three weeks ago and arranged for some pullets and a cock to come up.

They arrived on Tuesday evening and they are wonderful - 6, 2-3 month old hens and a cock. Rhode Island Red crossed with light Sussex.

I have had to do odd jobs to the runs, feeding troughs, drinking fountain etc. They are healthy specimens and feed very well. We are thrilled to bits with them. Unfortunately we had a lot of trouble with the two cocks and the turkey and they have all had to be in separate places to prevent fights! At the moment we are reading up about the diets of chicks in an endeavour to give them a properly balanced diet. They have learnt how to go up the ladder into the house at night and now come to the trough for their food when it is put in.

On Good Friday it felt like a Sunday. We were busy in the morning, but in the evening had a service for the nurses at which Pastor Williams preached. That night, I was wakened by Enid and Joyce, as they had had a burglary. Enid woke up and found him in her room and he took her watch and torch. I rang up the police and they came to look round. They think they know who it was but I doubt whether they will catch him. A most disturbing event.

Yesterday I had a letter from John Billinghurst, an old Londoner – now at the military Hospital in Lagos. He is coming up next weekend with another M.O whom I don't know - it will be very nice to entertain them.

Do hope you are all fit - we are very well indeed.

Much love from us both, David

April 17th 1955
Another week has passed and Sunday afternoon is here again. You will all have finished lunch by this time, have cleared away and perhaps are writing letters also.

We were very pleased to receive your letter on Friday- you seemed to be having as busy an Easter as usual, with early communion and breakfast and so on. We look forward to hearing how you all spent Easter Monday.

Last Sunday evening we had a musical service, items by the choir, a quartet and a solo by Jean who sang 'I know that my Redeemer liveth' unaccompanied - very difficult and would have sounded much better with an accompaniment of some sort Andrew gave a short address. Two records were played, one of some Easter music with oboe solo by Leon Goosans at which the nurses just laughed - couldn't understand or appreciate it at all.

I haven't done any carpentry- but have got together the things for the tray of the work box, so that I can complete it this week if all is well.

Yesterday was an interesting day. Work, with a bit of shopping in the morning, and accounts in the afternoon and then about 4.30 we went to visit Mrs. Cowan and her new baby. They seem quite well and have a lovely house.

The chickens are flourishing on a well balanced diet and come running when anyone appears with food. It is fascinating to watch them grow though it will be some time before they lay. However we are hoping for the best.

We are very fit and well, going up to Ifaki and Ikole on Wednesday for one night. Hope you are all well, Henry should qualify soon.

Much love from us both, David

24.4.55

Another very hot Sunday afternoon. So hot that it feels as if it may rain and we very much hope it will - because it is over a week now since we had any and the garden is very dry indeed and all the seedlings in are struggling to keep alive. Some have been eaten by large grasshoppers - every leaf - so I feel they will not live. The cucumbers are continuing to do well.

Monday and Tuesday seemed ordinary days except that on Tuesday Joyce got her parrot. It is grey and red and a most attractive little thing. It is quite young and does not talk as yet. On Wednesday we set out for Ikole. We had good journeys despite the fact that six bridges are down and the mud crossings of the streams are very bad. We stuck once, but got out with a push from Margaret and Mr. Abe. We found Jonah looking well but he had not heard that Alan had been received into membership. Jonah is going to be acting Chairman when Mr. Angus comes home on leave next month. On the Wednesday evening we went on to Ikole and were welcomed by Louie who looks well though she has some pain in her arm very similar to Margaret G. She is going to have it seen to at home. She is flying home on May 5th so you may see her at Westminster ere long. We haven't any relief so the nurses are carrying on in a limited way themselves, but it means the doctors will have a lot of checking up to do when they get there. We came back through Abo Ekiti to call at the CMS Hospital there. We had a letter from them asking us to supervise them for two months

(August and September) as they could be without a doctor. They wanted weekly visits but the state of the roads and the amount of work we have makes that rather impracticable   However we talked it over at it seems as if two visits in September would be ample, so we shall probably come to some arrangement.

On Friday Enid went off to camp at Imesi with the Guides - quite an undertaking. Apparently two more senior Guides were going and Enid was hoping to pass her company license. Unfortunately the District Officer went the previous day to occupy the same quarters, so what happened we shall have to wait and see. On Friday evening Dr. Ogan looked in on his way from local leave - he seemed very well. I fear our local leave in Dahomey will be off - roads impassable to a small car, but it looks as if we may be going with our lorry to Eastern Nigeria to deliver an engine we have sold so we shall see.

This morning we went to Otapete and at lunch time a Dr. Langley of the CMS from East Nigeria looked in on his way from leave and asked us to stay with them when we go over. Do hope you are all fit and well. We are in the best of health though Margaret says I am getting fat!

Much love from us both   David

May 1st 1955

Your letter arrived yesterday this week instead of Friday and we were delighted to receive it and to hear that you are having some good weather after the very cold and wet winter you have had. It is a pity we can't parcel up some and send our weather to each other to make a change.

Very glad to hear Michael had a good time in the Lakes. He will be with you today, and we are wondering how his interviews are going and which way his mind will be made up. I shall be writing for his Birthday when I have completed this letter.

We are at the moment both rather depressed and rather excited. Yesterday Skates our beautiful cat killed and ate one of our more wonderful hens! So rather than have a rapidly disappearing flock we have had to dispose of the puss. We have found some Apostolic folk who are willing to have him so we do not actually have to put him to sleep which is a mercy. Rather upsetting and in one day we have lost one hen and a very nice cat Skates the aristocat!

The more exciting thing is that tomorrow we are going on local leave for two weeks. The school to which we have sold the engine wants it before the school term starts in two weeks.

We have just had a letter from John to say that Sylvia is ill and in bed and it is not likely that they will be ready for the boat next Thursday. Andrew says that although he will be alone it is better if we get off.

As far as travelling goes it will be very cheap, as the hospital pays for the lorry to go. It is to Oran. I don't know if you have your map still but it is on the opposite side of the Cross river to Calabar and 20 miles beyond Ituk Mbang. If all is well, we shall see the Cundalls just before they go. It is 500 miles which we hope to do in two days. Mr. Lanyian is coming to install the engine and share the driving. The lorry is packed with a generating set that weighs over a ton, a control board, tripod and tackle for unloading, and the cooling system etc. Then there are our things including camp beds, nets, mattresses, linen, clothes, pans, pressure cooker, food etc. What fun it is!

Mail takes a very long time from here to there so the letters will remain till we return in two weeks time.

On Wednesday we had the Premier of West Africa to look round. He thought our home very nice as well as the hospital. Last night we were out at the District Officer's for chop - a very nice evening. Do hope you are all well and fit. We are very fit and looking forward to our trip.

Much love from both, David

Oran, 7.5.55

Here we are in Oran on the Cross river, in the extreme east of Nigeria, and a delightful place it is too. As I write this I can see monkeys playing in the trees not 30 yards away – small ones, although the older ones are quite big. They are black and white with a white spot each side of the haunches.

We left Ilesha at 10am last Monday in our lorry with Mr. Lanyian, our engineer and his boy. We took it in turns to drive and reached Asaba, on the Niger, just before six (246 miles). We stayed in the rest house there and were quite comfortable. The next morning we left early and caught the 8.15 ferry

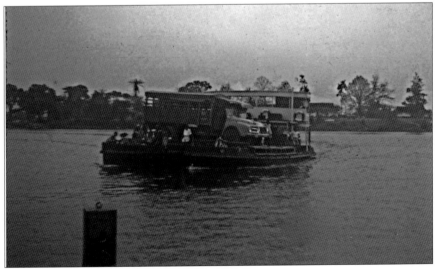

Niger ferry

across the Niger to Onitsha, a three mile trip. We then pressed on through the east hills and came to Ituk Mbang, which is only 20 miles from here. We had a cup of tea with Helen Hooper and then a proper tea with Mr. Gower. Marjorie Gower was not at all well and he is alone for several months, and is incredibly busy. I looked round the hospital which is much more 'bush' than ours, especially the new one. Margaret stayed with Mrs. Gower who, due to an infected centipede bite, is unable to walk, so she has not seen around yet.

Lanyian began work on the installation of the engine, which is now nearly complete, but has taken longer than expected because of the slow labour at our disposal. On Wednesday morning we went to the hospital here (Methodist), run from Ituk Mbang (like Ikole), where Ivy Taylor is in charge. There was a woman requiring a forceps delivery, which I did for her. (Fortunately the patient is doing well, unfortunately the baby was dead when she came in.)

On Thursday morning we went down to the local saw mill, which is run and owned by a European, George Allen, a most self opinionated and garrulous man. He works overlooking the Cross river, a very large and beautiful situation.

On Friday we took the lorry from Oran to Calabar – a trip in a launch of fifteen mile. It was a wet day but we enjoyed it thoroughly. We did some shopping first, then went to see Mary Slessor's grave, and then went up to the rest house for lunch, during which a chimpanzee climbed onto Margaret's chair (a semi-tame one) and the owner of the animal played hide and seek whilst we tried to eat our lunch. We got the ferry back at 2.30 arriving at Oran at 4pm. Yesterday we went to see Bob Judkins and his wife whom I knew at Selly Oak and he was most surprised to see me!

Whilst there I felt my temperature rising and when we got back it was 102 and I felt rather the worse for wear. However it is down this morning – a bout of malaria.

Tomorrow we hope to go to Aba, then after that to Umuahia and so home next Saturday. Your letter will await our arrival.

We are having a wonderful and most enjoyable time.

Much love from us both, David

May 15th 1955

Here we are once more safely back in Ilesha and enjoying being back in our own home once again and one of the great delights was to receive and read our home letters. Very glad you met Eileen Searle and heard of Sylvia's thrombosis. Apparently John is flying back at the end of the month and Sylvia with the three children is returning by sea, leaving on June 2nd I think. We feel very sorry for Sylvia who will just have finished six weeks in bed and will be in no state to cope with three bouncing children.

We were very glad to receive the packets of Punch and Housekeeping, which will provide us with ample reading material.

Last Sunday evening whilst at Oran my temperature was slightly up still but on Monday morning awoke very fit, bounced out of bed and went to see how Mr Lanyian was getting on with the engine. It was practically ready - then the great moment came - the engine started first time - the voltmetre registered 230v. When we switched on however there was a short circuit in their wiring system, which is very primitive. We found several bare patches of wire and their man is going to overhaul it. However the engine and generator are fine, so we earned the hospital £350 by our trip. We left on Monday morning and had lunch at Ituk Mbang with John Gower. He and his wife had both been unwell, and looked very tired. Helen too looked tired though she said she was keeping well. We then went on to Ikot Ekpene where there is a Weaving Guild, that makes lovely mats of various sorts. We bought two for our bedroom. Later we went into Aba where we spent the night with the Bennetts and had a very nice evening. The following morning we went to Umuahia where Ken has been at the new Union Hospital. It is excellent, 120 beds but costing £160,000 when ours cost £75,000 for the same number of beds. It has every convenience and piece of equipment that one could wish for. John Gower is going from our mission. In the evening we went to Uzuakoli the world famous settlement for leprosy patients and research into the condition. We first visited the school and met Howard Ashley who was in Guernsey. We then went on to the settlement where we stayed with Ida Robinson. The next day I sat in on the clinics and was shown round and I hope when I have a few moments to work up a deputation address on the work there. Mr. Lanyan refused to come into the settlement for fear of leprosy.

On the Thursday we came over a beautiful road on which we had a picnic and primus etc. and we might have been in the Lakes - no tropical trees, as we are quite high up. We called at Enugu to have a tyre mended, then stayed the night at Aruba with some CMS friends of Margaret's. On the Friday we called at the big CMS hospital at Lys Emi and looked round. It is about the same size as ours but they have more staff.

We crossed the ferry, having a picnic by the waterside of the Niger. That night we spent at a Rest house and then yesterday came straight through arriving soon after one o'clock having had a wonderful twelve days. We found all well on our arrival and were in time for the Birthday party at the Pearsons' for Joyce. Rather a lot of office work to be done! Andrew is off to Ikole on trek on Wednesday.

Love from us both, David

May 22nd 1955

We were very glad to hear from you on Friday and to learn that Henry had qualified and we are very pleased indeed and send him our congratulations. We sent a cable on Friday afternoon and hope it arrived safely, should be interested to learn how long it took. I expect he will get a job on the House at the Royal Free.

We had a letter from Michael this week also, he seems in good form and has taken quite a part in the Campaign about which he speaks enthusiastically. He has also been applying for student research appointments and I do hope he finds the job he is looking for.

This week has been busy catching up on things whilst we were away but we are straight now. Andrew went to Ikole on Wednesday, returning on Thursday and is going to Lagos this afternoon to get fittings and equipment for the new Private wing, returning on Tuesday, which is a Muslim holiday, when all the shops are closed. It will make a busy week. Then the following Monday he is going to Ibadan for a committee, and again I shall have a rather busy time, as Monday is our heaviest days at the moment.

Enid was unwell last weekend and had to go to bed again yesterday feeling very down. During the night she was in such distress that Andrew had to get up to see her and gave her morphia. However she is a little better today.

Last Tuesday we had a meeting of representatives from the Mission Hospitals in the west - to discuss nurse's salaries and so forth - a most interesting meeting. Afterwards Dr. Salisbury of Ado Ekiti stayed the night with us rather than push on to Ibadan his next destination.

The hens are doing quite well and we have just had proper door put on the runs - so that they are all complete and in fact all set for brood time. However we shall be well pleased if we can get some eggs!

The garden too is looking up. The cucumbers are doing well, and we hope to pick the first tomorrow. We have been enjoying some of Jeans - delicious in this hot climate. The radish also, are doing well and the spinach is colossal.

Our latest news of the Wrights is that John flies on May 30th, Sylvia sails with the children on June 16th, so the Pearsons' will have left by the time they arrive.

The private block is progressing, but unfortunately the door and window frames are not square or plumb, and the donor rather resents it being pointed out. We shall call it, I fear, the Folly!

We are both very well indeed, and my weight shows a slight increase again 9st 3lbs!

Much love from us both, David

May 28th 1955

Another Sunday afternoon is here and a very hot one it is too besides being very hectic! On Thursday we were asked if we could put up two evangelists who are here on a crusade under the Christian Council of Nigeria - both Americans (though only one has come) and that evening John Billinghurst and his friend rang to ask if they could come so you can imagine how hectic we are at the moment.

We had a letter from Henry also, on Friday, full of his Scotland trip, which seems to have been wonderful, and also the trip to Wembley to hear Billy Graham.

This has been a very heavy week here. Andrew went to Lagos last Sunday to do some hospital shopping. He returned on Tuesday evening so I had two full days alone- and then he went to Afon on trek on Friday and returned on Saturday - and tomorrow he is going to Ibadan for a committee, so tomorrow our heaviest day I shall be alone again. However all has gone well so far. John should be with us by the end of this week - I think he flies tomorrow, so for a fortnight there will be three of us again, Oh happy thought.

The week has been a heavy one surgically, with a ruptured uterus, an intussusception, a baby with exompthalus, a gangrenous appendix, a strangulated hernia and sundry other minor operations for good measure.

Friday night was Nurses class, which I took, then a very busy morning yesterday, and then at 5.30 John Billinghurst and his friend, another John arrived. It is very good to see them after all these years. They seem to be struggling at the military hospital in Lagos and most envious of our work here and wish they had something like it to do. They are counting the days till their National Service is complete.

Last night we had a very nice dinner party and were afterwards a little late to bed I fear! Our other guest a Mr. Petergross from Kaduna, half American and half English is a very nice man indeed - he is with us for a week.

This morning we looked part way round the hospital and then went down to Otapete and sat through the service (1 and 3/4 hours), We had coffee when we came back and lunch. There are quite a number of Africans in the team, but the leaders are three Americans, one from Kaduna, one from Igedi and one from Ibadan, of the American Baptist Church. They all have marvellous cars!

The Johns are looking around the town at the moment and when they return we are going down to the garden and then the stream. Tonight there is our hospital service. You must be looking forward immensely to your holiday - close now.

We are both very well and very happy. Much love from us both, David

Sunday, June 5th 1955

It was a lovely surprise to receive your number two letter of the weekend before last on Monday and to learn of your activities. Your item of news re our new Sister arrived the same day as our official intimation. This would suit us well as Elsie sails the first boat in September. We are thrilled to hear that Uncle Stanley and Auntie Theda will be at home from Jamaica next year - which part? We should be due for furlough at the beginning of March.

Very pleased at Mr. Maltby's word of praise for Stanley and if the latter wants any more building experience we have a hospital chapel to build sometime!

This has been a very hectic week. John Billinghurst and his friend went on Monday, having had a very good weekend indeed. Andrew had a committee in

Ibadan, so I had a great deal of work to do, about 180 outpatients. Mr. Petergross, an American and one of the Crusade team has been with us the whole week and we have greatly enjoyed having him, and he in his turn has been a great blessing to the hospital - helping several of the nurses to make a decision to become a disciple of Christ.. He left yesterday and has gone on to Ife to take part in the weeks campaign there.

On Thursday there was a meeting of the Nursing Subcommittee and it was our hospitals turn to act as host. So at 10am Nursing Sisters converged from all the Mission Hospitals in the West - practically all American, our quota was three for lunch, one of whom brought her little boy, so with Mr. Petergross and all the others Margaret and I had quite an American twang.

On Saturday-last night- John arrived. He reached Lagos on Thursday evening, Elsie went down to shop and they got back last night. He is well but Sylvia is in hospital in London with some odd tropical disease and they do not know when she will be out again. The children are with her parents in Northern Ireland. It is most unfortunate, and very plucky of John to come out and leave her in bed. They have not yet diagnosed it, so the future is very uncertain. Andrew has a court case at Ife tomorrow and I have one in Ilesha so we are likely to be rather hectic.

We are both very well, Margaret's birthday is on Wednesday and I have almost finished the work box. Next Sunday it is our first Wedding anniversary!

Much love from us both, David

12 June 1955

We were very glad to receive your letter this week. It arrived on Saturday, so was not held up by the rail strike, as we feared.

I have extended your invitation to Andrew. He does not envisage Jean and the children down in London much but he himself will have to come to see Dr. Bolton periodically and would be glad of a resting place I think.

The Pearsons' leave here next Saturday, sailing on Tuesday and will in fact be in England three weeks tomorrow! They feel that the tour has gone very quickly and they have all kept very well.

We have had quite a hectic week here, one way and another. John has had fever and has been in bed for several days, but he was up and about yesterday and is back to normal I think now. However Andrew and I have not had the slightly easier week we anticipated. This week John is going to Lagos to examine so we shall be much as usual.

Wednesday was Margaret's Birthday and the work box was duly presented and with great satisfaction. We had a very nice day. Elsie took fellowship in the evening.

On Thursday the Philips X-ray people came up to see us. Our X-ray machine has become faulty again and Andrew may be bringing it home again with him. Anyway Andrew wired Mr. De Nye (Dutch) and asked if he would give us some advice even though it's not their machine. They brought up a very nice portable machine to demonstrate and we almost bought it but when we brought two patients along to X-ray it would not work!! The atmosphere got a little tense and Andrew and I left them to it. They struggled to put their machine right but eventually took it away with them, and hope to return this week. We are seriously thinking of getting a new one and selling our old one.

Today is our first Wedding anniversary - we have had a wonderful year. We are both very well indeed and very happy, though Andrew's departure will come soon and gloom fall temporarily. Much love from us both, David

June 19th 1955

The wet season is truly with us now, at the moment we are having some heavy rain and we have had some very heavy storms in the last week. Unfortunately the roads will be rather treacherous and we are due to go on trek next Wednesday.

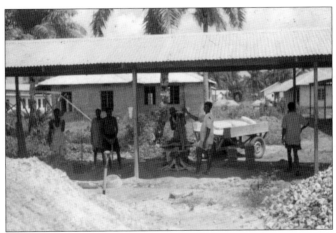

Making lancrete blocks

This had been an eventful week. The most significant fact being that Andrew and family went to Lagos yesterday - sailing on Tuesday, leaving me holding the baby so to speak. However if we take the tasks one by one as they come we shall pull through, but at the moment it feels quite a responsibility.

They have been very busy packing all the week and Andrew has had to do a great deal in putting the affairs in order in home and hospital. John has been examining in Lagos for three days and so it has been a little heavy for me. However we shall soon settle into the routine again. At our last hospital committee on Wednesday it was agreed to start building a garage come

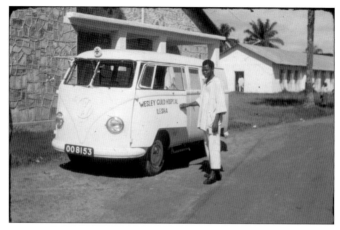

Ambulance

schoolroom. The estimate tendered was £188, which was only for walls and floor. This was felt to be too much to pay and said it would be cheaper by direct labour and agreed to it that way. This means really that I have to do the contracting, employ the different workmen and supervise construction. However I have got some men making landcrete blocks, having first hired a machine, and we have got a tree down and started to peg out the foundation.

In addition the management committee agreed to the starting of the Hospital Chapel! However that is in the hands of a contractor but will never the less be quite a responsibility.

Our first year nurses have been to Ibadan for their final general Nursing exams. They quite enjoyed the papers but did not like the practical examination.

Last night we had Vernon and Doreen Woods from the Otapete church in for an evening meal. They are a very nice couple, and we had a most enjoyable evening together.

The ambulance given to us by the government has arrived and very nice it is too, most luxuriously finished and will hold two stretchers, two sitting in the back and three in the front. It is almost too good to be true

Our tomatoes are doing well but are not yet ripening but we have some very big trusses. We are both very well, love from us both, David

26.6.55

Very glad to receive your letter yesterday. Our fruit trees are growing slowly, I think next year it will be time to get them budded if we can. Our interest at the moment is in some teak seeds, which have been planted. We had hoped to have a grove of Cassia to cut for firewood, but the forestry department was unable to supply us with young plants but sent teak instead, which is apparently also good firewood! At the moment they are about an inch high so have some way to go!

We have had quite a busy week here, and as you say with the Pearsons' away it is very quiet with a lot more work. Still we have got on quite well so far.

In addition to the usual work we have our garage/classroom. It has progressed fairly well and we have got the foundation pegged out, dug and filled, and they are now at work on the footings. A second group of five men have made the 2000 blocks with a machine that we hired, so next week should see the start of the walls. Our carpenter, meanwhile is getting on with the window frames. It is most interesting to have a hand in it but it is something more to cope with.

The contract for the chapel is yet to make out and the consent of the committee to obtain. I shall be glad when that is started and under way also. The private block is a little slow, in fact nothing has been done to it for several weeks and I hope it doesn't conk out and we are left to finish it. I have ordered some equipment for it in faith.

On Wednesday it was our turn for trek but unfortunately the roads were in very bad conditions and with two bridges down so we had to go a long way round - 110 miles-instead of 60- rather tedious. However we found Jonah in good from and all well at Ikole. The nurse in charge had collected £78 in fees in the month so I was able to pay salaries and have £40 odd to put in the safe. By the time I got back on Thursday evening I had driven over 150 miles which is quite enough for these rough roads.

Friday was a busy day and so was Saturday with several operations. I got the accounts done in the afternoon as well as one or two letters, and in the evening we went across to John's for dinner and had a nice time. Next week will be busy I expect. On July 1st I shall have to get out the under eighteen returns for the first three months working of the scheme and send up for re-imbursement.

To complicate matters at the moment I have to take the service for the leprosy patients this afternoon and take the Sunday evening service here next Sunday evening. John is in good form just now - he is looking after the compound. Elsie is rather tired and will be ready for her furlough in twelve weeks time. Margaret has some toothache at the moment but otherwise we are keeping very fit. Much love from us both, David

July 3rd 1955

Another Sunday afternoon and a huge storm is blowing up at the moment so that we have had to close up the windows. Here things have jogged along. The garage building has taken quite a bit of time and energy but is now to the point of having the concrete lintels placed over the doors and windows.. Then later this week we hope to get the roof put on so that the masons can work inside, laying the floor and plastering the walls inside and out. Then there will be the electrical fittings to put in and then the decoration.

The management committee have sent in their notes of agreement so it is now a case of getting the contract drawn up for the chapel and then the contractors can get to work on the site. The District Engineer has the plans at the moment and is getting out the specification to be incorporated in the contract, which will be a great help.

Last Sunday we went down to the leprosy village where I took the service and this evening I have got to take the service here. Next Sunday I have the service for the leprosy patients again. Tomorrow Margaret is taking the English-speaking group at Otapete.

The hospital has been as busy as ever with large outpatients and all the beds full. We have just come to the end of the first quarter for under eighteens and are getting out the statistics and as they are going I think we shall request £2,500 on the first three months - quite a lot, but it will just about cover the cost of treatment.

We have used the ambulance twice so far to fetch patients - I used it for the second time yesterday to fetch a patient from down the road. I went to the house to see her, got the stretcher out but she apparently refused the stretcher and preferred to walk!

Yesterday we had an interview for drivers and I have taken one on. Last night Margaret went to see 'Ascent of Everest' at the training school. I was on duty and I had my service to prepare so very unfortunately could not go, but Margaret enjoyed it very much indeed.

We are both very fit now though Margaret had toothache and went to Ibadan on Wednesday and had a tooth out.

Love from us both, David

July 10th 1955

Here we have had a busy time as usual. Last Sunday was my service here and quite an ordeal, but safely over. We have had quite a number of visitors the largest number yesterday with two in the morning, Allan and Hanbury's representative and his wife and Bill Mann and his wife, he teaches at the Methodist Girls High School. They let us know they were calling and had tea with us, they are on their way to Owa where a church has collapsed and they are going to assess the damage.

Last Wednesday we had the first staff committee since Andrew left, it went quite well, nothing very startling.

Last evening we had John and Sister Mabayaje in to evening meal and had quite a nice evening, though Mrs. Mabayaje stayed rather a long time, she is very nice though and talks quite a lot. We did not play any games.

The garage is progressing, we have got to the point where the roofing slates can be put on and, if all is well we shall start that tomorrow, then when the roof is on we shall have to plaster inside and out and the floors to lay. In addition, there are the windows and doors to make followed by the decorating. It will cost quite a bit more than we expected, but I don't think it will make us bankrupt

This week I have had to get out the returns for free treatment and I have sent in a request for £2614, which will help us a little when it comes. It is considerably more than we anticipated because of the vast increase in work and I hope that there is no trouble over getting it.

Affairs with the private block have reached a head with a letter from the District Engineer saying there are many faults in the building which should be rectified otherwise it is likely to fall down. The donor came on Saturday to borrow the lorry to get wood for the roof and start roofing tomorrow so perforce I had to raise the matter and suggested he went round to the District Engineer to seek his advice. I don't know whether he will or not.

Affairs are progressing with the chapel. I have got the specification back and made out the contract. Mr. Martin has a copy, which he is reading over. We hope to get it agreed this week and then he hopes to start work on it. It will take some time to get the site cleared and so forth. Then we hope that Elsie will turn the first sod and make a ceremony of it. We shall have to get on with this this week if we can.

Sylvia is at last on her way we believe and by cargo boat to Takoradi, stay there the weekend and then pick up the mv. Aureol, and arrive here on the 27th of this month. John will be going down to meet her.

Joyce has had her two weeks local leave and went by lorry to the East. She stayed in a school in Umuahia but was not able to get around much and arrived back safely yesterday. The other sisters have been very busy without her. Enid goes to examine this week so the sisters are back to two again.

Ambulance not used much yet but had notices read out in all the churches today so we hope something will happen.

We are both very well and very happy amidst all the work. Looking forward to hearing from you. Much love from us both, David

17.7.55

The two letters you sent arrived this week. The large travelogue on Monday and last Sunday's came as usual on Friday.

This morning I got a telephone message to inform me that our pupil midwives have to train for eighteen months and not for a year. The Ministry of Public Health has made a mistake! Naturally the nurses concerned are upset about it. In addition our new salary scales for nurses were read out in Otapete in a notice requesting applications for the new Nurse year. It was greeted with most unpleasant laughter. We, with a struggle, have raised their salaries almost up to Government levels and then, just this last week, the government have put theirs up again. A bit depressing, however we shall see what happens.

Our weather has gone quite cold! In fact resting this afternoon had to put a dressing gown on to keep warm! In the mornings have long trousers and jackets - very like England in fact it has been down to 70F. It is delightful - we feel full of energy.

Last Sunday was Hospital Sunday and the services went well with Nurses reading lessons and so on, and my service with the leprosy patients went well too.

On Tuesday Margaret and I went out to dinner with the District Officer and the Resident was there. He was brought up a Methodist, though I think he has lapsed now, but knows all the personalities

On Thursday we went out to tea at the Hammonds who are Apostolics at a small village two miles from the town. They are a nice couple from Bradford so we were able to talk about the West Riding. It made a very pleasant change.

One night when we went to bed we found a stream of ants crossing the ceiling, some dropping onto the mosquito net and getting into the bed! We got into bed but having been bitten we got out again and went into the spare room, where one single bed was covered with them. We got into the other - slept fitfully for three hours and then with relief found the ants had gone and returned to our own bed!

The garage progresses and is now being plastered. The chapel site is levelled and a heap of sand accumulates. The private block remains the same!

We are both keeping well, much love to you all from us both, David

31.7.55

Just five minutes ago Margaret and I went down to feed the hens (their mid-day feed) and we returned with our first egg and we are just about as proud as if we had laid it ourselves! It was laid by one of the brown hens that we have been given. The egg is small and William says that the brown hens are rather old therefore. However if it produces some eggs until our hens begin to lay they will have done their part and then we shall have them for a special meal sometime.

Your letter came on Friday this week as usual and we are very glad indeed to receive it and hear all the news. Glad indeed to hear that Michael has accepted the scholarship and look forward to hearing more about it

Our passage is booked on the Aureol for February 28th, we heard this week but we have been wondering if we should take the opportunity of flying via Rome, Geneva and Paris on KLM and spend a day or two in each place. It will be more expensive of course but is an opportunity whilst we are still more or less unencumbered and feel that if we didn't take the opportunity whilst offered we might well regret it later. We should be home sooner than boat and without the two weeks of uneasiness, besides the opportunity to see these places. Bill Mann is making enquiries for us and we will let you know as soon as we know definitely.

We have had a hectic week here. Sylvia and the children arrived on Monday evening and all looking very well and they seem to be settling down into their routine. They had a good journey out but I imagine it must have been hard work for Sylvia because on the cargo boat there are no facilities for children, playroom or nannies to keep an eye on them.

Wednesday night was fellowship led by Margaret, but during the night I had to sew up a perforated peptic ulcer - only the second that can be remembered for several years!

On Friday mid-day our guest arrived, Eric Roberts, a Methodist who is an engineer to one of the printing firms in Lagos. He is a nice fellow but has no conversation at all! He is going tomorrow.

Yesterday I had a long day in the office, with rather complicated accounts due to the fact that it was payday.

Last evening we had Enid and Joyce in to chop and then played 'Pick up sticks' Unfortunately maternity was very busy and later during the night I had two forceps deliveries and a D&C to do.

The garage now waits for its doors, windows and paint but is otherwise complete. The chapel foundations are being laid, so progress is being made there too.

We are keeping well. Hope you are all well at home.

Much love from us both, David

14.8.55

It was good to receive your letter on Friday and to learn that all was well at No. 1 even if a little hectic! Glad to hear that Louie Trott is with you - she is a live wire!

Stanley seems to have had a very nice thirteenth birthday and the long trousers would be a thrill. I am afraid that we failed to send greetings for the day, but do wish you many happy returns old chap.

This week seems to have been quiet one as far as visitors go but has been busy from the hospital point of view. Wednesday we had our monthly Hospital committee, which passed uneventfully.

One of our hens has laid thirteen eggs now but the others seem to have no inclination to lay. No doubt in time they will. Have you any suggestion for getting them to start? Friday is our turn to go up to Afon, where we may stay an extra night to have a short break.

We are both very well and send you all our love, David

21.8.55

It is 10.30pm and the latest I have let the day get before writing this letter, but I must finish it before going to bed.

On Monday this week our drain blocked up! so we had an excavation behind the house, and it was soon put right fortunately.

On Tuesday we had seven folk drop in from Eastern Nigeria on their way to Ibadan for the Christian Council of Nigeria meetings. It was the chairman, Paul Kingston with some others. We had them to coffee and enjoyed showing them our hospital.

On Wednesday it was the Medical Board of the Christian Council of Nigeria in Ibadan. Margaret and I and Elsie and Enid went. We left at 6.30am and dropped Margaret at Ibadan, where she had the other un-erupted wisdom tooth out. We went to the Board where we met many new people of other missions and had a good day. Returned to Wesley College and picked up Margaret rather the worse for wear and arrived home at 9pm - a long tiring day.

On Thursday our first white hen laid its first egg - and a lovely one too, and since then it has laid two more and we are thrilled to bits. Another good piece of news is that the money for the under eighteens has come - a great relief.

On Friday afternoon we set off for Afon. We had a good run up and found the Rowlands well. I shot a bush fowl whilst we were having tea and so helped with the menu. There weren't many patients and we stayed two nights - a pleasant change.

This afternoon I got the office done and this evening John took the service - sermon heavy (40 minutes) but good.

Next week looks like being very hectic - estimates to get out for the new leprosy village. Doors to alter in the chapel and an engine out of order, fourteen electrics not functioning. Still strength will be given for the tasks. Margaret's father is much better. We are both very fit except for slight colds.

Much love to you all, David

Sunday, August 28th 1955

As our pens do not seem to run well on these air letters I am writing this one with the typewriter so that there can be no complaints on that score, though the number of errors may well be increased.

I wonder why Ken did not stay at CAV? The last letter we had he said that he was working there, and I assumed had got a more or less permanent job, but he seems to have moved into the opposite camp for Perkins are their rivals!

We have had a busy week. I have been on night duty, which fortunately was not heavy, but on Tuesday and Wednesday nights we had Bill Mann and Rowland Hughes with us, they were up examining the accounts of the Supervisor of the schools in the District. On the Wednesday afternoon we went up to Imesi, the very nice village 26 miles from here, which Bill had never seen. It poured with rain and we got soaked to the skin to such an extent that we men took off our shirts and borrowed towels from our dispensary there to have a rub down. Margaret couldn't and shivered all the way home, but fortunately none of us suffered any ill effect. In the evening we played Scrabble, a fairly new game, and we enjoyed it so much we have bought a set (wholesale price) and also bought one for the Sisters for a Christmas present.

On Thursday after they had gone we had a series of visitors in cars all returning from the Christian Council in Ibadan to their stations in the East. Whilst Bill Mann was with us we talked of selling our little Morris Minor. This I did to Paul Kingston, the Chairman of the Eastern Nigeria, and we have bought another Opel Olympia, for the hospital. It came up from Lagos last night and will do us very well indeed, I think. That evening we had another visitor passing through, a Miss Russell of the Church of Scotland missionary who is a Women's Worker, stationed at Itu. She is a Scot, and quite nice. She was a bit late arriving unfortunately, which made our arrangements rather difficult as we were expecting some of the Apostolics in to borrow our electricity to work their projector and show some coloured films. However it all worked out fairly well.

In addition it was trek week and John and family went up in the ambulance, having rather a hectic time as they picked up a man who had shot himself in the chest by mistake and who unfortunately died before they could get him to hospital. Fortunately the children were all in the front and unaware of what was going on.

Friday was a busy day. Margaret is catching up with the jobs that visitors make it impossible to keep up with, and the hospital took up much of my time. Yesterday was a full day. It is drawing near the end of the financial year and I began to work on our annual accounts. To my great joy and no little satisfaction, they came out exactly which is not bad on a turnover of £45,000, which is what it has been since the 1st of December. There will be other items to add in and payday on Wednesday, to complicate matters, but it is reassuring to know that it is 'all square' so far.

Our largest white hen is continuing to lay, and we have hopes that the second largest will soon start. One of the brown ones is broody, have you any advice about broody hens? We haven't any eggs for her to sit on. It is too late in the tour for us to start a batch. The chapel is going on quite well, and work has started again on the private block. The garage is short of only of solignum on the main doors and so it goes on.

We are both very well and enjoying the tour very much indeed. Hope you are all well and settled down again.

Much love, from us both, David.

4th Sept 1955

Another Sunday is here again and the week seems to have flown by due to all the palavers we seem to be having at the moment.

It has been a very busy week in hospital, but we have not had any visitors at home except today when Joyce has been here for her week end off.

Hospital has been rather hectic. It has been the end of the financial year and I had to do much accounting.

One piece of news has come - that all our finalists (eleven) have passed their exams, so that they are now Nigerian Registered Nurses. This means that we shall have a total of seventeen pupil midwives. Unfortunately though, this week one of our senior nurses has left without warning, I understand she is going to have a baby and has left to get married. These things occur occasionally and are very distressing.

Eileen arrives in Lagos next Wednesday and Elsie will be going down for the boat next weekend. She is very tired, she has done 21 very long months and will be very much in need of her holiday. Enid will be over looking the work.

Our new sister - Miss Lethbridge comes out on the next boat - in two weeks time-so again we shall have four sisters in the compound and that is how it will be until Christmas.

We are hoping that we shall be able to get down to Lagos to meet Miss Lethbridge, as there are many things the hospital needs, which really have to be bought in person. However we shall have to wait and see.

The chapel is going on well - up to the top of the windows in places and is going to look very well. It should be finished about Christmas time, I think. Unfortunately Elsie will be away at the time it will be ready for opening and only this evening she was saying that she would like to be at the opening, very difficult, as she would not be due back until March.

We are both very well and very happy, though up to the eyes in work and problems. Hope you are all fit. Our love, and prayers for Stanley especially, as he prepares for Kingswood School.

Much love to you all from us both, David

11.9.55

A very wet Sunday afternoon! It has now been raining solidly for three hours and everywhere is under water. Margaret has just (yesterday) put in some seeds for Jean and the boxes are swimming so we fear they may all be beyond hope. The roads will be very bad indeed for a day or two, but I think Enid is due to go to Oshu tomorrow, which is a tar road all the way.

I am wondering what kind of projector you have obtained and if it will take both slides and filmstrip, shall be most interested to hear, and also how your photos have come out. I understand that the black and white filmstrip of the hospital is also ready so I will try and borrow a copy for furlough.

We have had a busy week here, again with quite a number of visitors. Miss Gwen Davies and Miss Kathleen Wood of Shagamu Girls School stayed in the compound for three days as part of their holiday. We had them in to dinner on Thursday evening, after which we played Scrabble. There is an African Principal being appointed from next September (in one years time) in Shagamu and Miss Lazelle and Miss Wood are leaving. Jonah too is giving up as Principal of Ifaki and Mr. Ajayai (of International House) who taught me Yoruba is going to be Principal I think.

On Saturday (yesterday) we had five visitors in the morning, two of whom stayed for lunch - Rev. and Mrs. Alan Ashley. They are stationed at Owa 83 miles from Ilesha towards Benin. They were married last April. Margaret Ashley trained at St. Hellier with Mary Broad and knows her quite well. She apparently came over to Tooting with her on one occasion at least. In the evening we had Margaret Grant and Margery Clarkson from the Women's Training College in to dinner and afterwards we again played Scrabble. They stayed rather a long time so that by the time I had done the round it was well after midnight. Still, though on duty, I had a quiet night.

Then the great event of the week is the arrival of Eileen Searle on Thursday and Elsie's departure yesterday, ready for the boat on Tuesday. Eileen has never looked so well and fit and is already down to work. Elsie looked very tired indeed. Our new sister Miss Marion Lethbridge arrives in two weeks time, if all is well and Margaret and I are hoping to go down to Lagos to meet her and do some shopping for the hospital and for ourselves to see us through the next 5 and a half months.

The hospital has been busy, but manageable despite the fact that John has had a day in Ibadan.

The Chapel building is going on well, one of the walls up to the roof level now and the place is beginning to take shape. I shall be starting the carpenter on the furniture in the next week or two. We are very well, despite our damp weather.

Much love from us both, David

18 Sept 1955

A very hectic and rather worrying week is over, and I am looking forward to this afternoon when I am off call and able to relax.

We are all very thrilled to hear of Ken's engagement and look forward to meeting Audrey next year sometime.

Here we have had a number of palavers with the nurses, which have been rather worrying. On Monday six girls missed the meal, which was put out for them but probably eaten by others. Enid put a notice on the board, which included the words 'animal appetites.' They took exception to this and went on hunger strike for 36 hours. Eventually I had to intervene and settle it. Then we had to dismiss one of our nurses, which went reasonably smoothly, but then another senior nurse argued and fought with one of the clerks. This involved two hours of deliberation, neither party telling the truth. Finally each was fined £2 and bound over to keep the peace. However we seem to be out of the wood now.

Yesterday John went to a Student Christian Movement conference at Oyo taking some of our nurses. It was a very long day for him leaving at six and returning at 10.30. They seem to have had a good time, and incidentally John was able to get his eight Rhode Island hens, so the compound has a selection of poultry.

We have been given two ducks a male and a female! Thus we are hoping to rear ducklings - but it seems rather off our beaten track. We have put them in Jeans' run, with the antelope in case they have some strange disease.

The chapel is going on well, now up to the top of the walls. I have bought the timber to make the main doors and the Communion table and on Wednesday we are taking our carpenter to Ibadan to look at some pews, which are very nice I believe. There will be a great deal of furniture making involved and it will take a lot of maintaining in the polished state. By Christmas it will be complete perhaps and I shall be quite glad when it is finished, though the contractor is very good indeed.

We are having John Crossley to stay tomorrow for ten days or so. He is on his first tour and is having a holiday. Sylvia will feed him for the 48 hours we are away. The following week he will be coming on trek with us.

We are very well indeed and busy as ever. Much love from us both, David

25.9.55

Another Sunday after a very hectic week, but one which although busy has been full of interest. Unfortunately Margaret has a very bad boil on her back, which is most painful and is developing very slowly. Quite why it has come we don't know because it is the first that she has ever had - perhaps it started from a bite.

On Monday of this week we welcomed Rev. John Crossley- who has been out just a year now- and had experience of work with Muslims. He is a quiet fellow, who can I believe, be very humourous. He arrived rather late in the day so we were unable to get down to class.

On Tuesday Margaret and I set out with a driver for Lagos at 2pm or so in the lorry. We called at Wesley College and saluted the Days who were in rather a hole as their house boy has just walked out on them.

We then went to the United Missionary College, looked at their pews had a cup of tea and then pressed on to Shagamu where we called at the Girls School had some squash and then went on to Lagos arriving about 7.45pm, rather a tiring run down.

We met the Mellors at the Mission, where we stayed with Mrs. Mann. Mr. Mann was in the North reviewing teacher's salaries. The Mellors have spent their leave in South Africa. Mrs. Mellor seems far from well with blood pressure trouble and will be a semi-invalid I fear. They are doing one more year I believe and then retiring.

On Wednesday morning, armed with formidable lists we went into Lagos and bought what we could. At 2.20 I set off for the docks and arrived at 3.00 and went on to the boat. There I met Marion Lethbridge, the Boshiers and Rev. Masters.

On Thursday we picked up loads at various shops and then drove home very heavily laden. Since then we have been busy sorting out our accounts. John Crossley went to Ifaki yesterday and we shall bring him back after the trek on Wednesday. Tomorrow we expect Miss Rance (CMS) for a night or two. Hope all well and safely gathered in. Much love from both, David

1st October 1955

It is Saturday night and I am waiting for Margaret to complete her toilet before going across to the Sisters for a dinner party. It is to mark the arrival of Eileen and Marion and is the first party we have had for a very long time and we are all looking forward to it.

It has been a very hectic week indeed and the one ahead looks as busy. Having come to the end of the second quarter we are about to get out the returns for the under eighteens - a gigantic task, not made any easier by the fact that John has not filled in any of his in-patient charts for the quarter. However we hope for the best!

We have had another visitor for the week - Miss Rance, a CMS a 'Supervisor of Schools' who usually stays with Elsie, wrote and asked if she could come and so she arrived on Monday and left yesterday. She is a very nice person indeed and we enjoyed having her to stay.

On Wednesday I went on trek. Margaret stayed at home because her boil was very sore and we had Miss Rance.

I left in the ambulance with a clerk and went to the dispensary at Ija District Office where I saw the patients and then went on to Effon where we found a tree across the road - a colossal tree and they said it would take two days to cut it through. There was nothing for it but to retrace out steps (15 miles) to the main road and then go the long way round to Akure and Ado Ekiti. On the road between the latter two towns two men waved me to stop but as it often happens because folk think the ambulance is a bus I took no notice. However in rounding the corner there was a European gesticulating wildly and obviously I was to go back. I reversed the ambulance round the corner and just as we got round there were two explosions - they were blasting rock by the roadside - no notices - no red flags- no barrier! truly Nigeria! We were very fortunate, 15 seconds more we should have been in a mess - there was rock all over the road.

After this incident we pressed on from Ado to Ifaki and had lunch with Jonah. Unfortunately they are surfacing and widening the road and have just chopped down two trees so we had to wait half an hour whilst these were cut and rolled

217

away! We didn't get to Jonah's until 3 o'clock, two hours late. Then we had the clinic and John Crossley came down to give me a hand and gave out the medicines.

In the evening we had a good chinwag and then in the morning, set off for Ikole where we found all well. We had to deliver a message to a village 2 miles away for Jonah and bought 180lbs. rice (£5.10.0) for the hospital. On our return to Ikole nurse said she had locked her keys in her store so I had to break in to get them out! Again we were late in getting to Jonah's. A quick lunch and I set off for Ado but found that they had cut another tree and we couldn't get home that way however we went home a third very poor route and had to cross streams where there is no bridge! We arrived home safely and found Margaret much better. That evening we had a coffee party to say goodbye to Mrs. Mabayoji who is returning to Lagos as her husband has returned from England. She is very sorry to leave the Hospital.

This is being finished Sunday morning. We had a nice party last night, though no games so it was a bit slow afterwards. This morning I got through the hospital letters and this evening we have been to church. We had a new teacher (Anglican) in for lunch, a Miss Taylor of Lancaster, who arrived on Friday.

We are both very well and hope you are all keeping well despite the advent of autumn. Love from us both, David.

9.10.55

Another Sunday morning is here and at present peaceful and restful, but it is our turn for coffee, so shortly the peace will be shattered by the Wright children! It has been a hectic kind of week and may well have another hectic week ahead so we will make the most of the oasis of calm.

Margaret's boil is completely better I'm glad to say though there is still a mark at the site.

Glad to hear Louie Trott is on the way, she should be here within a week or two now. Andrew will be with you this week and I expect you will go to the Kingsway meeting - shall be interested to hear your impressions of it.

Requests for deputation are beginning to come in! I have had two very pressing letters from Methodist Youth Department, asking me to go to a weekend youth conference at Squires Gate, Blackpool - a combination of Guilds and Senior Club members (500 altogether). The thought of having a Whit weekend used up is not an encouraging one, but the invitation has come so early and so insistently that I feel I cannot refuse. However I shall keep Easter as free as I can.

Last Monday I went to Ife to give evidence in the High Court. The Judge was a European, the Council was African - all were wigged and gowned and were most pompous. However it is a more or less open and closed case so there was no cross-examination. Three other doctors were there giving evidence in different cases. The judge takes all the evidence on the one day and gets it over for us. I was subpoenaed for next Wednesday at Ado but it has been cancelled.

In November we have been asked to have the Moderator of the Church of South India and the week after that the Bishop of West Africa.

We are both very well and hope you are too. Much love from us both, David

16.10.55

This is Saturday evening and Margaret is just having her bath, so I am improving the shining hour before chop, by starting the letter home.

We have had - are having a hectic week! The office work is particularly heavy at the moment - the government wanting detailed costs of the hospital for a period of three months - which takes a bit of getting together. The auditors have the books too and are proving very slow unfortunately. In addition the Under18 figures for the last quarter have to be produced. However we are gradually getting through. In addition Ralph Bolton has asked me to call a special meeting of our Management Committee to decide about getting Dr. Morley out. Dr. Morley is the pediatrician whom we have recruited to research the causes of death amongst children. We have found only half the children born reach the age of five years. Once again this means considerable palaver, letter writing and so forth. However at the moment I have done all I can do so perhaps after dinner, Margaret and I will have a game of Scrabble!

In the compound we have our two overseas brethren, who have come to Nigeria under the Christian Council of Nigeria to organise a youth leadership course. At present they are going round the whole of the country meeting young people. Mr. Witney Dalrymple is a Canadian theological student in one of the United Church of Canada colleges. He is a very nice fellow of 33 or so. He is staying in the guest room of the Pearsons' house and eating at the Wrights.

We are entertaining Miss Leonora Flores who is a Filipino with a marked American accent. She is a graduate of one of the universities of the Philippines and teaches in the secondary school. She is petite, Asian in appearance -about 24 - engaged to a theological student now at college in Canada. She is very nice, but certainly has a tongue in her head. They arrived last Thursday and are staying until next Wednesday.

Next Wednesday I have to go to Wesley College, Ibadan to medically examine all the students - a very heavy task. The same day the Archbishop of West Africa comes to the compound for the night and we are all invited to the reception on Thursday afternoon to meet him officially! He will stay in the guest room - the Wrights are very keen he will have meals with them. Then in a months time we have the Moderator of the Church of South India.

We are now having the latter rains - not to be confused with any religious body and very stormy it is too. It is wonderful to have really fresh eggs for *breakfast. We think that one of the hens is going to be broody again and we hope to set some eggs and rear a batch of chickens.*

By this time next week we shall have Louie Trott with us perhaps and have all her news and down to earth views!

We are both very well indeed and very happy though busy.

Much love from us both, David

October 23rd 1955

Another Sunday is here, and it has arrived after a very hectic week. Last Sunday night John had another 'attack' the first being some weeks ago and which we thought was due to sensitivity to croton. I was called at 3am by Sylvia who was very worried, and found John in a state of shock due to a very severe pain in his chest. In 20 minutes or so it passed off, but very alarming for us all at the time. On Monday he rested and went to Ibadan on Tuesday where he was kept in for investigation. A note from him yesterday states that they have not found much wrong with him but think that it is due to filaria, the cause of Sylvia's illness when they were on leave. However he is returning on Tuesday, but is going up on the Ikole trip the next day, so it will be altogether ten days that I shall have been alone! Needless to say we have been very hectic.

We, and the whole compound were very thrilled to hear of the fourth baby Pearsons" safe arrival, Bryan John. The nurses especially are very excited.

Margaret is not very well today, a little bit of fever, but it makes one feel unwell. Except for this we have been very well despite the extra work.

Last Monday I had a gruesome experience. The inspector of police called and asked if I would go with him to a postmortem examination some ten miles away. As there is no question of refusing and John was still in the compound though in bed, I went. We travelled by Jeep for five miles then turned off the road to a track which said 'road under repair No Way', However we pressed on for another ten miles until it petered out in a very primitive village. Then we had to walk through the forest. Fortunately I found a lad who spoke English and who carried my box, apron and gloves etc. On rounding a bend in the depths of the forest we came to a large stream. I hesitated to take off my shoes and wade across it as there is always the danger of bilharzia, and water snakes. The lad said jump on my back - so I was pig-a-backed across! The Inspector saw this (he is Nigerian) but he weighs about twelve stones and it took several men to get him across!

After 20 minutes brisk walk in single file we reached the Oshun River, the largest in our area and across it a frail bamboo bridge - 60 feet long. I plucked up courage and crossed this swaying insecure contraption with the murky waters only a few feet below and crocodiles around the corner? We were then in sight of the object of my investigation - a man who has been missing seven days and spent them in the river - I will spare you the details.

The next day John went in to hospital and the following day we welcomed the Archbishop of West Africa and his wife. We were greatly honoured to have them, and very easy to entertain they were. They stayed in the guest suite in the Pearson's house and we all had the evening meal in Sylvia's and then they had breakfast there and came to us for coffee. They were very tired after their tour of Nigeria and then they were returning to their home in Sierra Leone. He was at one time the Principal of the Furah Bay College and his wife was on the staff. He is a double honours man in mathematics and theology. Both were remarkably homely.

The same day that they arrived our other guests went, Miss Flores and Mr. Dalrymple. They were a very nice couple, naive as far as Africa went, taking very much on trust. They too were going to have a very busy time whilst they were in this country.

Our hens are laying quite well, we have had 25 eggs this week, it is marvellous to have fresh eggs for breakfast each morning.

Hope you are all keeping well. Much love from us both, David

30.10.55

Another Sunday is here after a hectic week - but John is now back so things should ease up a bit - at least I hope so!

John returned on Tuesday evening. Monday was a very hectic day and Tuesday also. On Wednesday John and family went on trek to Ikole so you can see he is quite fit. It did mean though I was still alone Wednesday and Thursday. However we are now back into routine I am glad to say and next week should be easier, though we are likely to have a number of palavers with the nurses tomorrow.

Looming up is the Hospital Management Committee annual meeting, due next month. For it I shall have to produce the Medical Superintendents report as well as the annual statement of accounts and the budget for the coming year - all rather a lot of work.

The chapel is progressing. The ceiling is now in place and the majority of the walls plastered. Meanwhile we are trying to get the wiring done but unfortunately there is a bit of friction between the contractor and Mr. Lanyian. However I hope that it will soon sort itself out.

Margaret's fever is better I am glad to say she is feeling much more lively. I am keeping well though a bit tired.

Hope you are all well, much love David

PS We are all very thrilled to think that the Queen is coming to Nigeria

5.11.55

We are very sorry indeed to hear that Father is confined to bed for a week or two with suspected ischaemic heart disease. The normal X-ray and screening are re-assuring and I feel that there is nothing very much to worry about. It is a factor to be thought of though and perhaps a slower tempo is called for in the future. It is a good idea to have the bed downstairs it saves all the traipsing up and down stairs with trays and what not. It is providential that Michael is at home now.

The current concern is the Hospital Management Committee held twice a year. It is due at the end of this month and requires quite a lot of preparation for it. However I have got out the Medical Superintendents report, the Agenda fixed and the date and time so it is now just a case circulating the members.

On Tuesday and Wednesday we had the Nurses entrance examination. Margaret and I set and marked the General Knowledge papers and got some very strange answers! – 'book of revolutions' for instance.

On Monday we as good as expelled three nurses for their poor behaviour and lack of interest in the work, and since then we seem to have had a much happier spirit abroad - they were real trouble makers

Work is a busy as ever but we are looking forward to seventeen weeks today when we shall be home. Our revised trip is as follows:-

depart Ilesha Sat. by train to arrive Kano Monday

'Kano Tuesday arr. Rome Wednesday

'Rome Monday arr. Geneva pm

'Geneva Thursday arr. Amsterdam

'Amsterdam Saturday March 10th arrive Liverpool Street 8.06pm

We do hope that all goes well with the family invalids and that father will soon be up again. Much love from us both, David

November 13th 1955

We were very glad indeed to receive your letter, opened by Michael, and to learn that the domestic scene is being restored to order.

We have had a hectic week again, with one thing and another and the next two weeks look equally busy. In passing, my deputation in Doncaster is in the North East Circuit, May 10-17th, a Rev. Kerridge has written about it.

Very interested in Henry's car at £27.10! and wonder how it is going? Might consider a similar priced one when we are home, though preferably to go a bit faster than OW used to travel (32 miles an hour though downhill with a following wind 35!)

Excitement grows for the visit of the Queen in January/February. Already I believe there are disputes as to who should meet her and what she should do, for in the brief time she will be here she can do very little indeed. The sooner they publish her itinerary the better. On Thursday afternoon we went down to a function in the town to say farewell to Charlie Harding, the Bank Manager, who is going on leave and not returning to Ilesha, but will be posted elsewhere. He is a very nice fellow who is very well liked in the town. The folk were most sincere in their speeches though had some quaint phrases to our ears 'he is lovely to look at' and so forth. Then yesterday we had to go to the Town Hall to receive the overseas organiser of the British Red Cross who is visiting Nigeria. She is a Miss Wittington MBE quite a personality. We first of all had a group photograph, as at all such functions, then speeches, then refreshments a la African which consist of dry water biscuits and either Krola (our form of Coca Cola) or beer which ever you fancy. After another small speech we went to the Hospital where we showed her round very quickly and then she went up to the Women's Training College. The Red Cross branch here is a new one, and spends its time raising money with raffles.

In the evening Margaret and I went out to chop with Miss Clarkson and played Mahjong (not sure of the spelling). It can be used for gambling as it is in China, or of course can be played as a game.

At the moment there is an all Nigeria Jehovah's Witness congress, in Ilesha here. There are thousands of them all over the town and one cannot go anywhere without being accosted by them and given tracts.

Next Friday Margaret and I are welcoming the Moderator of the Church of South India into our home for four days - a great honour. He is touring Nigeria and the hospital has been asked to entertain him. We shall have folk in from the town for most evening meals therefore. He has come under the auspices of the Christian Council of Nigeria.

The weather is getting much warmer 88F today in the shade, the garden is still flourishing, the hens are laying a little better and our broody brown still sitting on ten eggs. We have acquired a kitten of undetermined sex called Patch, a most attractive handful, which we hope will get rid of our mice. We are both very well and hope all well with you. Much love from us both David

November 20th 1955

Another week has flown by, brightened by your letter, which arrived on Friday. We were most alarmed to hear of Ken's' broken engagement

We are in the midst of another busy spell. The local Student Christian Movement branches are having a conference at the Women's Training College. We have two folk up from Ibadan, who are staying in the Pearsons house and feeding with the Wrights. In addition a commercial traveller for British Drug Houses who has only been in the country two weeks or so has descended on the compound. He seems a most unsuitable man for the job and simply cannot stand the loneliness of travelling from place to place - new towns - new rest houses each day. He should have gone on but I think he will stay here for a week and then cable them to say he is coming home.

Our guest of honour is the Moderator of the Church of South India. Bishop Sumitra who is staying with us. He is a very nice man indeed, very humble for one in such an exalted position. He has been invited by the Christian Council of Nigeria to do a tour of the country and see what his impressions are concerning church union. He is an easy guest to entertain, but he spends a long time in the bathroom - a little disconcerting!

On Friday I had to give evidence in Ado Ekiti and went afterwards to the CMS hospital where I had lunch with the staff and the Bishop and then brought him back in the evening. On Tuesday he will be going on to Ibadan for a few days and then on to Lagos.

Next Tuesday it is our turn to go up to Ifaki and Ikole. Jonah will be away so we shall be staying with Louie.

Next Saturday is the Hospital Management Committee. I shall be very glad when it is over - it has meant a great deal of work, and will mean much more to get the minutes out and circulated. The director of Medical Services is coming so we shall have to be on our toes.

The various branches of our family are in good health. Our hens lay about two eggs per day at the moment. The broody one is sitting well on the ten eggs. Incidentally William had a broody hen some weeks ago and Margaret gave him six of our eggs and they have all hatched so we are hoping! The kitten is a bit refractory and at night seems to want to return to its' mother.

Mr. Easton of Mission House has written asking me to be a delegate to Missionary Medical Conference at Swanwick in March towards the end for three days. I think I shall have to go - Hey Ho!

We are keeping very well despite our various duties

Much love to you all from Margaret and David

Sunday, November 27th 1955

Another Sunday is nearing its' close and somehow I don't seem to have got done as much as I hoped. However the management Committee is over and went quite well I am glad to say. The big item of news is that the hospital is going to engage locally Dr. Morley, to help with the free treatment of the under eighteens so we shall have four doctors on the staff, though at the most three out at a time.

We have had another busy week. The Moderator was here last weekend, we had a very good service last Sunday night at Otapete, and then on Monday evening we saw the film 'South India Journey'. The Bishop had brought it with him but we have no projector, so I rang up the Baptists in Ibadan and they very kindly came along with their equipment to show it to the churches here. It was shown in the open air, in our compound here. The two Baptist ladies who came stayed the night, so last Monday evening we had nine in for the evening meal, so a very mixed bag, but a most interesting time. On Tuesday the Moderator left us for Ibadan and today we heard that he was involved in an accident on the way down but was unhurt. He is a most humble godly man and it has been a real benediction, as well as an honour, to entertain him.

On Wednesday we went up to see Louie on trek. We had a very good and uneventful trip but returned to find that John had been unwell with an attack of swelling of the whole body so that he has been unable to do any work. I had to operate on a strangulated hernia when I got back, which he was virtually unable to undertake. However it only lasted 48 hours and he is now well again, though it is a bit worrying for us all.

Yesterday was our committee, Mr. Angus and Bill Mann coming up from Ibadan where they had been for the November Committees. Jonah came also but he has had a smash in his car that has tilted the body on the chassis and so has to drive very slowly. He arrived late and went at the end so didn't have a word with him. The committee went without a hitch. I must have everything in order for Christmas time, and Christmas will soon be here.

This morning we went down to the Harvest at Otapete a very hot and noisy service, but we managed to get out after two hours, it would go on another two I expect, but there is a limit.

We went out to lunch with Dorothea Taylor the new Church Missionary Society teacher who has come to the Anglican Girls Secondary School. It is a hot time of day to go out and one feels very sleepy after a heavy meal.

The next week looks a little quieter I'm glad to say though on Tuesday a Dr. Nicholson is coming to look at the new leprosy site. He was a Methodist and his brother went to Kingswood School, even if he didn't.

The chapel is almost finished, and the paint, which we are waiting for should be here this week. Andrew has got a big bell (weighs 82lbs.) and some lampshades and so forth, which we look forward to receiving. We are both very well, though at the moment a bit tired.

Much love from us both, David

4.12.55

Another Sunday is here and at the moment we are trying to develop an appetite for lunch, though it is not easy in this heat, but before I go any further we must thank Michael very much for his Christmas present to us 'A Doctors Casebook'. I got into the first chapter when Margaret reminded me it was a Christmas present, so it is put away until Christmas day.

We are rather worried because Sylvia's hens have got Newcastle disease, which is very infectious. We are hoping that it won't reach ours, but apparently the causal virus can be transmitted on shoes and so on. So far they are all right though one of Sylvia's is dying and they are all affected. It is a sort of paralysis of the legs and lassitude.

Now we think about it, my raincoat is in Liverpool. I went up in it by train and left it there, using only my old one for the boat and here, so Margaret has asked

Thea to send it to Andrew.

We are going to have our Christmas dinner in the Sisters House on Sunday evening after the evening service, which Enid is taking in Otapete. We are jointly responsible for lunch and tea on Christmas day with Sylvia.

On Monday evening though we are having a fancy dress party in the Sisters House, cold chop to which each house is contributing.

The office work has been heavy, getting off the minutes of the Management Committee and latterly I have been getting ready the Medical Report for Synod. There are one or two small reports to be incorporated and as soon as I get these I can get them duplicated. At the end of this month there will be another batch of under 18's returns to get off and the annual statistics for the government - it never seems to end. However in six weeks Andrew will be here, though plunged immediately into Synod.

The weather here is changing. The rains have ceased and the harmattan is coming. One's lips feel dry and there is a haze in the air, fine dust blowing down from the Sahara and it is still hot, but much more comfortable.

The chapel is virtually finished, though there are still some pews and the pulpit to make and it all to polish.

Thirteen weeks today and we shall, at this time be having Sunday dinner together! Much love from us both, David

Sunday, December 18th 1955

A very Happy Christmas to you all. I hope this arrives on Christmas Eve to bring our up to date good wishes to you. At the moment we are in Ikole having a very lazy and restful Sunday morning writing letters and this afternoon return to Ilesha.

We are all looking forward to the fancy dress party we are having on Boxing night, though there is a considerable amount of mystery attached to it, and nobody knows what anybody else is going as. Our guests arrive on Friday afternoon and we hope to decorate the house on Friday evening. The Hospital will be decorated on Saturday. I heard too that the film van from Ibadan will be coming on the Friday after Christmas, so that will be something for the staff to look forward to.

Mr. Angus has been through during the week, up to Jonah's for the end of year service. He brought up the invitations to synod, and I see I am down to preach one of the Synod sermons. A letter from Andrew this week indicated that he is intending to stay in Lagos after his arrival - for synod - so once again it looks as if I shall not be able to get.

The weather is getting very hot and dry with cold nights, real harmattan weather. Yesterday we had breakfast at 6.15am and set off for Ikole bringing up Joyce Tomkins who has a weekend off and wished to come. Before we had gone ten miles we were all frozen and shivering it still being very early, with a damp mist which made driving difficult. We hadn't got any warm clothes! When we got to Jonah's we found him in long trousers and pullover, and he immediately got me one of his pullovers and gave us some hot tea for the remainder of the journey. We found Louie well, arriving at 10am so we had travelled well. Jonah came on later, and brought up two African ministers. We had the committee that lasted about an hour and a half, had lunch and were about to set off for a picnic when a woman came in with an unusual maternity problem. Louie gave the anaesthetic and I operated. A doctor is never off duty!! We had a nice picnic, some 40 miles away, though M. began to feel tired and unwell before we got back and went to bed after a bath. The rest of us were tired and went to bed early.

Tomorrow John is going to Ibadan to take Gregory to the dentist so I shall have the very large outpatients to cope with alone. In addition a Dr. Warwick of the World Health Organisation is coming, so we shall have to look after as well. The hens and chickens are thriving though they are not laying very well at the moment, still perhaps they will pick up a bit for Christmas.

Once again a very happy Christmas to you all and only eleven weeks now! Love from us both, David

Boxing Day 1955

It was lovely getting your letter on Christmas Eve and to read how thrilled you are at our impending parenthood as Michael puts it! We too are very happy. I will write to Queen Charlotte's as soon as I get a moment.

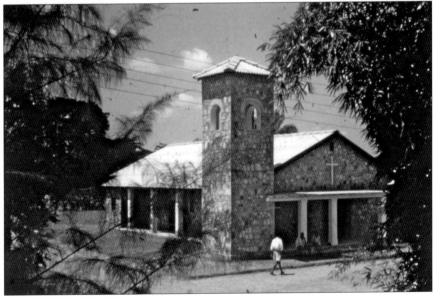

Stella Leony Chapel

On Christmas morning we had a wonderful surprise - at the bottom of the Christmas tree was your parcel to us. Some of the guests must have brought it up from Lagos where it had been left by Kathleen Ormrod. It was slipped in without us knowing anything about it. Thank you very much for the tie it is just right and as for Margaret's brooch and earrings, they are perfect.

We have had a very hectic week of preparations. Last Sunday we had a good run down from Ikole and a good service in the evening here. On Monday John went to Ibadan to take Gregory to the dentist, so I had a busy day in Outpatients and then at mid-day we had Dr. Elspeth Warwick - a World Health Officer visitor to Nigeria. We entertained her for lunch and tea and the Wrights for dinner and breakfast. She is very critical (and rightly) of some of our places here, latrines and children's ward especially, and so we shall have to try to improve things!

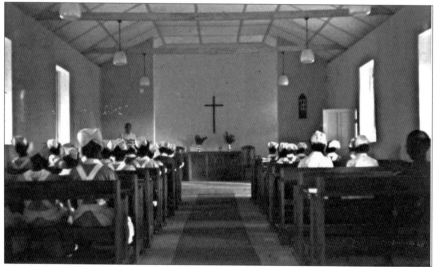

Stella Leony Chapel inside

On Tuesday Kathleen Moore of United Missionary College, Ibadan our first guest arrived - she is staying with the Sisters. She has done a lot of painting of little animals for the ward walls and so on.

Our guests arrived on Friday evening Jan and Arthur Hands - lecturer in ancient history at the University and the Rev. Frank Morton. We are a very happy household!

The Becketts, the Wrights guests arrived on Christmas Eve. Margaret has made a cake and mince pies- very nice. Joan brought up some mince pies and we had a turkey given by the senior Methodist in town!

On Christmas Eve we sang carols on the wards. On Christmas morning we started with Communion at 6am in the chapel, which we were using for the first time and it was a very good service - 50 taking Communion.

Then followed breakfast and the opening of presents - we gave each other the first volume of Churchill's book - to start our library. We have had several other books given 'the struggle for Europe', 'Florence Nightingale' amongst them. We had ward services at ten and our guests took the service in the leprosy compound and gave them their gifts. Then presents for the patients, lunch and listened to the Queen and tea and then the nurses nativity play!

We are having a lovely Christmas, but have often wondered what you are doing! We are very well indeed, Much love, David.

This has been a wonderful Christmas and the wearing of the brooch and ear rings put the final touch of happiness to the Christmas dinner party. They are really lovely. Thank you very much indeed. Margaret

Jan. 1st 1956

A Happy New Year to you all - and 'ere long we shall be home again - in eight weeks we shall be in Rome.

Last Sunday evening seventeen of us sat down to Christmas Dinner and a lovely dinner it was - though I still prefer goose to turkey! Boxing day was a busy day, though throughout the whole week the hospital was very quiet and did not intrude itself upon us! We spent part of the day in preparing our fancy dress. Margaret and I went as a Tyrolean couple, Frank Morton as Long John Silver, three of the sisters as Chinese ladies, Enid as an angel. John and Sylvia changed, Sylvia going as John and John as Sylvia.

Arthur and Joan Hands went as Dr. Morley and a sister. The Becketts - he went as Sherlock Holmes and she as William of Richmal Crompton fame. Margaret Grant came as a Yoruba woman.

Tuesday was a quieter day but again we had to prepare for the nurses party in the evening. We rigged up a string of lights between two palm trees on our lawn, played games and then had sardine sandwiches, biscuits and squash. Arthur Hands directed the games and we all thought how well they had gone. I am sure the majority enjoyed themselves, though a few weren't very enthusiastic.

Wednesday we were back at work again and the Hands and Kathleen Moore returned to Ibadan. They had had a very nice time I think and we certainly enjoyed having them.

On Thursday by special request from the nurses, Marion arranged a service of nine lessons and carols - a good service.

Friday we should have had a film show from the Public relations folk in Ibadan, but for some unknown reason they failed to turn up. The place was full and so the folk were most disappointed.

Yesterday the Becketts returned to Lagos, so our sole remaining guest is Mr. Morton, who is taking our Covenant Service tonight.

Last evening we took down our decorations and put them away for another year, and I drained the sump of the ambulance as there is something wrong with the oiling system.

This morning Mr. Morton and I have been to Otapete. Margaret was not feeling just 100% so stayed at home.

We are looking forward to hearing from you to learn how you all spent Christmas. We have had a real harmattan - down to 58F during the night and three blankets on the bed.

Andrew and family should now on the way. I shall be going to Synod a week on Tuesday if all is well.

Much love from us both, David

8.1.56

We have had an interesting week, though there has been a great deal of office work to get through - all the annual returns for the government and the free treatment of under 18's figures for the last quarter. However they are now all finished.

We had a very good Covenant Service last Sunday evening about 50 took Communion afterwards. Then on Monday Mr. and Mrs. Perry of the Nigeria College of Arts and Technology came up to fetch Frank Martin home again. They are Methodists and have two children.

On Wednesday evening we had a Committee - a most amusing one on the whole but we got a little worked up over sanitation, about which we shall have to do something. It will be my last as chairman for a while.

On Thursday we had a visitor for the night - a Miss Owerkirk (phonetic spelling) a Dutch lady who is teaching in the Anglican Girls School in Abeokuta - an interesting lady, but one who talks almost incessantly. She was on her way to Akure.

This weekend John has a Dr. Heindrich (South African) staying with them, with wife and three children, He is the pediatrician at Adeoyo Hospital, Ibadan.

On Tuesday I am going to Lagos for synod and shall be there about ten days I think unless plans are changed. Margaret will stay here and prepare for the Pearsons' who arrive in Lagos on Wednesday.

We are both keeping well, Margaret has recovered after a very hectic Christmas. Love from us both, David

Lagos, Sat. Evening, 14.1.56

As you will see from the address, I am in Lagos for synod. I came down last Tuesday and expect to return on Thursday. Unfortunately Margaret is not down - no room, and as you will see later, she had to be at hand for the Pearson children!

Monday was a hectic day getting as prepared as I could for Synod, but our *plans were complicated somewhat by a telephone call from Bill Mann to say he had heard from the boat that the Pearson children have chicken pox!*

However on Tuesday afternoon I set off - after a tender farewell to Margaret and arrived in Lagos four and a half hours later - a record trip. I did not stop at all on the 160 mile trip.

On arrival in Lagos I found that I was staying with the Mr. Steinman - a friend of the Bill Mann's- a Swiss shop owner in Lagos. A very nice man, his wife and family are in Switzerland. He has a lovely house and is glad of some company. Unfortunately it is five miles out from the Mission, which is a complication. In addition it is incredibly noisy - ten yards from the main road into Lagos and 100 yards from the main railway line! The first night I found it difficult to sleep - but since then have slept like a log.

On Wednesday morning I attended the pre-synod finance committee, then in the afternoon went to the boat. Poor Jean and Andrew - what a tottering trip - ten days, four children confined to the cabin, with either Andrew or Jean with them 24 hours out of 24. They were glad to get off the boat! I whisked the family to Yaba where they stayed with old university friends, then on Thursday morning they shopped and travelled to Ilesha Thursday afternoon. They had a good journey and arrived about 7.45pm.

I have done odd bits of shopping mostly for the hospital and attended the property committee and the Christian Citizenship committee. The big worry the last few days has been the Synod Medical Meeting. It is left to the hospital staff - and as I am the only one down - it fell upon my shoulders. Unfortunately I had decided to show the slides and it was fixed for 5.30 in the afternoon in the church and so I went along to see if it would be possible to make it sufficiently dark. I shut up all the shutters and hung curtains over some stained glass windows. It made it relatively dark but the pictures did not show up as well as they might have done. The Chairman failed to materialise, so Mr. Angus took the chair and the meeting as a whole went quite well. I showed pictures of the building, opening day and the new hospital in action. I am glad it is over. Now I shall have to think about the medical business to present to synod on Wednesday next week and then I hope to get back to Ilesha and Margaret on Friday.

Lagos is not so hot and sticky as I have known it on previous occasions and almost pleasant. Great preparations are in hand for the Queen - road making and painting and so forth. I doubt if we shall see anything of her at all.

We are both keeping very fit and not long before we are home now much love from us both, David

22nd Jan 1956
Once again, back in Ilesha, and very glad indeed, to be back with Margaret. I was away nine days and at the time it seemed interminable but in retrospect hardly

any time at all. Margaret had kept well except for one day when she wasn't very fit, but is well again now.

Two letters have arrived whilst I was away. One from Queen Charlotte's-booking Margaret for June, and for the antenatal clinic, which is very good news - and the second letter from Mr. Kissack in Rome saying that he had booked accommodation for us at the 'Mission Theological College' at 1100 lire a day for bed and breakfast plus evening meal (about 13/6) each which is very good indeed! So we are very pleased.

Glad to hear of Elsie Ludlow's visit. Incidentally, nursing sisters prefer to be called Sister Ludlow.

Last Sunday evening I went to one of the Lagos churches and heard Alan Ashley preach and then in the evening went on to the Mission House, where we had hymn singing and then on to Mr. Steiner's to bed.

Monday was the opening of Synod, with communion first and then opening, business, and then the voting for chairman. To everybody's surprise, Mr. Mellor (who is retiring) put up, but after three votes Jonah got the majority. I expect Alan has told you though. The question now is - will Mrs. Jones come out next tour with him? I think she may if Mr. Jones father can be cared for.

On Monday evening I took Charles, Margaret and Christopher (18 months) Day down to the beach where we bathed and played on the sand for an hour or two, then in the evening went to the ordination service of John Crosby

On Tuesday there was interesting business - Synod agreed to united MMS and CMS theological training starting in 1957. This will be a great step forward - largely due to Charles Day's efforts. Also Synod agreed to pressing for a West African District Conference as well as church union.

On Wednesday the Medical business was discussed and I presented the medical report. Several questions were asked, one rather persistent brother queried the accounts but was put in place by the Chairman. The synod hall was so noisy that Bill Mann suggested that I got hold of microphones and loud speakers. I rang up the Nigerian Film Unit and they were installed the following day.

Thursday morning - I finished off the shopping I had to do, and had intended to return at 1pm but Enid was not ready so we did not get away until 3.30, however we had a good run up arriving about 8pm.

Friday - I settled down to the accounts, yesterday I operated, then in the evening we entertained the staff to a welcome party for the Pearsons' who are well settled in and fit except for Alison who has many spots.

Five weeks today we shall be very excited indeed and shall travel to Lagos five weeks tomorrow

Hope all well with you all   Love from us both, David

Sunday Jan 29th 56

Thank you very much indeed for your birthday wishes! Michael's letter arrived the day before and your letter arrived the following day and it was good to hear al the home news.

We have had a quieter week than many, and very glad of it too. Thursday was of course my Birthday and Margaret gave me a book of Reptiles of West Africa and a bowl of shaving soap - a most attractive container.

To my surprise the Pearsons' came round with a booklet for a baby's cot and an Agatha Christie book - most welcome presents. Margaret made a very fancy sponge cake for tea and in the evening the Pearson's came in to dinner. Unfortunately, Andrew, who was on duty, was called away several times, but Jean, Margaret and I played Scrabble. It was a very nice evening. In the morning I had a bit of operating to do - including a hysterectomy, but the rest of the day was quiet.

We are already thinking of our trip home. We shall have to pack all our things in boxes, as the Morleys will be here in the house for a few months whilst their house is being built. Aileen Morley is bringing out her own crocks, cutlery etc. so we shall put all ours away.

John and family have gone for their local leave to the Cameroon. It will be a delightful break.

Thus Andrew and I are on our own. Payday comes on Tuesday and we are anticipating a spot of bother as we shall be expected to give a considerable increases to the staff in view of the vast government increases in salary given during the year.

The Queen has arrived safely - I doubt whether we shall see her. We are both well, but ready for a rest and change! Love to you all from us both, David

5.2.56

It was good to get your letter with Michael's note on Friday and to learn that you are fit and intend to keep so with molasses! I understand also that Guinness is good for you - but please do not turn vegetarian! The thought of no sirloin or shoulder of lamb is enough to make one offer for the extended tour!

We are expecting infant Cannon prima around June 16th.

Interested that you saw the Queen and Duke of Edinburgh pass. I don't think I shall see her, but Margaret may go down to Ibadan a week on Tuesday. We have got tickets for the Nurses in one of the enclosures and Andrew is going to ask Mr. Bury which would be the spot to go to.

The last two nights I have had difficult cases in Maternity, so I too am a bit short of sleep, however tonight I am not on call so hope to make up for it.

Last night we had Vernon and Doreen Woods to dinner and killed the sole surviving duck of the pair we were given. One died earlier this week of a *mysterious unidentified disease.*

One piece of news - I nearly forgot I have been nominated as a Mission House representative to the Methodist Conference in July! This ought to be most interesting - I believe it is in Leeds. Alan Birtwhistle asked if I required accommodation and I said yes. If we know of anyone there we can always cancel. Will Daddy or Uncle Stanley or you be going?

We are a bit at sea at the moment as our back verandah is being re-sloped but by tomorrow that will be complete but then we are having a low wall built around with a trellis on top to give us a bit of privacy, so once again we shall be in a bit of a mess. At the end of next week we are entertaining a Government Nursing Sister who is coming up in connection with the proposed welfare scheme. We are very fit and looking forward immensely to Rome and home. Love from us both, David.

Saturday, 13.2.56

It is Saturday evening and I am not on duty, and we haven't anyone in so I am taking the opportunity to write this letter. Tomorrow we are expecting Colonel and Mrs. Walters. They were to have come on Thursday but wired to say it would be Sunday and they would not be staying.

Have booked April 15th for Jordan's - you will see that the Tuesday following, I have put down for Chiswick. It should be fairly satisfactory I should think - if we wanted to we could go to Jordons soon after the Easter weekend.

Yes we are sorting out and getting ready. The week after this will be 'operation pack' - just now it is operation preparation.

We have a piece of news I can keep bottled up no longer. Margaret and I have been invited to the Royal Garden Party at Government House, Ibadan on Monday 13th! It arrived by a court messenger on Monday last! There will be many, many folk there, so the opportunity of speaking to her will be very small, but we should certainly see her well.

The one slight embarrassment is that we are the only ones from the compound and we think we must have been invited because we entertained Lady Rankin when she was ill. However the others are as excited as we are and have taken it in good part.

With the invitations are instructions as to what we should do and wear and so on and where we are to have tea and so forth. We are going in our 'going away' things - very fortunate to have them. Margaret has borrowed a white handbag, bought some white shoes (very lucky to find them in Ilesha) and so we are all set.

We are going down in the morning and having lunch with the Days and then getting ready in their house. I don't think that it is broadcast - nor are photographers allowed in - but should there be any chance of us appearing on a news reel we will have cabled you before you receive this.

John and family arrived back safely from the Cameroon last evening having had a very good time, though the journey took five days going and four days returning.

This last week has been very hot indeed - some of the hottest weather we have known and in addition to being over 90F in the shade it is very humid and one wilts like a flower in the afternoon.

We are both keeping very well and both as excited as children!

Much love from us both, David.

Sunday, February 19th 1956

Time rushes on apace and it is once again Sunday morning. Great preparations are afoot as Bryan John is to be christened at the morning service at Otapete, and everyone is clucking around their children getting spruced up! My task has fallen to one of chauffeur to the Christening party. The Fathers are taking their offspring down earlier! According to the programme the service begins with the Introit.

The morning of the Garden Party dawned cloudy and fears stole upon us that rain would arrive, and cancel the little get-together. However it remained fine, even sweltering so little further need be said on this topic. I did the morning round and out patients and Margaret got the house straight and so on. At 10.30 Jonah looked in complete with MBE with which he had been decorated the previous Saturday. He was in ecstasies! We drove down to Wesley College where we had lunch by arrangement, with the Days who were all well, and packing up ready to come on furlough in March. After lunch we had a rest and then at 3.45 began to dress, Margaret in her going away clothes plus a pair of white shoes she had managed to buy in Ilesha, myself also in going away clothes. At 4.30 we got into the car and said 'Bashola (the driver) - Government House' and away we went. The car was parked with some difficulty as the driver got a bit flustered, however no harm was done except to our nerves. We had left the house spotless but were now faced with a 300 yard walk through almost solid dust. However - perspiring not so gently in the fierce sun, and dust on shoes, we seemed to arrive in the garden, past sentries and guards in the same condition as everyone else. We went to the tea stall and got glasses of squash and some rolls, fruit cake and so on, and took a couple of seats under the shade.

After tea we saw Frank and Jessie Longley of Oyo who were there and together we sat on the edge of the path along which the Queen would walk. The garden is divided into two upper lawns and a larger lower lawn and most of us were on the lower one. Promptly at 5.30 the Queen and Duke came out of the House and began their perambulation. We could follow their progress on the upper lawns from the top of the Royal Standard, which was carried with her.

About five minutes later she descended to the lower lawn, where we could see her easily for about 20 minutes as she gradually got closer. Some folk were presented to her - some very close to us so that she was about four feet away for five minutes or so. Margaret will be able to tell you what she was wearing, but she was a truly Royal figure. In fact she was so close for so long we got rather embarrassed looking at her. The Duke approached from the other side, chatting very informally to folk. He stopped at Frank Longley next to me who was wearing his clerical collar and had a few words, so we had a very good view of the Duke too. They then wended their way back and appeared on the balcony of the house, The National Anthem was played and the Garden Party was over. We went up to look at the house and upper terrace more closely and then left the grounds and set off for home, as you may imagine thrilled to bits.

We called at the Baptist compound on the way and were given a snack. We had really called in for a drink of water to take a couple of aspirin, for what with the sun and the standing and the excitement we had the beginnings of headaches.

On our arrival, we were mobbed by our colleagues, to find out how we had got on. On Tuesday, Andrew and the family went down and saw her pass twice in her car - and Eileen took down seven nurses to an enclosure, where again they had a good view of her in her car, so one way and another we have all seen her.

Andrew was up to Ikole on trek this week, and found Louie well. We have been sorting out drawers and so forth this week and tomorrow start putting everything into boxes. It looks like being a very busy week. We must have it done by this time next week as we travel to Lagos a week tomorrow. We are keeping very fit indeed. It seems almost impossible that in three weeks we shall be home!

Much love, from us both, David.

Rome, 4.3.56

Sunday evening and we are sitting in our room at the Waldensian Faculty, waiting for the evening meal with healthy appetites and a little apprehension.

We have been comfortable here - but the continental breakfast and the rather hostelish food are at times a trifle inadequate. We have seen a great deal - though not overdone it, but by walking rather than any other form of transport have found our way around quite well.

Yesterday afternoon the Kissacks took us in hand and we went out to the catacombs and then back to a very nice evening meal, after which I showed our hospital slides, which were appreciated.

I hope that you have received the card I sent on our arrival by now - after I had written it we went to St. Peters and saw the Michael Angelo ceilings and so forth and the devout Catholics kissing the toe of the statue of Peter. We visited the Vatican treasury, where there are the most beautiful golden chalices, crosses and so forth.

Each day we have set off about nine - seen the ancient Rome Forum, Coliseum, Capitoline Hill, Palatino Hill, temples and so on. In the evening we have had the meal about eight, after which we have been ready for bed.

We have been very fortunate with the weather, most of the time it has been sunny and out of the wind it has been warm although today has been pretty nippy and overcast.

This morning we attended the English service taken by Mr. Kissack and then being in the neighbourhood of the National Museum went in and saw some of the most marvellous mosaics from baths and sculptures - really breathtaking when one considers it is over 2000 years old. We really felt to have rubbed shoulders with antiquity and wished we had a greater knowledge of ancient history.

On Sunday afternoon the Kissacks have 'open house' and invited us to tea - there was one other English person there. Mr. K is taking us to the air terminal tomorrow morning for nine o'clock. The plane leaves at 10.20 and we are in Geneva at 1.15.

We learn that there is not a great deal to see in Geneva itself and are going to make enquiries about a day trip out into the Alps for the second day we are there.

On Thursday evening we fly to Amsterdam and on Saturday morning start the last leg of the journey - train to the Hook, boat to Harwich, then train to Liverpool St. arriving just after 8pm.

We have had a wonderful time here and have taken 30 photos, so hope to be able to share it with you more fully.

We are both very well. Much love from us both to you all, David

THIRD TOUR, 1956-58

aboard the cargo vessel 'Sherbo'
2.9.56

Another Sunday is here and at the moment we are jogging along past Cape Palmas, which is, I think, in Liberia. Although the sea is the calmest I have ever seen it there is quite a bit of swell but the roll which we have had since we started is not so marked

We were very thrilled to receive your letter when we arrived at Dakar and to hear how your Edinburgh holiday went. I hope that it was fine in the dale, but rather fear it has been pretty wet.

Today is the first Sunday of the new Church Year and we shall be thinking of you all as we often do. I have just done Peter's vaccination dressing. It has been rather messy, but today is much cleaner and in another three days or so it should be cleared up. The inflammation has been localised and he has not been too fretful. He is developing now and seems much more awake for much longer and after a feed will smile and chuckle at the smallest provocation. He has just learned how to pull up his nightdress and often pulls it up over his face leaving his tummy quite bare! He is quite a favourite with the passengers and the little boy Ken (2 years and 4 months) comes and says good morning to him each day. Peter seems entirely unaffected by the motion of the boat - except at Dakar, when we stopped for a few hours he was unhappy.

Margaret and I are well, though stopping at Dakar destroyed our sea legs and we had an unhappy 36 hours following our visit last Thursday. However once again we are OK. I took one or two photos

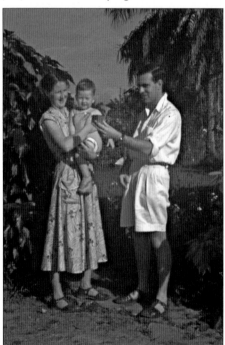

Margaret and David with Peter

of a very picturesque market and then bought an ivory necklace to bring back for Margaret. It was very pleasant to be on land again but just as we left Dakar we had 24 hours of rain and high seas that were most unpleasant.

Since then we have settled down again, eating sleeping and reading and occasional games of quoits and table tennis - very lazy. We hoped for a while that we might be transferred to the mail boat at Takoradi where we shall meet, but the captain cannot transfer passengers without very good reason, so no doubt we shall remain on board for a full week off Accra - only 18 hours sailing from Lagos.

We reach Takoradi, when I hope to post this, on Monday night, reach Accra on Tuesday night and then we have to unload 2000 tons of cargo into small surf boats that hold one and a half tons each! Each boat does 8 trips per day so you can see what a job it is.

Well space has gone, do hope all is well and look forward to hearing from you. Love from us both, and a chuckle from Peter, David

On board MV Sherbo a cargo boat with twelve passengers
Accra, 9.9.56

Another week has passed and here we are anchored about a mile off shore, rolling steadily from side to side - but we are finding it quite pleasant and our appetites are unimpaired. Peter is flourishing and is looking very sweet - but Margaret is going to add a note about him!

It was decided that we should not stop at Takoradi because a Dutch boat was also making for Accra and we wanted to get there first. We arrived on Tuesday morning and had some 2,200 tons of cargo to unload. There is no port, and every ounce has to be unloaded onto surf boats, which hold a maximum of one and a half tons - so you can see what a terrific job it is. They start at 6am and the noise of 70 crew boys on the boat and 30 or so boatmen is incessant until 6pm, and no chance of sleeping at all. They have seven derricks working at once but with the swell it is very difficult to land the cargo onto the boats. Already I have seen four boats capsize and each load sink! One day it rained all day so they packed up work at 10am. However up to last night 1500 tons had been off loaded so we are hoping that it may be finished by tomorrow night, followed by a day at Cotonou and then on to Lagos - perhaps on Thursday.

By now we have got to know the members of the crew quite well. The captain is a keen fisherman and even as I write this he is about two feet away with his rod over the side.

On the wet day one of the passengers and the captain caught sufficient mullet for them to put it on the menu for breakfast the next morning. It was delicious. I spent several hours unhooking the fish, as Mr. Jones did not like the job very much! Unfortunately today the fish are just too far from the boat to be reached easily. I have been knocked out of the table tennis, but Margaret won her first match last night. In the evening we have had several games of Scrabble and Cludo and with knitting and reading the time passes quite well.

Accra looks quite an interesting place but I have no desire to go ashore in one of these surf-boats - three lost yesterday alone trying to land.

Peter is just dropping off to sleep in his carrycot on the deck after an exhausting time with his small rattle. He has just learned to hold it and can shake it vigorously It is quite impossible to keep a sheet over his legs while he is awake as he kicks everything off and pulls dress and sheet up over his head. In spite of all this exercise he is putting on weight faster than ever and is looking really bonny. The chief steward helped me to weigh him yesterday - 10lb 12oz. He even enjoys his bath now and is sleeping from 10.30pm to 5 or 6am.

With love, Margaret and David.

Lagos 14.9.56

Here we are in Lagos - safely arrived and installed on the Marina. Tuesday night we sailed and arrived in Cotonou in French West Africa the next morning. Again we anchored off the coast and unloaded into boats, which were then towed ashore with tugs, 60 tons of salt - and by 11.30am we were off again - the last lap to Lagos. We arrived at 4.30pm but were told there was no berth in the harbour so we had to anchor outside Lagos for fourteen hours with the boat rolling terribly. We all felt a bit giddy but not sick - but the night was most uncomfortable - one of the worst I have known - one had to be ready to hang on to the side of the bunk to stop falling out. Many pieces of crockery were broken and at the evening meal you had to tip your soup bowl appropriately to stop it spilling and even then the plates were less than half full.

We entered the harbour at 7am on Thursday - were tied up at 8am through customs by 10am and at the Marina by 11am - no trouble and only £4.6.0 to pay on our goods.

Peter was wonderful and he has settled down to a mosquito net without any trouble. Fortunately it is very cool at the moment considering it is Lagos. The hospital lorry arrived tonight and we are going up tomorrow if all is well.

Margaret has practically finished my pullover- only three rows to do and then sew up - but wool has run out! Could you send one ounce by airmail of Greenock Brand double knitting wool Shade 87 Dye G 7763. If it is declared as knitting wool we shall only have a few pence to pay customs.

We shall be glad to get to Ilesha - we seem to have been en route long enough. Peter makes new conquests every day, bless him and he is very well.

Love from us both, and a big smile from Peter, David

Ilesha, Monday, 18.9.56

A hurried and probably brief note to let you know we have arrived safely in Ilesha, and are all very well. It was lovely to find your letter and Michael's awaiting us and to learn that all is well.

The lorry came down to Lagos on Friday night - again with one or two shopping requests. These we accomplished before 9.30am Peter then fed and we set off at 10.30 arriving in Ibadan at 1.20pm where we had lunch at Wesley College with Rowland Hughes and Frank Morton

We left again at 2.40 and arrived in Ilesha about 5.20 having had a very good journey indeed. There was not room in the front of the lorry for the carrycot so Margaret had to nurse him the whole way, which was a bit hot for both. However Peter is fine and so far doesn't seem troubled by the heat.

The other members of staff were on hand to greet us and since arrival have had all the members of the compound to salute us, all being very thrilled to have a peep at Peter.

Our loads have all arrived safely - though the pram case was battered - the pram itself is in good condition - Peter is out in it from 10am to 6pm in the shade. The house is beautifully clean and the garden is absolutely marvellous - more next week.

Yesterday we spent most of the time unpacking our cases, trunks and boxes, a real task. However we have got everything out now and most things put away. The boxes have all gone into the store and the fridge is to come over this afternoon. The Pearsons, Wrights, Morleys and Sisters are all well and the children are all rather noisy - but come very quietly when they come to see Peter.

This morning we went to Aileen's for elevenses and looked round their house - very nice indeed - the largest of all the houses.

Do hope all is well with you all. I have got a lot to do - Margaret even more! Love to you all from us all, David

23.9.56

Another week has passed - a busy one for all of us without doubt. Margaret especially. Last Sunday we felt a bit overwhelmed by the quantity of work to be done but we have got through it now. It was exciting to unpack all the new things we had bought and show off the hair drier - and the electric fan is a very dinky little one indeed, with rubber blades.

The Acme wringer also is lovely and works very well indeed. Joseph the carpenter made a stand one morning and we have made a little plastic cover for it, so it looks very neat as it stands next to the bathroom, where Margaret runs through the nappies - very convenient.

By Monday evening we had the boxes and trunks stored away and most things in drawers - but it has taken the rest of the week to get the spare room straight.

On Wednesday I began work in the office on last years accounts (till Aug 31st) attempting to balance them. It took until Friday night working on them continuously before the errors were sorted out and then when I had a balance to carry forward I had to start this years. However they are up to date now - but there are a large number of invoices and so on to sort out. Still this coming week I am not on either afternoons or nights so I should be able to get on quite a bit. In addition Andrew is not on duty at all so he should be able to get things sorted out a bit.

The garden is wonderful, cabbage, cauliflower, runner beans and lettuce ready for eating, with tomatoes, radish and onions coming on. The hens though are a bit of a disappointment. They are right off laying and there has not been an egg for three weeks from any of them. However Margaret has them in hand and we hope that, with more scientific feeding, they will begin to lay again.

Last night we had Elsie in for chop. The Pearsons' were coming too, but were prevented at the last minute, however came in to coffee afterwards. Tomorrow evening the Morleys are having a house warming party - there are 35 folk invited - quite a lot of folk from the town - a buffet supper followed by games.

So far the weather has been quite pleasant though it is getting hot just at the moment. With love from us all and a smile from Peter, David

Sept. 30th 1956

It is Sunday afternoon and the temperature is well in the 80s and it feels as if we shall have a storm before evening. It has been our turn for morning coffee and even though the Morleys are away till evening it is quite a job with seven children and ten adults! I did an early round and then came home to make the scotch pancakes - which I did on the griddle over the primus.

We are very glad for your letter on Friday and for the wool, which arrived safely and no customs duty to pay - on Saturday. I am sorry it was so expensive to send by air!

We have had a full and interesting week. Margaret has been busy in the house and with the hens. The new plastic curtains are up in the bathroom and toilet and look very nice indeed and now some larger nighties for Peter are in production - taken from a pattern of Jeans. From the carpentry point of view - the clothes rack is complete and fixed - a great success and clothes dry overnight with the residual heat from the stove. I have put in quite a lot of time on the ironing board - and it is nearing completion, all that remains to be done is the fixing of a piece of asbestos and covering with cloth. Sylvia was mentioning that the recent ones have clips around the sides to hold it in position, yet easy to remove for washing. Last Monday night was the party - part home warming for the Morleys, part welcome for us. It was a very good party, with competitions to start with - then buffet of cold meats, salads, fruit blancmange - followed by games. Margaret won a prize of half a pound tin of treacle toffee -most acceptable!

On Thursday Mr. and Mrs. Glass of Oshogbo came over with their projector to show some films taken by John (he has borrowed a cine camera) to the staff including nurses. We had just got nicely going when the hospital engine broke down and we had no light at all in the hospital. Andrew and I fiddled without any success. The situation was complicated by Marion, who filled the storm lanterns from a drum containing soap solution instead of kerosene!

I began in the wards and have been kept busy - had to do a caesarean on Thursday and a hernia yesterday and several fractures to stabilise so I am getting my hand in. We had a sad case of an ex-nurse who died of an acute crisis in sickle cell anaemia - a rare condition.

We are all keeping very well with plenty to keep us going in every way.   Love from us all with a coo from Peter, David

PS - We had a letter this week to say that Mrs. Mellor died on the 20th September

14.10.56

Another Sunday has come round - very quickly - we have finished breakfast, I have looked around my wards and there is half an hour before it is time to go down to Otapete for service.

We were most distressed to hear of Stanley's trouble - We do hope that he is better by this time - we are anxiously looking for your next letter. It is most unfortunate that it should have happened just at this time so far as school work goes - and I fear that it may stop his swimming too, though his learning should be unaffected.

Henry does seem to be at low ebb. When does he sail for Antarctica? We had thought that he had more or less made his mind up about which girlfriend to marry when we left but apparently not!

We have had another full week - and all is well. Peter has gained again - henceforth we are only gong to weigh him every two weeks. He drank his orange juice out of a cup for the first time yesterday and really made a very good job of it. He is very good indeed - sleeps all night and if he wakes up in the morning just lies and kicks until Margaret feeds him at 6.30. He is playing well with his beads, rattle and fluffy ball. Last evening we pushed him up to the netball pitch where we watched the nurses playing - next Saturday the staff are going to play them - it should be very good fun.

Last Sunday night we had one of the members of the Apostolic Church preached - he was very good indeed and on Monday night we went to chop with the Morleys, a very pleasant evening. Wednesday night it was my turn to take fellowship - we had the Pearsons' in to chop which went quite well. John and Elsie had gone down to Lagos to meet Miss Woodland, the Sister who is to be part of the Imesi scheme. Enid Blake and I had met her at the Mission House.

She came out on the 'Hilleary' a boat that E.Ds have chartered to take the place of the Aureol, which is going to have a re-fit. Apparently conditions were awful - and Miss W and her fellow passengers were unable to have a bath the whole fortnight! The washing up was done so badly the passengers offered to do it and a very strong letter has been sent to the directors of the company. It was this boat the Wrights were to have sailed on but their passages have been cancelled, so it is possible that they will be with us for Christmas - if so there will be 23 (including children) without guests who are coming. John, Elsie and Miss W (another Margaret) arrived rather late on Thursday having been delayed by a tree across the road. Andrew and David M had gone to a clinical meeting in Ibadan - so I was left (I am on night duty) to hold the fort and had a strangulated hernia to do for my pains.

On Friday morning the Anguses had coffee with us on their way back to Lagos and Mr. Esan our new minister looked in.

Last night we had the Wrights in to the evening meal and today the Sisters are coming in to lunch. On Wednesday a Mr. Ekundayo arrived with a scrapbook and ball for Peter from you - most unexpected. He came down to the house for coffee and told us about himself and then on Thursday we went round to his house to see him and had coffee there. He seems a nice lad but finds Ilesha too slow after England and is going to settle in Ibadan. He seemed very grateful to you both for your help.

Our hens are coming into lay; twelve eggs during last week and one yesterday weighed two and a half ounces! I had it for breakfast this morning! Margaret is now having to pay 3d for the very small market eggs so it is much better to produce our own! Space gone and time for Chapel. Do hope you are all well and Stanley is better.

Love from us all, David

21.10.56

We were glad to receive your letter from Doncaster - but we were most distressed to hear of Mr. Ranger's death.

We have had another full week - I don't think that any of us could complain that our lives are dull! Last Sunday we had the Sisters in to lunch and then Mr. Onaeku, the Head Master of the local Methodist Secondary School who was the preacher in the evening, came in for coffee afterwards.

Monday evening I went down to class at Otapete but no leader arrived so we had a short prayer meeting.

Tuesday evening we had a welcome for Margaret Woodland at the Sisters - coffee, refreshment and games - a happy evening. We now have a visiting dentist - on tour from Akure, and he visited us so was at the party, with his wife also. A rather odd couple, who have been out here for six months.

Wednesday evening was committee. There did not seem much on the agenda but went on until 11.45!

Thursday I spent trying to get the minutes completed and letters written. At lunch time the Pearson's set out for Lagos for their local leave for two weeks. They had a very poor journey down a puncture before Ibadan and solid rain after and it took them about seven hours - most exhausting for the children. David Morley went too, to see the folk in Lagos about the Imesi scheme and while he was there final agreement came, so we are at the moment buying a car, microscope etc.

Friday evening I took part in a Brains Trust in the Wrights house and last night we had the Morleys and Miss Woodland in to dinner. Unfortunately I got held up with a caesarean section so they had started when I got down.

John has gone to Otapete this am and I shall go to chapel this evening with Margaret and one of the others will baby sit.

Peter is very well and has just learned how to put his feet on the beads stretched across his pram and push on them. He is discovering he can bring his feet up to his hands but he has not yet got hold of them himself. He is keeping his colour very well despite the climate and is almost podgy! He has his orange juice from a cup just finished off with a spoon and still sleeps very well and has to be wakened at 10pm so it should not be long before that feed can be dropped. He had his second batch of injections (whooping cough, diphtheria, and tetanus) on Tuesday without any reaction.

The hens laid eighteen eggs this week - so once again we are we are relishing new laid eggs for breakfast., We are all three very well, very busy and very happy. Love to you all, David

28.10.56

This week your letter arrived on Wednesday - having been posted on Monday - which is a record I should think and it is also very nice indeed to receive news so soon. Glad too, to hear of the Medical meeting - and you sitting with the Souster's - how is Jack getting on? Sorry to hear that Henry is still in low water - he will have to make up his mind sometime!

We have had another busy week - but nothing very outstanding has occurred. It has been made more difficult by John being in bed for the last four days - his leg ulcers again - and is likely to be there another week yet, in addition to Andrew still being away on local leave though back next Thursday. However David Morley and I have managed so far, but on Wednesday coming it is our turn to go to Ikole on trek.

The main interest this week has been the visit of Dr. Porterfield from the Vines laboratory in Yaba. We have had a number of unusual cases in the wards which we have termed 'Ijesha Shakes' The virus people are interested and we rang them up when we had a fresh wave and Dr. Porterfield drove up at once with 108 white mice! We took blood from the patients and then injected it into the mice having first anaesthetised the mice. In a month or so they may show some signs of disease - or they may not!

Next Friday Professor Brown - Professor of Medicine from Ibadan is coming up for a night to see the patients. At the moment they are all getting better - I hope one or two more acute case turn up for him to see.

Yesterday we held a netball match - nurses versus the staff. David and Aileen, Sylvia, Margaret Woodland, Eileen, the warden, a nurse and myself played for the staff. Margaret was referee. The nurses won 6-1 to their great jubilation. We were all exhausted in the extreme at the finish and are all determined to get in some practice.

Last night we all went to David and Aileen's to a musical coffee party. There were gramophone records to suit every taste - it was a most pleasant evening.

This morning I went down to chapel - Margaret is going this evening. It is another very hot afternoon indeed and we are all very short of energy - even the children seem subdued.

Peter is in good form. Margaret weighed him on Friday and he is 12lb 2oz and looks very well. He has discovered how to make a new noise - a very deep sort of throaty growl. He employs this when he has had sufficient food and growls away after he has been put into the cot after the 2pm feed.

He is almost too big now to sleep in the carrycot and we are waiting to get one of the compound cots from Aileen who has her youngest (Andrew) in it at the moment.

The hens are still laying quite well - fifteen eggs this week and the little black and white native hen has gone broody so she is sitting on eight eggs. In three weeks time if all is well there should be some chicks.

We are all very fit and hope all is well with you all and Stanley quite better again. Love from us all, David

4.11.56

Another eventful week has passed - and no doubt in a few hours you will be writing to us on the topic of the Egyptian news. It is terrible isn't it? but I feel we cannot judge yet because we haven't all the facts. And Russia shelling Budapest - it looks as if 'ere long there will be a showdown between Russia and the rest.

Here we have had a busy week, John has been in bed all the time but hopes to begin a little work tomorrow, which will be a great help. However, Andrew, Jean and family arrived back on Thursday looking very well, and in good spirits. They had bought quite a lot of things for the Imesi Scheme and we have a house chosen so things are really on the move.

On the mail boat, which arrived on Wednesday, there were many missionaries including Mrs. Jones and Enid. Jonah and Mrs. J. and Enid arrived on Friday evening so the Joneses stayed in the compound - had evening meal with the Sisters and had breakfast with us, which we enjoyed. They both looked well and went up to Ifaki the next day. The trek has been cancelled - owing to John's illness last week, we just couldn't have got away so we shall be going up on November 28th if all is well.

During the week we have had several visitors. Professor Brown of University College Hospital Ibadan - the Professor and his wife came up for two days - we entertained them to dinner. Very easy to entertain, and a humble man (aged 46) for his position. He seemed very interested in everything.

On the Wednesday David Morley took them to Imesi, which left me the hospital and also the paying of the men, which was a very full day with our usual Wednesday evening fellowship at 8.30.

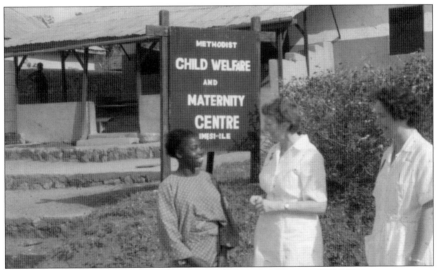

Imesi sign

Enid is looking well and full of energy and will be starting work tomorrow I expect. On Wednesday also we had a visit from the Consultant eye specialist from Ibadan and he came to tea, so it really was a day.

Last night we went out to chop - Eileen also - to Margaret Grants at the Women's Training College. She is well, due for leave in April and undecided whether to come back or not. I advised her to, as if she does one more tour she gets a pension of £80 pa for life after only five years in the country!

Today it is our turn for morning coffee - eight children and thirteen adults - so I have been giving a hand in the kitchen with Margaret and they are all due any time now.

We are all well and flourishing, Peter is in good fettle and always laughs when wrapped up in his towel! Kicks wildly in the bath. He is a bonny lad with large blue eyes - and has caused, so Jonah was saying, quite a stir in the District. Apparently in Lagos they are saying - have you seen the beautiful baby the Cannons have?

Do hope all is well with you all and that the world news improves! Love from us all, David

18.11.56

Another Sunday afternoon is here and again it is very hot indeed - however the news, what we have heard, it seems a little improved. The sooner our troops are out of Egypt the better.

We were glad to have your letter and to learn that all is well at home, Stanley and Michael - even if Henry has been a little exasperating!

Peter is doing very well we think - he comes out on the rug on the floor when we have tea, and he is able to roll over from his front to his back and vice versa, though occasionally gets stuck and becomes most exasperated with himself.

We have had a very busy week, one way and another, with my being on afternoons, David Morley on local leave in Lagos and this weekend John has gone up to Afon on trek with the family. It will be the last time they go up I expect.

On Wednesday we set out for Ikole, had a good run up to Ifaki where we had lunch with Mr. and Mrs. Jones. Mrs. Jones being there makes a big difference! Then Margaret fed Peter and popped him in his carrycot. He was cared for by Mrs. Jones, whilst we went down to the dispensary and I saw the patients. We got back in time to give Peter his orange juice, have tea and then we went on to Ikole where I had a busy time with the patients. On the return journey we called at Iddo, where a new Government hospital has been built - it is beautifully finished - but as yet they have not the staff to open it. On the way back we passed a place where an accident had taken place half an hour before and I was called upon to certify death. We then stopped for a crowd of people by the roadside and found they had someone who was mentally unbalanced! Finally we stopped and gave a lift to a lad who was fetching petrol for a passenger lorry that had run out. With these various stops we did not reach home till nearly seven o'clock - but Peter was very good and settled down well after his feed.

On our return, Jean told us that our hen family had increased by two - then during the next day two more so we have four baby chicks! Two are from our own eggs and two from eggs that we bought from the agricultural department, two Light Sussex and two Rhode Islands. Now comes the problem of deciding if they are cocks or hens!

On Thursday a Government Sister arrived from Lagos, named Mary. She is coming for a month to help us to get the Imesi scheme started. She will fit in *quite well I think. The Morleys returned last night from Lagos before going up to Ikole for their second week.*

On Friday Andrew and I left at 5pm for Ibadan, where we had dinner with Prof. Brown and then went to a lecture by Prof. Paul Brand, of Vellore, India, on the surgery of deformed hands by leprosy. We returned by 12.50am a most interesting if exhausting outing.

We are all very fit and happy - with too much to do! Love from us all, David

25.11.56

Another Sunday is here - morning this time - relatively cool - Peter having his feed in his nursery! Earlier this week the big change was made and Peter has gone into a cot in the spare room, which is now called the nursery. The cot is one belonging to the compound and fits well under the single mosquito net. I think the first day or two he was overawed by the size after his carrycot - but he seems used to it now. I have just watched him having his bath - he loves it, splashing away with his legs and he can hold himself sitting upright by holding on to the sides of the bath. We weighed him last Thursday - now just 13lbs. 6oz. so he seems to be doing well. He takes a little Farex before two of his feeds now and enjoys it. He has it in the bath so that he can be washed easily. He wore one of his nylon dresses last Sunday and will again this! He looks very nice indeed.

Henry sails for the Antarctic tomorrow - we shall be thinking of him. I hope our card arrived in time.

We have had quite a busy week without anything outstanding. The Morleys have been away at Ikole for the week, returning last night having had a nice time though Aileen has not been very well, I fear.

Wednesday was our staff committee, and one of the matters raised was that of the swimming pool. For several months we have been debating whether the hospital could build it (£120) but feel that it is not right that the hospital should pay for it to be used mainly by the missionaries. However the committee did agree that the hospital should pay half if we could raise the other half. It would be so wonderful to have a pool but £60 does take a bit of raising! Enid and Eileen are not interested and it is going to fall largely on the Pearson's and us, with perhaps the Morleys as the Wrights are leaving the hospital. I don't know whether you would care to assist or anyone else you think may contribute for the welfare of the 'poor missionaries sweltering under the blazing sun'! This is an entirely local affair and any money subscribed should be sent as a cheque to me here - Bill Mann can negotiate it for me.

Eileen Searle sails on Tuesday and is going down to Lagos tomorrow. Margaret Woodland is going down also to buy one or two more things for her house in Imesi and she will make odd purchases for us too

Elsie is due for local leave and is going away with Louie to the north in Louie's car. It will be a very nice trip indeed, going up as far as Jos and coming back through the Eastern Region.

For some weeks I have been debating or rather we have, whether or not to buy a new wireless. We have decided to send ours down to Lagos and see if the firm will take it in part exchange for one which works off the mains, but even if they will, it is quite an expensive item which we haven't budgeted for. However with the international situation being as it is I think it is important to get the news easily.

Next week would seem to be a busy one as we look at it. Andrew has a committee in Ibadan tomorrow, so the family is going also. Then the experts from the West Africa Council for Medical Research in Lagos are coming up about the Imesi scheme so we shall have to be on our toes.

We are all keeping well, looking forward to Christmas - only a month today. Love to you all from us all, David

December 2nd 1956

Another Sunday is here after a rather hectic week, but it finds us all well and thriving, and in the midst of a photographic session. So far I have taken eighteen of Peter in pram, bath, and on the rug and I hope to take some of his Sunday dress soon.

I do hope you have had a good time in Doncaster and a good run down again - it could be quite a family gathering! Very sorry to hear of Uncle Edward's impending surgery

Henry's departure seems to have been in true Henry style. At my suggestion we prayed for him at our fellowship last Wednesday night - I feel sure he was in need of our prayers!

We were most distressed to hear of Mr. Patterson's accident, I do hope he is alright again by this time.

Another busy week is past, mainly for us on Tuesday and Wednesday as we entertained the accountant from the West African Council of Medical Research (WACMR) who are sponsoring our Imesi scheme, and went over the accounts he wishes us to keep. I fear that it is going to mean quite a bit more work for us - me especially at this time when Andrew is having to spend quite a bit of time at Imesi getting the house ready for Margaret Woodland.

Friday was a very heavy day with Andrew and David at Imesi and to complicate matters I had a caesarean section to do during the morning, then an antenatal clinic in the afternoon. I was only home for fifteen minutes from 7.45 in the morning till 5pm and then we had nurses fellowship and a couple of hours in the office to do.

During the week, we have had a visit by Mr. F. E. G. Pearson the Treasurer at the Mission House, a most unprepossessing person. Made worse by the fact that he stated that he did not travel like missionaries - he travelled first class in a single cabin so he could do some work! A very poor attitude and a poor advertisement for the Missionary Society.

The week ahead looks full. On Tuesday we have the Hospital Management Committee with Bill Mann and Mr. Angus and the Joneses to put up for the night and also a Malaria specialist coming up from Lagos for three days, arriving the same day! In addition the pundits from WACMR are coming up on Friday- a most inconvenient day for a conference.

In addition John is gong up to Borgu by lorry thus we shall not have his help here at all. Incidentally they are booked to sail sometime between Christmas and January 7th.

We have got a new wireless that works from the mains! It does very well and we can get the BBC without trouble direct from England! We gave our old one in part exchange and feel we have done quite well out of the deal.

We are very well and fit - looking forward to hearing more of your Doncaster trip. Love from us all, David

9.12.56

It is Sunday afternoon, a little disorganised because I have just had to do a caesarean section so have missed my rest and also letter writing time.

It has been a busy week, but a happy one. Thank you very much for the decorations for Peter's Christmas tree and the promise of £5 for the pool. The decorations came without any trouble and no customs to pay. They are grand and will make all the difference to the tree. We are all wondering where we are going to get them their gifts from this year but no doubt we shall find something from somewhere.

Henry seems to have been truly Henry to the end! What will happen during the next two and a half years I don't know - I should love to have seen him in Antarctica on the television.

Glad the Christmas fair was so successful £112 is a goodly sum and should help to pay off a bit of the loan.

We are well - Peter now 13lb 10oz and still a very happy little boy. We got out his chair today one that fits on the back of an ordinary dining chair. Margaret put a cushion down the back and he sat up beautifully - but he cannot sit up alone yet without any support. He has his Farex to supplement his feeds and Margaret is introducing him to the taste of Heinz soups - very slowly- they are definitely an acquired taste.

Peter received two other presents this week one from Bill and Dorothy Mann, a woollen cardigan for his first holiday in England - a most thoughtful gift and the second a plastic parrot that squeaks - from Miss Dalton one of the teachers in the WTC here in Ilesha. We shall put these in his stocking. Having Peter makes

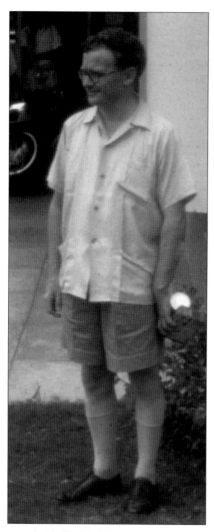

Roland Hughes

Christmas seem more exciting somehow.

We have had a very busy week - John has been away in Borgu where I went with Mr. Angus - so we have had to share out his work. Last Monday, a Specialist from the hospital in Ibadan came, so slowed up outpatients considerably. On Tuesday we had our Medical Committee with Mr. Angus and Bill Mann and Roland Hughes. Margaret and I were expecting Jonah and Mrs. Jones to come to stay the night with us but they had a farewell function near Ifaki to go to, so they did not come to the committee. The committee went quite well, though one or two objections were made to the budget that we will have to revise. Also on Tuesday the leading expert on malaria in the country came and stayed until Friday. He was most interesting and did certain tests on 300 Ilesha infants and he will let us know later the results. He went to look at Imesi and was very thrilled to find a type of mosquito that he didn't expect to find! We had him to an evening meal and found him easy to get on with. He is Polish, but his wife, I believe is English. On Friday we had a visit from the WACMR clan - six of them so we had two of them in to lunch both around my age I should say and nice folk one an entomologist and the other a malariologist - they seemed most interested in the hospital.

Yesterday was a long day, though I had a game of netball in the evening but the accounts took longer as the sisters had not done theirs.

This morning I went down to Otapete and this evening I am preaching in the chapel here, and next Wednesday taking the Wednesday fellowship. Thank you for the Punches and Readers Digest - most welcome

No doubt you are all busy with preparations for Christmas. Margaret made our cake yesterday. Much love from us all, David

252

Dec 16th 1956

A very Happy Christmas to you from Peter, Margaret and David! You will all be in the midst of many preparations - making and doing, and arranging many things. We do hope all goes well with you - we shall be thinking of you and wishing we could be home to share it with you.

Home news from the Ilesha front is good. Peter has cut his first tooth - right lower incisor. It announced its presence by rattling on the spoon! He has certainly been dribbling more recently and now is making real chewing movements. He is very well and taking the Farex, orange juice, a little soup, both William's and Heinz. He is making a number of new noises - largely in the upper register and he bangs his legs on the bed and chuckles at the noise he makes. He is thinking about trying to crawl, but has not managed to get his knees under his tummy yet.

Our baby chickens are doing well and last week we had a record number of eggs from our five laying hens - 21 eggs - very welcome indeed. In addition our pineapple plantation is doing well - with 20 ripening or due to ripen in the next six months!

We have had a busy week. The service I took last Sunday evening appeared to be satisfactory - then Monday was a very heavy day, with outpatients going on from nine until 2pm - hundreds of them. In the evening we went round to the Pearson's for chop and played Scrabble afterwards. Tuesday was again busy and on Wednesday I had to take the evening fellowship. Andrew went to Ikole and brought back Elsie from her local leave. She and Louie have been to the North and had a very nice time indeed.

On Thursday Margaret, Peter and I went with Margaret Woodland to Imesi. We had an early lunch, packed some sandwiches - filled up my tool box and set out. It is the first time I have been to the house, which is truly African with a number of smallish rooms opening one from the other. Our painter has been there for a couple of weeks and a bricklayer is putting up a shelter for the car. I spent the time - as intended - unpacking the fridge and getting it going and unpacking the 'Elsan' - indoor sanitation, which likewise was put into going order.

Friday was a full day with a first meeting of the missionaries over the play we are going to do for the nurses over Christmas - based on 'Call me Florence' a humourous book about nursing.

Saturday was very busy. Andrew, John, David M., Elsie and Rebecca went to the opening of a new school at Imesi, and Margaret Woodland moved into her home. All who went to Imesi helped to clean and bring the furniture upstairs and so forth and David and Aileen and their family have gone this pm to see how she fared the first night. Whilst they were all away a woman was admitted with a gunshot wound of her abdomen and also is 36 weeks pregnant and very ill so I had to undertake a rather involved operation during the afternoon. She has improved a little but her condition is still critical.

This morning it was our turn for coffee twelve adults and nine children - but probably our last big one as the Wrights should be off soon.

The private block is nearly finished and the swimming pool has been started! The weather is real harmattan - dry and very hot in the afternoons - cool at night. We are all getting sore eyes and throats with the dirty atmosphere. Once again a Very Happy Christmas to you all. Love from the three of us, David

23.12.56

Only 36 hours to Christmas! By the time this reaches home it will be time to wish you all a very happy New Year! I expect that you have had a busy but also a very Happy Christmas.

We have been thrilled to receive two parcels during the last week - one from Michael - we think and one from you containing the transfers. We have also received a parcel from Gladys, so we have saved them all up for Christmas Day!

Glad to know all is well at home. I am glad the Ilesha reports have arrived - we haven't seen them yet. I slipped up and should have let you know they were coming. I asked for them to be sent for distribution in Rivercourt.

Today is a busy sort of day. I was up at 5am with a face presentation, then a caesarean, then a retained placenta and finally a forceps delivery, so at the moment (4.30pm) I am feeling a little tired!

The harmattan has persisted this week - it is very cold at night and very hot and dry in the afternoon. I have been on night duty this last week and have been up each night so am very glad it is over.

Last Thursday we had a hectic day - it was our turn to entertain the Medical Meeting of the four neighbouring hospitals - Ife, Oshogbo, Ogbomosho, and ourselves. Five doctors came - I spoke on maternity records, then the Tuberculosis officer from Ibadan on tubercle and then John on the Ilesha shakes, a full day. Then at 8pm the wives of the Ilesha Doctors, shared in the Christmas dinner they had provided.

Grapefruit or tomato juice, turkey, roast potatoes, carrots and sprouts, Christmas pudding- a delicious one, American ice, coffee and mince pies. I think that our American friends were quite impressed - and it was a delicious meal.

Margaret has iced our Christmas cake - it looks beautiful, four colours of icing with holly leaves and berries as the main motif.

Last night I potted our tree and we decorated it with the decorations you sent - looks very nice indeed, and those strips which, appear to go up and down are wonderful. Peter has been gazing at them. He is very well - 14 lbs and two teeth! and still an angel.

This evening is the Carol Service, then tomorrow decorating and last minute preparations. Our guest a Mr. Frogget of the Public Works Department, a

Methodist arrives tomorrow evening.

We are all very well indeed and looking forward to our first Christmas with Peter. Much love to you all from all three of us, David.

30th Dec 1956

We were very thrilled to open your parcels on Tuesday morning last - my pencil is just what I wanted - have needed for a long time and Margaret's bracelet is lovely and she is very thrilled with it and will add a note at the end.

Peter was on Margaret's knee when we opened it and looked with wondrous eyes at his Nursery Rhyme book! The animal cut outs for the wall are good too. I haven't got round to sticking them yet but they are most realistic.

Then on Friday Michael's letter came with the pictures of Peter - we think them very good. The book Michael has sent has given us much pleasure - the drawings are excellent and one can just see oneself in the same position.

We have had a lovely Christmas - Peter has been very good, though he has had a little cold and had few snuffles for a couple of days. Peter received lots of presents and watched very carefully whilst they were all being opened. We have put most of the toys away as he will grow into them.

On Christmas Eve our guest arrived - Norman Frogget of the PWD just as I was setting out Carol singing, so Margaret gave him his meal and settled him in. I went round the hospital and then helped Andrew drive the nurses round the town

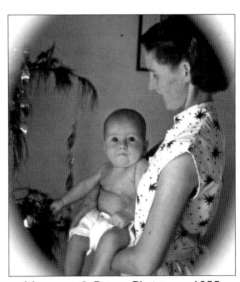

Margaret & Peter, Christmas 1955

Christmas morning began with Communion at 6.15 - a nice service, then breakfast and presents followed by services in the wards. I spoke in the male ward helped by our guest and then coffee. Preparations for lunch took quite a time. The day before a shelter had been built of bamboo and palm leaves but on Christmas Day we had to get out tables and chairs for 70. The meal of rice, chicken, kola, and biscuits was nice and a very happy spirit was present amongst the nurses. Almost straight away it was time for the Nativity play in the wards then tea and the Queen's speech which came over quite well on our wireless.

Tea followed and the Christmas cake is wonderful and the icing and decorating very well done indeed. Then the evening meal - tomato juice, or grapefruit, Turkey, cold ham and vegetables - plum pudding, coffee and sweets, Margaret had made some coconut ice and Turkish delight which was very nice indeed.

Then we had a rather sad little ceremony - presenting the Wrights with a work box. They have now left (27th) and are on their way home. They had a frantic last two days packing and drove down on Thursday, getting straight on to the boat. Andrew went with them and came back the same day.

Love from us all, David

Just a note, to add my thanks for the Christmas gifts, especially the bracelet, which is very beautiful will be just right with my nylon dress. Peter is already taking an interest in his toys and will enjoy the animals on the wall - they will really turn his room into a nursery.

With love, Margaret.

13.1.57

Sunday is here again - but at the moment it is Sunday morning - Peter is just having his bath. He loves the duck that floats and holds the soap, which we bought at Barker and as soon as he is sat in his bath he makes a grab for it and makes it squeak!

He has his cod liver oil whilst in his bath and takes it very well indeed! Andrew has taken the nurses to church and I have a maternity case to cope with so will write this whilst the opportunity offers.

How has the petrol rationing affected things and Michael's tube travel for instance? Very distressed to hear of Grandma's trouble, but agree that liver spread is the best and there is unlikely to be much discomfort. I shall be writing to her today.

Henry seems to have had a most uncomfortable voyage - the John Briscoe is a small ship - and I hear that sailing has been bad recently. No doubt his uneasiness of body has been aggravated by uneasiness of mind, which would certainly not help matters - I am sure that he cannot be very happy. Perhaps when he has some work to do when they reach land, he will settle down.

We have had a full week without any major events except in the poultry line. Last week I mentioned one of the little chicks was ill with pneumonia - unfortunately it died that evening. We had recovered from this loss when on Thursday we were having tea - a teacher Miss Saunders had dropped in for a cup of tea- and a hawk swooped down and took one of our nicest young chickens and despite shouting and running towards it, it made off.

The egg situation has been good though, 25 eggs this week - we have not had to buy any for several weeks now though we have recently bought some more laying hens. Since we came back though they have run at a profit, (small).

We are settling in to a routine without John - but this last week, it was David Morleys trek, and with his Imesi trip has only been in outpatients one day. On Wednesday Andrew goes to Lagos for Synod for ten days so I really will be busy.

Yesterday we had a visit from a skin specialist from World Health Organisation, who saw a number of patients that we had collected for him. He was from Portuguese East Africa and spoke little English and so communication was difficult.

We have had a really cool spell of nights - down to 54F, so cold that Peter was able to wear the sleeping bag from Monica and we had three blankets last night. It is one of the coldest spells of harmattan that Elsie has known, though in the sun yesterday it was over 110F.

We have got back a lovely transparency of Peter - in Margaret's arms, looking at the Christmas tree. David M took it at my request and has given us the transparency. When we have projected the ones that we have got I will post them off for you all to see and keep.

Margaret has had a bad cold earlier this week but I am glad to say it has cleared up very well and neither Peter nor I have caught it.

We are all very fit now, and busy but very happy though we could wish for a little more time off to be at home.

Do hope all is well with you, Love from the three of us, David

20/1/57

Another Sunday - about lunchtime - weather moderately hot and sticky. Andrew is in Lagos, as is Elsie, for Synod, so David and I are holding the fort- though tomorrow is going to be the heaviest day. We are all well now I am glad to say but Thursday morning Peter vomited his 7am feed and was very limp, refused glucose water so I asked David to have a look at him - and he had a sore throat and by afternoon his temperature was almost 102F and he looked rather unwell

Friday he was a little better, though still reluctant to feed and Saturday he was almost better and today is taking his feeds normally, though still a little out of sorts and crying off and on for a little comfort. However he is very, very much better and more like his old self, though a little pale. We have been a bit anxious. It is his first setback, but are now very relieved he is better.

Later: It is now evening time. Margaret has gone along to Chapel and I am baby sitting, a peaceful occupation I am pleased to say.

We were very pleased to receive your letter on Thursday and to hear that all is well with you all. We have had a busy week. Andrew went to Lagos on Wednesday leaving Bryan far from well - worse than Peter, but Bryan has picked up and although very pale indeed is back on his food again and trotting around.

With the very dry, dry season we are having, with a big variation in temperature, there is a great deal of sickness about - pneumonia - and now we seem to be getting some meningitis - all the ward beds have been full and we have had to have some on the floor. Today it is a bit better and things are slackening off a bit. The lorry went down to Lagos on Friday and Andrew loaded it with things that he had already bought and it arrived here last night. We had to unload it first thing this morning in order to take the nurses to church. I took them down and then came back, as David had gone down to the Anglican service. He and Aileen are Anglicans. It was our coffee, so Margaret was very busy - made some brandy snaps filled with cream on Saturday - as the speciality! As the next few days are likely to be busy I have unpacked most of the crates including £370 worth of penicillin and streptomycin.

Last night we had Margaret Grant and Marjorie Clarkson in to chop - a very nice meal and evening - they did not leave until 11.35 and then I had a ward round to do.

The coming week is going to be very busy, especially tomorrow, with a large outpatients in the morning and Tuberculosis clinic in the afternoon. I shall be very glad to see Andrew back on Thursday.

Margaret and I are keeping very well and Peter is more like his old self again today. Hope all is well with you all - new premises etc. We have a new king in Ilesha a most unpleasant fellow and the Premier of Eastern Nigeria has dissolved the Eastern House! Love from us all   David

27.1.57

Sunday and here is a composite letter to you all in reply to your letters for my Birthday. As I sit in this chair and write, Peter, who is quite recovered is just completing his orange juice sitting on Margaret's knee. In a few moments he will be put in his little chair and for a while will survey the room with a definitely Churchillian air, occasionally hitting the tray in front with his fist. He is perfectly well again and today we can see his top two teeth coming through. Aileen has lent us a swing for him, that we have put up in the doorway. We hope that he will soon learn to push his feet on the floor and make himself move.

Thank you very much for the two letters and Stanley's circumlocutory congratulatory phrases. We were interested in all the news and glad that Grandma has arrived safely and in good order. I wish we could send you a bit of our heat - it is really very hot indeed today.

I had a letter from Dr. Bolton - on the same day as yours arrived- and he too wished me Many Happy Returns of the day - the first time I have had a Birthday letter from him. He too speaks of the staffing problem and says he does not know what is going to happen at the end of the year.

As may be expected we had a busy week this week with Andrew away and even so I did not do any cold surgery - that is patients who wanted hernias done and were not emergencies - but if at the end of this year no one is coming out *to relieve, then I shall have to do the routine surgery as well, which will make me very busy indeed. Still we won't meet trouble before it comes.*

Thursday Andrew returned. He had had a very busy time in Lagos shopping for the hospital. All I asked for was an aerial for the wireless - which I have put up but not tried yet. It is 80 feet long excluding the wire down to the set so we should be able to pick up a number of stations - perhaps too many!

When Andrew came up from Synod he brought a visitor, Mr. Glasspool, a member of the General Committee who is trotting around West Africa at his own expense. He is staying here until tomorrow.

On Thursday evening David M and I went to a meeting at Ife hospital on premature babies at which the specialists from Ibadan were speaking. It was quite a good do - with a nice vegetarian meal, and only water to drink.

Last night we went over to the Anglican Girls school for dinner with Dorothea Taylor, a pleasant evening. The rest of the day was very busy and a major operation at 6.30 made us a little late for the meal.

In view of some research, which I am starting in a few weeks, I am seriously considering buying a new microscope. The hospital would buy my present one and I should have to put £80 to it to get a new one. It would be an investment and should not depreciate in value much in 20 years.

We are all very fit and hope all is well with you all. Much love, David

3/2/57

We were very pleased to have your letter on Thursday. Glad to hear that things are all in order and Michael going strong with his many interests! We are all well here, Peter, Margaret and I and in fact all the compound. We are very busy at the moment with one thing and another - many people are sick

At the moment Peter has been put down and Margaret has gone to give the hens their evening food, 30 eggs so once again we have been able to let the Sisters (who don't have hens) have some eggs. However all the other hens have been inoculated so we hope all is well - if it is not one thing it is another.

The week has been quite busy! Mr. Glasspool - the visitor accompanied me on the night round last Sunday and was very thrilled to watch a small operation - no doubt it will be circulated round the home districts in due course! He left on Monday morning and was spending a few days in Ibadan with Rowland Hughes. Tuesday was a Gala night - Margaret had a home perm being operated on by Jean and Aileen - it has taken very well and looks very nice.

Wednesday evening was fellowship when Elsie told us about Synod matters - nothing very startling I think except that Jonah has done well as Chairman.

Thursday was the first payday of the new year. It went reasonably smoothly though we have had a mass of letters regarding increases in salaries. It is always a difficult time but has been one of the quietest yet. Friday was the nurses

Fellowship night. We now have a new batch, they seem a nice bunch and it was my turn to lead.

Saturday we had the Pearsons' and Morleys in to chop - a very pleasant evening. Apple juice and ground nuts as we sat down, then soup, steak and kidney pie with beans and potatoes, followed by a lemon whip, a soufflé with ginger shortbread then coffee and sweets - smashing.

Have just returned from evening service in the chapel - Marion preaching and the chapel seemed quite full-a very nice service. The next day or two will be very heavy as David M is gong to Imesi on Monday and Tuesday which will leave quite a bit to Andrew and myself, still no doubt we shall manage.

Hope your plans for summer holidays work out and that all is well

Love from us both a gurgle from Peter - four teeth now! David

Feb 10th 57

Another Sunday afternoon is here and a very hot one it is indeed. Each afternoon this week it has been over 90F - most prostrating! Still we have kept going and are all well. I am having a lazy day as I woke up with a bit of fever, but no doubt it will be better by tomorrow.

Thank you very much for your letter and cheque. I am in the midst of enquiries about a microscope, as it would seem that the hospital is quite keen to purchase mine - however nothing is yet fixed,

The swimming pool itself is practically finished a wire netting fence is being put round to stop the children falling in and there is the handrail round the inside at the top to put in and the water to lay on. None of these jobs should take much time except that we have been badly let down by the pipe from Lagos.

The advert in the Times! Overland in Nigeria sounds most interesting but I should not consider it at all if it crossed the Sahara Desert - too many people have lost their lives doing it, it needs much skill and knowledge to cross 2000 miles of desert for there are no roads! To come around the coast is much more reasonable but I believe there are only six miles of good road in Liberia!

This week we have been up to Louie's on trek. We called again at Ifaki but the Jonahs are now in Lagos so it was not quite the same. They are making the road up so we got there in good time and went to Mr. Ajayi's house, the new principal. You recall he was at International house in 1952. Margaret stayed with Peter in the afternoon whilst I went down to the clinic - over 100 patients and then we pushed on to Ikole. Louie was well and in good spirits. They have pegged out the new dispensary, which I drew out last time It is going to be a longish building.

Louie seemed very taken with Peter, who was as good as gold, though coming home he was a bit restless because he missed his afternoon sleep. I was able to unblock the pipe to the cistern in the house so at the moment she is well pleased with us!

Yesterday was the Agricultural Show. William entered bread and biscuits and got a first and third prize respectively, a kettle and a machete - so he is very well pleased. Last night the Morleys gave a campfire party to all the Europeans in the town, 24 of us were able to be present. We had sausages, mash, beans, mince pies and coffee and then rounds and songs around the fire. It was a cool night and a wonderful evening. Hope all is well with you at home, much love from us here, Peter is a wonderful boy! Love David

17 Feb. 1957

Sunday morning and I have just returned from chapel - a two hour service in memory of the Baba Zo - the father of the church, who died around Christmas time - six ministers were present including Rev. Dada who was chairman of the District before Mr. Angus. I took Michael Pearson and he stayed the two hours and behaved very well indeed.

We were glad to have your letter on Thursday though it read a trifle like the deaths column of the Methodist Recorder in parts. We also received a letter from Grandma in a very cheerful vein - she seems very happy and thrilled to bits with the Recorder.

Most interested to hear of Michael's jaunt to the 'Skiffle Group' I think the term must have appeared since August last! Pardon my ignorance, but what is a 'Skiffle group'?

I am glad to say we are all well, though there has been an odd 'one day' illness amongst the missionary families. I had it last Sunday and was quite upset - spent the day in bed - then on Monday, Margaret and Peter had it so I had my hands full - but by Tuesday it had passed us and affected the Morleys. However we are all free of it I am glad to say. Peter is very well but feels that now he has teeth he needs more attention! Around 5.45 I try to be at home to play with him, and the last evening or two we have been for a walk together to look at the swimming pool, or the hens - he is most interested in everything. He lifts (when on the floor) his chest well clear but does not seem to have the idea of getting his knees under himself. He can sit up alone for a few moments too now, though his sense of balance is not quite up to keeping him upright for long.

This week we have had another disease amongst the fowls - our cock took ill and died. Margaret called in the vet and he said he thought it had fowl pest and was very worried because they had all been inoculated. However he looked at the cock after it had died and said it had died of something it had picked up- whilst on free range- which was a relief in a way. It rather reduces the profit on this tour though.

It has been a very busy week with large clinics and outpatients. I had 240 patients to an antenatal clinic on Friday.

Yesterday the Morleys went down to Lagos. Tomorrow David has to attend a

WACMR Council - then they will return on Tuesday. However I am looking after the Children's ward in his absence and was on duty last night and had a very bad night with a caesarean to do and a curettage with several other patients coming in and the engine going wrong!

I hope to have a rest though this afternoon. Tonight is a special Student Christian Movement service in our chapel so expect there will be quite a crowd there.

This week has been exceptionally hot 90F + each afternoon - most enervating. Oh to be in England! Do hope all is well at home

Much love from us all, David

24.2.57

Another very hot afternoon (94F in the shade) and in our living room as I settle down to write this epistle - but despite a busy week and one of the hottest I have experienced, we are all perfectly fit and in good health and spirits.

We were very glad to hear that you are well when your letter arrived on Thursday - Grandma's room sounds most attractive - and you all sound very busy with your comings and goings.

Margaret has just got Peter up from his afternoon rest, given him his orange juice and now he is in his chair, one of his plastic sheets under it on the floor 'eating' a biscuit. From the time he should have had rusks, he was given them but showed no interest at all in them as things to be put in his mouth. However Margaret got hold of some Ovaltine biscuits and he has a portion of one to follow his orange juice.

This last week has been busy. David and family arrived back on Tuesday evening, after a particularly hot time in Lagos. I had a very busy day with two caesarean sections and a forceps delivery. On Thursday evening we had dinner with Elsie, one of the teachers - Miss Saunders was also there - a pleasant evening, but I was very tired having had a very bad week of night duty - every night disturbed.

Yesterday was however a memorable day. Our hospital engineer, Lanyian, has been away nearly a month and we have been waiting for him to return to lay the pipe to the pool. He hasn't come so Andrew and I decided to lay the pipe our selves. So with the aid of three men we have laid a one and a quarter inch pipe, joined it to the mains and have taken it 50 yards, within six feet of the pool. Sheer fatigue caused us to give up at 6pm but we feel to have got most of it done, including the rather tricky bit that goes through the wall of the pool and opens near the floor in the shallow end. I have learned how to put a thread on the end of the pipe and jolly hard work it is too!

Trust all is well with you - if Michael cares to take up plumbing I shall be happy to undertake a postal course! Love from us all, David

From Dr. Henry Wyatt (the Henry mentioned in the letters.)
Base West, Antarctica, 25.2.57

Dear Auntie and Uncle,

I do feel a long was away in time and distance, from when I left in the taxi all loaded and you waved me away from the door. Thank you Auntie for your letter in Montevideo. I have made up my mind - yes but the emotional problems are still by no means solved. The saddest thing of all was saying goodbye to Mary at Liverpool. However I have had a letter from her and she sounds to be enjoying her job very much.

We are on a small island here very close to those I showed you on the map, at the mouth of a fjord just south of Darbel Bay. To the east about five miles away rise the mainland coastal range, to the west the mountains of Rouse Island, and to the South the fjord, again ringed round by mountains, and snow and ice and sea - no green at all, just blues and whites and blacks and greys. But it is very, very beautiful and most especially at sunset. Being so low in declination the sun takes ages to set, and so the colours change and change and are reflected from the snow and clouds most beautifully.

The island itself is quite small with a high rocky crest at the far end and mostly covered in snow and ice. There is quite good skiing, and there is a little climbing and some excellent bathing spots only one tends to stay in only a very short time!

We have about 35 dogs and dozens of puppies. They all stay out in all weathers. But when it is blowing really hard I can quite see that it won't be any more nuisance than was looking after Stanley's silk worms!

I have some stamps on a letter franked in the Antarctica, which I have sent to Stanley. They should be quite unique, for each of these bases is a Post Office and there aren't many visitors!

The research programme is well under way and I have as far as I can see forgotten nothing in the way of equipment, which is a very good thing and rather surprises me. I have sent several films home to Mother and Dad and I hope they will send them on for you to see.

It is a great pleasure to be rid of the boat at last, although the trip was very interesting - Montevideo, the Royal tour, several weeks in Stanley including a flight out in the ambulance plane to see a patient, and then a complete tour of all the bases except three. Certainly the days come and go very quickly and each one past is a day nearer home - not that I don't enjoy this life - I am very happy here. But the thought of coming home is very pleasant too.

The work this year will involve climbing as many mountains as possible to build summit cairns for the triangulation survey and there will be a great deal of dog sledging to be done later in the year.

It is a wonderful, clean open air life and I am amazed how pleasant it is to be away from the hurry and bustle of town life, where everything is set by the clock. We work here by the weather and by the daylight and don't have to worry about catching buses and trains. This will be the last letter until the end of the year - the ship leaves today. Please give my love and best wishes to all at Rivercourt, and to David and Margaret and Peter. I wanted to write to them but haven't managed it. I hope all is going well with you. I wonder if you have found a place to retire to yet? I think about you so often, and think how grand it will be to come home again.

With all my love, Henry

3.3.57

Another Sunday afternoon - I am duty and have just had to go up to see a patient, so am simmering gently. However today is a great day - we have started filling the pool. During the week we have had sessions on it - first laying the pipe, then making the rail round the top and finally fitting it in. It took a whole day to chisel out enough concrete to let it in, and a second day to fill up all the holes

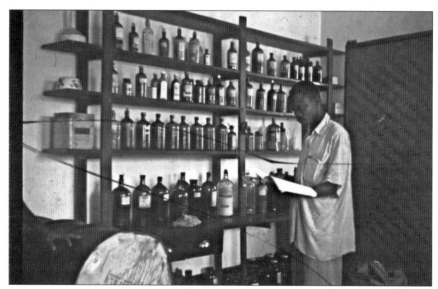

Dispensary

again - yet another day to get the wire netting up and then today all had dried out. After I got back from chapel this morning I found them all waiting for me to turn on the tap - the official opening!

We were very glad to receive your letter with Michael's musical introduction - much appreciated by us, and all the compound in fact! We were very thrilled to think that Father was amongst three nominated for Chairman, we send our love and congratulations to him.

We have again had a full week, my spare moments have been put to the pool and Margaret has been busy with Peter's new menus and with the hospital dispensary!

Peter has gained again this month - he was weighed on Friday - now 16lbs 4oz and he is really very well indeed. We are very thrilled with his attempts to crawl - he can get his knees up under his tummy but as yet has not really connected this movement with his hands, so despite vigorous agitation of his legs he only moves a few inches! However it is obvious that it won't be long before he is well under way. We have got out a playpen that the Wrights left behind - it has been scrubbed and I hope to get some more screws into it in the next day or two, for Peter will very soon need it. He is not really safe in his pram now, he heaves himself up and looks over. He has just graduated onto two courses - potato and gravy followed by custard.

On Tuesday evening we went to the Pearson's for dinner and have a very nice evening. Mr. Mellanby was up last weekend for a short visit - by now he will be home I think. He looks unwell and much older than I remember him before.

Last night we had Elsie Ludlow and Rev Esan in to dinner - quite a successful evening Elsie was a little late because one of the European teachers at WTC is ill and is staying in Elsie's house for a short while until she gets a bit better. Nigerians don't stay long - about 20 minutes after the meal is over, so we had a reasonably early night.

Two further items this week - we have had a tractor in the compound to plough up an acre of ground, which is going to be the hospital farm and farmed by the lad Ismael Awe who we sent to the Rural Training Centre. It has a special plough for use in the virgin earth.

The second item is that a large family of 'weaver birds' have settled in the tree outside our house. The noise they make is appaling and the speed with which they build their nests is amazing. There must be 30 nests in what is quite a small tree. Both Margaret and I are very well (PS 30 eggs this week) and Peter flourishes. Much love from us all, David

10.3.57

Sunday evening this time - another hot day but am glad to say we are all well - Peter especially so. We were very glad to have your letter on Friday and to know that you are all well.

We have had a busy sort of week - I have been on afternoon call and second night call last week and go into first night call this week, so can anticipate some broken nights. There is a great deal of sickness about just now and we are very busy indeed on the wards. Andrew was up at Ikole on Wednesday and Thursday and then up to Afon on Friday with his family, getting back a short while ago. Andrew seems rather cast down about the work up there. The dispensary (started by Joyce Ludlow) is outside the village and although the fees are kept minimal there is very little response indeed - and we wonder if it is really worth us keeping it open. The week has been enlightened by the swimming pool. Monday evening it was first used - absolutely wonderful - cool and refreshing and excellent exercise. As David M says it is the only way that you can get adequate exercise in this country and climate.

Three nurses have been in so far. Costumes were a problem, so Margaret and Jean helped one of the nurses make one up - a simple design and so they have started. The vast majority have never seen a swimming pool before and have never been in the sea so it is quite a new experience and they seem to manage very well. The shallow end is a good four feet deep and the deep end a good six feet, excellent fun. Could you obtain 'Teach yourself Swimming 'if there is such a book in the series, and send it out please because whilst there is the opportunity I should like to learn to swim well and to be able to teach others.

Stanley Hull has been staying with us for a few days - he was bursar at Igbobi College at Yaba, and seconded for a tour of all our West African Districts advising circuits on book keeping etc. He married a teacher and they have a baby daughter - both now in England. Stan is due to leave next month.

This afternoon Margaret, Peter, Stan and I went out to the new leprosy village site for a picnic tea - it is getting on quite well half a dozen buildings going up - it should be finished in two months at the outside.

Last evening we had Marion in for an evening meal, with Stan, got settled down to Scrabble when I had a maternity case to cope with - only getting back for the Ovaltine at the end of the evening.

We are rather worried about staffing still. Andrew has again said that he won't go until a relief comes. He is due to go in July and if he doesn't, it will throw all our furloughs out. David M is due in September - he can go if Andrew is here but we shall still have to look after Imesi! We pray most sincerely that another doctor or two may come forward. When one thinks of all the Methodist doctors qualifying it is a bit frustrating.   Love to all from us all,   David

16.3.57

It is Saturday evening and somehow I don't seem to have very much to do at the moment so I am improving the hour by writing the Sunday Letter. It is a cool evening and we have had the second heavy storm running in the evening, so that all the grass is green again! The compound wives have become acutely garden conscious!

We were very glad to receive your letter yesterday and to learn that all is well at home. Your holiday certainly seems to be falling into place and the advantages of staying in the same spot as Michael with his linguistic abilities at your disposal are great! Stanley will be thrilled to bits I expect - and no doubt when we are home next year we shall hear Stanley say 'when I was in Germany'.

The week here has slipped by reasonably quickly despite some bad nights - last night I only had four and a half hours sleep - though I made some up this afternoon!

Last Tuesday evening I took part in a Brains Trust organised by the hospital's Student Christian Movement branch. A certain amount of disagreement showed itself on the Panel, on certain fundamental issues - but the chairman, Stanley Hall, stepped in gently over it.

During this week Stan has been doing the Methodist School accounts of this circuit and then gave two days to our accounts. He found my error of seven shillings (in a turnover of £40,000) in about 20 minutes and then we spent time in re-organising the system so that it can be 'Nigerianised' and yet have certain controls and security measures incorporated. We have thought through certain plans, but they will take a while to get under way - really we need an accounts office building!

Wednesday evening was our Hospital Staff Committee of which I am secretary, which meant minutes to write up and various letters to get off, in addition to the weeks accounts which I completed this afternoon. I have typed out the trial balance, which shows in comparison with our budget we are greatly overspent on drugs so shall have to economise over this item in the second half year.

Last evening (Friday) after the Groups (which met together and Stan talked on Lent) we went into the Pearson's and played Scrabble - I sat out as I had to do a round and see some patients, but Margaret won both games easily. We had just gone to bed when a woman came who has a severe deformity - she has had two previous caesarean, one by Joyce Ludlow and one by me, so I had to spend two hours doing her third caesarean. At her request and her husbands, I have made it impossible for her to have any more children.

Our poultry farm is up and down and one hen is rather sick and being nursed in the kitchen - it is a very wet night- but on the other hand we have a hen sitting on ten eggs so we hope to maintain our full compliment.

Peter is very well and now sits up by himself. He is a little wobbly, so when he sits up in his playpen Margaret puts cushions round him to flop into. In his cot he can change from lying on his tummy to sitting up all in one movement and he is so pleased with himself!

Margaret is giving him milk in a beaker with two handles. He reaches out and grabs it and pulls it to his mouth - unfortunately not to drink but to blow and a fine spray of milk shooting it all around. He breaks off to chuckle and then does it again. The phrase 'it's probably just a 'phase' seems to be on our lips daily now - but Peter really is a joy to us both - we wish so much you could see him. We are all very well - plenty to do and so many interesting things around. Our love to you all, David

24.3.57

This letter brings you all our love and our best wishes for your Birthday and we hope you had a good day and have managed to go somewhere or do something special. We are all well here and hope that you are all also.

At the moment it is raining and Peter in his playpen keeps gazing out at it - he has seen very little of it since he began noticing things. Peter is keeping very well, and is a very happy little chap. Two more teeth have appeared, making six altogether and they don't seem to have caused him any trouble. He sits up beautifully in his pram and screws himself round to see where he is going. We have to have his harness on because he kneels up and looks over the side, sometimes at alarming angles and a restraining influence is very definitely needed. Weaning has proceeded steadily - he now only has his 7am feed from Margaret and that is to be stopped within the next few days, when he is nine months old. Margaret has done exceptionally well to feed him so well whilst we have been here with the heat and so forth. Peter is beginning to appreciate a little fried bread and scrambled egg and toast and syrup. Today at lunch time he had gravy, mashed potatoes, cabbage, then custard, which he fair tucks away. At 10 he had cereal and egg followed by a drink of milk, which he now drinks if it is diluted a little with water and more sugar added!

Once or twice this week he has been in the paddling pool. Jean has passed on a pair of swimming trunks for him - bright blue and Margaret holds him in the paddling pool, which he quite enjoys! In the evening about 5.30 he comes in his pram to the big pool and watches the swimming there, from a safe distance and smiles away when we wave at him.

The large pool is a great delight, though we have emptied it today - a lot of algae has grown and it will take quite a lot of cleaning up. However yesterday I found that copper sulphate - one part per million will prevent the growth of algae. Re chlorination - the water we use is from the town supply, which is already chlorinated, but I have no doubt that standing in the sun the chlorine soon comes off.

Our most interesting item of news was contained in a letter from Dr. Bolton - and it seems quite likely that Uncle Fred Craddock will be coming out as a locum for Andrews leave, starting in May! and that a Murray Cox may be coming in September to act as a locum for David Morley and that our permanent member of staff may be Ceylonese with an English wife. Not often that one's uncle in law comes out to Africa!

The Pearsons' have some friends in Lagos, the Porterfields- who are going home for good and had a small first size tricycle they didn't want. All the other families here are well stocked so it has been given to us. We have got it stored away for when Peter is ready.

The pedals are on the front wheel. Margaret has been busy making some petite rompers for Peter out of the material bought in London. He looks very smart and as he has enough hair to brush he looks quite a little boy. I hope to get some more photos taken soon.

We are all very fit. Love from us all to you all, David

31/3/57

This letter will reach you on April 5th or just after and so we send you both our love and greetings on your wedding anniversary and we hope that you have had a good run up to Boston and back and enjoyed the family gathering. We look forward to hearing all about it in due course. I wrote a note to Rex and Dorothy which should have arrived in time. Very distressed to hear of Dorothy's op. but expect that treatment has been started in good time.

We have had another busy week - but without any outstanding events - except last night, when we and the Pearsons' went out to dinner with Archdeacon Jadesimi - the Anglican minister here, Mrs. Jadesimi was there, and the Anglican vice - principal of the Oyo teacher training college - so we were quite a party.

We are all keeping well - Peter is fit and lively and at the moment rather anxious for his dinner! which he has at 12.30 - before we have ours. Coffee this morning was at the Morleys and Peter nibbled away and ate ¾ of a plain biscuit!!

It was Andrew Morleys birthday, so Peter took a present and got a ball in return, which were given to all the children. It will be put away until he is a little older.

We are a bit disappointed with our poultry at the moment. However Jean had an English hen go broody three days ago so we have popped eight eggs

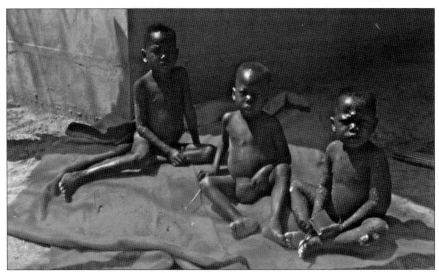

Children with smallpox

under her and time will tell. I can fully recommend keeping poultry as an interesting sideline!

I understand that the fact that during the past two or three months there has been a smallpox epidemic in Nigeria has reached the English press! This has been so but it is now on the wane. Lagos and Ibadan have been the most severely affected with thousands of cases and several hundred deaths. When we first heard of it in January we began a vaccination campaign in Ilesha and district, vaccinating altogether nearly 90,000 people about 50 per cent of the population of Ijesha Division. By this action we have prevented a major outbreak here and have only had about a dozen cases and two deaths, though in one of the villages about 20 miles away, they had quite a severe outbreak. However it is over now and there should be no further trouble. If the local health authorities vaccinated as they should - these outbreaks, which occur every 5-7 years would not occur.

It is now two hours since I wrote the last word above, since when we have had

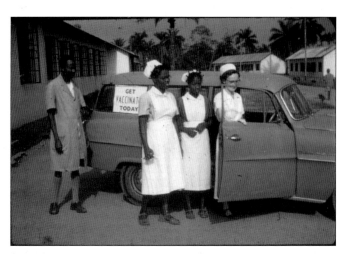

Vaccination Car

lunch and a really heavy storm that has cooled the air marvellously, and a post prandial nap! and it is now 3.15. Heard on the news last night that Cambridge won the boat race but that the London won the Hospital Cup.

The next week or two are going to be busy, and filled with statistics for the Government and returns of one sort or another for the under eighteen grant.

Trust all is well and Michael's singing and so forth on top form and Stanley pressing on at Kingswood School. Love from us all, David

14/4/57

It is Sunday evening, after a very hot and sticky day. The rain which we had expected, which would have cooled the air hasn't come so we are all rather damp. Peter has just had his bath and gone to bed, and will have dropped straight off to sleep. Margaret is looking at the garden and planning the next weeks activity as the light begins to go. It rained yesterday so there is no watering to do, which is most fortunate.

We were very glad indeed to receive your letter and to learn what a good day you had at Boston. I am glad that it was such a happy occasion, although sorry to hear that Auntie Sarah does not look very well, and still no word about Uncle Edward's operation. By the way - how is Ken Parker - any news?

Glad Stanley is well and trust that Lady Anne is well - no doubt the garden shed will once again come into its own as a rabbitorium.

Thank you very much for the book on swimming and the article on chlorination, which you have sent off. The pool is really marvellous This last time I added 8oz of alum, 5oz copper sulphate and 12oz bleaching powder. Certainly the water is clearer and it did not taste very much!

The week has been a busy one and even though I was not on either afternoon or night call I don't seem to have got much done and there are all kinds of returns waiting to be filled up and so forth.

On Monday the Manns and Jonah stayed the night en route for a board meeting at Ifaki. We entertained the Jonahs and we had a committee in the evening to decide what was to be done about a relief for Louie. We are very short here and so we are going to advertise for a sister (we hope with Mission House approval) and get her out here at our expense to act a relief for Louie at the end of this year. Don't mention this to the Mission House! Regarding doctors it looks as though Uncle Fred will be alone from October until February - it will be incredibly hard work for me, unless the other locum - Murray Cox can come out. Apparently the Ceylonese doctor is coming to us, his wife comes from a broken home and has no church connections at all. They are going to Selly Oak for a term starting in September and coming here in January.

On Thursday it was our turn to have the medical meeting of the four hospitals - we had not got an outside speaker, so Andrew, David and I spoke. It went very well and then we had dinner - we entertained Dr. Lamp from Ife and a lady Dr. Gilliband from Ogbomosho

We all had coffee in the Morley house and a pleasant evening. The visitors then had to set off for their homes. Just as they were getting into their cars, Margaret came over and whispered to me that Dr. Gilliband was locked in the lavatory and could not get out! A frantic five minutes wrestling with a refractory lock before it finally yielded. I doubt whether either she or us will forget the visit.

Yesterday we went to John Ambrose's for tea- he flies home on Easter Monday and in the evening we all went for buffet supper at Elsie's. We are all very well here and hope you have a very happy Easter. Peter thrives and can stand when he holds on to a chair. Love from us all, David

Easter Sunday

We are in the midst of a rather busy Easter weekend and I am seizing the moment whilst our guests prepare for the evening service to pen this note. We were very pleased to receive your letter earlier this week - on Wednesday and to hear that you had received one from Henry. We look forward to seeing it - any comments on his affairs of the heart? Glad to hear that the finances are in good state at Rivercourt - certainly the effort of reducing the loan on the house has been most successful - and as you say to repay £50 per annum for the principal is a different proposition to pay £60 interest!

Glad to hear about the music cabinet - it would seem though, that a disciplined clearing is also necessary.

The week here has been a busy one. David has been to Wesley College Ibadan for three days which meant quite a lot for Andrew and me. However since he returned on Thursday evening he hasn't been well. He spent Friday in bed and today he has been to bed for part of the time. However both Friday and Monday are Bank Holidays so we haven't any outpatients, which has made it easier.

Friday was quite a busy day though - with the Days arriving at mid-day. They are all well and their boy Christopher has grown into a fine lad and is very well. Charles has kept much better this tour and they seem well settled down.   The Theological department has obtained a vehicle which Charles can use so they do not feel so tied. They have invited us down for a few days so when it is time for our local leave we shall split it between Lagos, Ibadan and Ikole.

Friday evening Charles took the service in the Hospital Chapel -a very good thought provoking sermon - but a little above the heads of the nurses.

Saturday was another busy day - I had a major operation in the morning and then the Hospital accounts to settle for the week. We all had a swim in the evening. The pool is a real boon.

Today we had a Communion Service led by Charles at 6.15am. I forgot to mention that our guests – Mr. and Mrs. Garling, Ann aged sixteen and Lois seven, arrived on Saturday night. He is the administrative Secretary at West African Council for Medical Research. They are members of Kingsway Central Hall, London. Donald Soper is their minister, have a house in Dalling Road and know Rivercourt very well indeed.

I went down to morning service led by the Rev. Esan, taking the nurses, Elsie and Margaret Day. This afternoon I took a service in the female ward and this evening I am on duty. Margaret has gone down to Otapete where Charles is preaching. When they return we are going to have hymn singing at the Pearsons'. Peter and Margaret and I are all very well. Peter can now stand up when he holds on to the top of the playpen. He has won the hearts of the visitors and is really enjoying a spot of company. Do hope you have all had a happy Easter -

did you venture out for a run? I suppose with petrol coming down in price a bit, more folk would be out!

Much love from us all, to you all, David

28.4.57

We have had two letters this week - three really, and it has been nice to receive them and hear how you are progressing. We were most interested to hear of your variation of tennis with its additional hazards. The pool is still a source of great enjoyment yesterday we were diving for pennies - result two pence still somewhere on the bottom of the pool.

Sorry to hear Kingswood got knocked in the seven aside and Oxford in the boat race. Interested to hear of the Rivercourt party going to the continent and Ken - who incidentally is Sylvia? Sorry to hear about Uncle Edward's operation. It does seem very odd.

We are looking forward to seeing the pictures of the dog - perhaps by the time we are home it will be in the centre of the dining room! over the mantle piece.

We have had a busy week but we are all well and fit and well able to cope.

On Easter Monday we decided that we ought to go out somewhere so we all climbed a hill opposite the hospital about a mile away. It was quite an easy climb but as I carried Peter I was a trifle warm by the time we got to the top. The women and children went back and the men and Elsie explored further getting back rather late for lunch. There really is very little fun in walking here, which is a great pity.

Our guests went back to Lagos on Tuesday morning having had a good weekend I think. The Days returned on Monday afternoon and gave Christopher, their son a Quell because he is car sick. It obviously did not suit him and Charles rang up at midnight and asked what they should do. We haven't heard any more so presume he is well again but a most unfortunate ending to their break.

The rest of the week has been busy - Unfortunately David Morley has not been very well. We think that he has got Filaria, which is one of the banes of the life out here. We had thought that one only got this trouble after one had been here about five years.

The rains seem established now and the new batches of seeds are up and Margaret busy planting them out in the evenings. Cabbage seemed to get a fungus - most of them died- otherwise all the other usual vegetables are doing well. Incidentally this is the first week since Christmas we haven't any tomatoes in the garden.

Two baby chicks hatched out over Easter but one of our layers has died. The ups and downs seem unending.

Peter is thriving - he now has a small fresh egg for breakfast each morning and a bowl of his porridge and then toast - it all gets tucked away and he loves his custard for lunch.

He stands up frequently in his cot and playpen but unfortunately still cannot sit down so a wail of distress echoes round till he is sat again.

We have not heard yet when Uncle Fred is coming out but we have tentatively fixed our local leave in Lagos (the shops) Ibadan (with the Days to see the University and UCH) and then the rest with Louise at Ikole to have a rest.

We are all well and flourishing and send you all our love, David, Margaret and Peter.

May 3rd 1957

Dear Michael,

Just a line knocked off in haste as the postman is waiting to collect the letters, to wish you a very happy birthday on the 8th. Hope that you have a good day and do something a little out of the ordinary to celebrate!

We were very glad to receive the letter from home on Wednesday and to read of Lady Anne's somewhat surprising but fortunately safe accouchement - the diagnosis of the vets in Bath wasn't so far out!

We are keeping fairly well, rather Peter and Margaret are well but the three doctors are suffering from overwork and we have all been a little unwell, touches of fever and a few aches and pains. Andrew has been in bed for a day, now up, David has had sinus trouble and a touch of fever and I have had one early night. However we are all recovering but the thought of all the outpatients to be seen, is where I should be at the moment!

Thank you for the chlorination blurb. A trifle complicated for yours truly and even more so for our technicians, who are entirely out of their depths. Your earlier suggestion about tasting the water is much more to the point. Incidentally we have a little pool trouble at the moment as the outflow seems to be blocked.

I have a problem to set you - the production of a nomogram if I have got it right. I will send the details on Sunday. I have posted off the second report of the scheme here by sea mail -trust you find something of interest, would draw your attention to the last page.

Once again a Happy Birthday, Love David

May 5th 1957

Another Sunday is here - it is almost lunch time but I thought I would get this letter started. Have had to break off though to see to our fridge that has not been cold for about a week. William has 'tried' but I had a full investigation of same and it looks as though the last batch of kerosene wasn't very good and also the wick seems pretty well clogged - so have put in fresh kerosene, from another source and a fresh wick and hope for the best. Jean has been a little distant about the fridge not functioning but trust she will thaw as the fridge freezes! It was our coffee this morning and also my turn to go to church so one way and another it has been rather full. This afternoon I am on duty but not on nights, which is rather nice. I have managed during the last week to catch up with accounts, returns and so forth so at the moment am fairly straight.

There has just been a gap of nearly twelve hours. As I was writing a nurse came to tell me that a patient in maternity was in trouble so I had to do a caesarean, rather a difficult one and then there were a number of other new patients - then a visit from Dr. Salisbury from Ado Ekiti, tea, washing up (Williams half day) and the evening service followed by coffee at the Morleys and now down to letters again.

We were very glad indeed to receive your letter on Wednesday- a very swift one - and hear of your Easter outings, most interesting that Mr. Miller was with you - how did you like him? Your recounting of the viewing of the house with a boathouse was most amusing and we could just picture you all trooping down the garden. A boathouse on a Thames backwater would be rather nice! On Bank Holidays instead of getting stuck in traffic jams - could take a picnic up the Thames in our motor launch! Peter I am sure would have appreciated it. He has learnt to crawl and today when we were having tea he was out through the french windows on to the verandah and about to explore one of Margaret's large plant pots! He can now sit down again when he has pulled himself into the standing position which is quite a relief - it gets a bit tedious having to sit him down every time he stood up. He is very well and his legs seem to get stronger each day

The week past has been a busy one - we went out to dinner last night with Jean Saunders at WTC - quite a nice evening but the meal was a bit late, starting at 9.15 or so, so we were rather late home.

We have heard Uncle Fred's sailing date about May 28th on a cargo boat the 'Sansu' from Liverpool, so he should be in Lagos about the 18th of June. If this is so we may be able to arrange our local leave to meet him and bring him up which would be most convenient. However we shall have to wait and see. The Pearsons' have had their sailing date confirmed - July 16th it will very soon be here. Elsie is having her presentation of MBE at Government House Ibadan on Friday this week. She is allowed to take two friends so is taking Louie Trott and Enid Blake - if we can persuade them that we can manage the hospital for a few hours.

The two chicks are still with us and the garden is beginning to be something like one under Margaret's skilled hand. We are all well and flourishing though look with some trepidation to the months Andrew is away.

Hope all is well with you all. Love from Margaret, Peter and David

26.5.57

It is almost lunchtime and time Peter had his dinner. Margaret is busy with the Mouli Baby and Peter is making his presence known. Not actually crying but banging his rattle and jiggling his playpen and shouting - rather disturbingly for

Daddy who is trying to write this letter - but perfectly understandable. Peter is very well indeed - as are we all, and his diet has been enriched by the addition of a minute piece of bacon with his egg in the morning. Very soon we shall have to get out his spoon and pusher as he is showing signs of wanting to feed himself.

We were very thrilled to read of Michael's debut on the Royal Albert Hall organ and it must have been quite an experience, to put it mildly. Glad all went well. I may say that your stock is very high in the compound here, we are all most impressed.

We were very pleased indeed to receive the book on swimming for which we are most grateful. Unfortunately since it arrived we have had rain each evening and even though it is still quite warm a bit odd to swim in the rain. I have been in twice and though it sounds so simple and straight forward in the book it is far from easy in practice and I have swallowed more of the pool on these last two visits than ever before.

Glad to hear that Father's shoulder is improving and congratulations Mother on the Women's Fellowship District Presidency.

This last week has been an easier week for me with no afternoon or night calls, but this coming week, starting this afternoon I am on afternoons and second night call. In addition Andrew is off to Ibadan tomorrow for the Medical Advisory Board, so he will be away all day. It is likely to be very heavy indeed.

Last night we had Enid and Eileen in to chop, Enid was on duty and had to go but the three of us played Scrabble. I started and my first turn put out all seven letters - rather depressing that for the other two!

Yesterday morning Dr. Collis (he is Professor of Paediatrics in Dublin) and Prof. of Beirut in Lebanon came up to see Imesi etc. They stayed overnight with David and then we all did a ward round of the children's ward this morning. It is most refreshing to have such visitors who can give us ideas and assistance.

Peter has now had his dinner - three roast potatoes, peas, fish, followed by custard and lemon whip - but he seems just as noisy! Perhaps he has indigestion! He is due to be put down for his afternoon rest so he should sleep after such a meal.

We have had to move our chicken runs. They were put up before the Morleys house and are a bit of an eyesore to them so we have moved them behind the garden. It is quite a job - wire netting is frightful stuff when it has been used once. Still it is now chicken proof but needs finishing off. This week we have had a large turkey given to us - one of my 'private' patients, a lawyers wife who I have delivered twice, a most welcome gift, it is going to be used for a joint Birthday party on Whit Monday for Margaret 8th, and Jean and David Morley 15th.

Hope all well with you all - what about an advert in the Methodist Recorder for a house - using a box number? Love to you all from us all, David

2.6.57

Another Sunday afternoon- after a week that has been much cooler and much wetter so our gardens are really feeling that the wet season has set in. The compound people here said that Peter resembled me - but the Days when they were here said how like Margaret he is. His eyes are deep blue.

What a struggle for Stanley's passport! Once it is obtained we must keep it renewed so that we don't have to go through the same palaver again. Incidentally I have just got mine renewed - I got it just over five years ago. Bill Mann copes with it in Lagos for us.

The house hunting does seem to be a bit of a problem to put it mildly! I don't know if you could make yourself into a limited company and Michael and I buy shares! Money invested at 2½ or 3 per cent is barely keeping its value at all in view of inflation and it might be worth investing it in real estate. An extra £1000 to put down might make all the difference.

The week here has been a bit hectic - Andrew and family went up to Ikole on Wednesday back on Thursday. In addition Andrew went down to Advisory Board in Ibadan on Monday and so was away for half the week. The week ahead too is a bit hectic with Andrew having a case in Ibadan High Court again tomorrow. On Wednesday is our Hospital Management Committee and we are expecting Mr. and Mrs. Jones and Mr. and Mrs. Mann to stay the night. The committee should go without much trouble though one can never tell!

The week has been complicated by an attack of dengue fever in yours truly. Just after I finished the letter last Sunday my temperature went up and remained up more or less for three days since when it has come down. Monday I felt very groggy and Tuesday I stayed in bed and Wednesday was back at work again. Today I have a little fever again - tomorrow I should have the rash and then I shall be quite better again. Margaret and Peter are very well - at the moment Peter is vociferous waiting to come out of his playpen. He loves to be out in the room crawling across the floor, looking out through the French windows, pulling out the books, and newspapers from the shelves. His latest achievement is to wave 'bye bye' - with both actions and words - which is most engaging.

Uncle Fred should now be on his way - we hope to have a letter early this week giving us the approximate time of his arrival, if he wrote from the boat as most folk do. I fear Auntie Florence will feel quite lost won't she?

The number of outpatients here is as heavy as ever, especially with a very severe measles epidemic. The children become very ill indeed because it is a Yoruba belief that when they have the rash they should not be given anything to drink. Still I think the worst is over. Incidentally we had two new cases of smallpox this week so the outbreak is grumbling on.

The new laboratory is almost finished. The benches are in, the wiring almost complete and the plumbing under way. It will be a really fine room when it is completed - one of the best in the hospital.

We heard this week that we are getting another Sister in September who has been doing leprosy work in Eastern Nigeria which will be a great relief for our Sisters though someone has to relieve Louie at Ikole - a problem yet unsolved.

Do hope all at home are well - despite mild fever in me, we are all flourishing! Love from us all, David

9.6.57

Another Sunday is here - with a slight difference! I am writing this in bed! Last week I gave a firm diagnosis of Dengue to my fever, however it has turned out to be infective hepatitis so I am now a bright yellow colour and confined to bed. I fear it has meant a lot of extra work for Andrew and David and it will do for our Local Leave, which is due at the end of this week in fact.

Margaret and Peter are very well and I am improving daily though I have not got much appetite back yet. We were very pleased to receive your letter on Thursday, to learn that Fathers arm is improving and that all was well with you all except for some difficulties in finding a house - you certainly seem to have seen a few already. Why not obtain the most recent copy of Homes and Gardens - if I remember rightly it has many advertisements for houses and there just might be something suitable in it.

This week has been a busy one for everyone except me. Monday was very hectic. Andrew had to go down to Ibadan to the court - when he got there they could not find the accused! Thus he had to come all the way back again! However he managed to pick up cheaply two laboratory sinks which we were needing for the new laboratory. David M and I were busy all day in outpatients but got through most of the work. On Tuesday David M was at Imesi and Andrew and I coped with outpatients - but by Tuesday evening I was not feeling up to much, went to bed and remained there on Wednesday morning. Wednesday afternoon was our Hospital management Committee.

The Manns were in good form and we have arranged to stay with them a few days in Lagos when we go down to meet Uncle Fred. The committee went quite well - I got up to attend, not feeling 100% and fear I may have passed on my hepatitis. By Thursday tea time the jaundice had appeared and the diagnosis made. I only hope that Margaret and Peter don't get it too. Since then the days have slipped by. My appetite is coming back slowly, the nausea fading a little but am still lemon coloured!

Tomorrow is likely to be a very hectic day as Andrew is supposed to go to Ibadan for this same court case. The police have no realisation of the inconvenience they cause. It means that 250 patients or so will not be seen tomorrow, David could not possibly see all that will turn up.

If all is well we plan to go to Ibadan on Friday afternoon, then to Lagos the following Monday to meet Uncle Fred who should arrive during that week. We shall return then the following Friday for a few days until the Wednesday when we are due to go on trek to Ikole which we shall do and stay there for a week or so to have a proper rest. It will be cool and restful there especially compared with Lagos.

The garden is struggling against the odds; the hens are holding their own, 20 eggs this week. The two youngest chicks are growing up. Peter has had a good week - his appetite grows daily and he has grown another lower tooth. Margaret had a very busy Birthday receiving a colour photo of herself and Peter from the Morleys, powder and cake decorations from the Pearsons'. I fear my present has not materialised - I hope it hoves too in Lagos next week. We are all well and cheerful and looking forward to our holiday. Much love from us all, David

17.6.57

Another week has slipped by and I am still in bed, though now on the mend I am glad to say. Actually the time is about 7am. Margaret is getting up - Peter is awake in the next room and William is getting breakfast ready. It is cool, a pleasant sun shining through the window and breakfast should be here soon and for the first time for a week I am looking forward to it.

From my point of view the week has been rather uninteresting from a letter point of view as I have been in bed all the time becoming more deeply jaundiced until Friday when it began to lessen and though still present a little (which means remaining in bed) it is obviously getting less. I have just dozed and read throughout the week.

Peter and Margaret are both very well, Margaret has been doing my back and keeping the temperature chart and both Andrew and David have looked in each day to cheer me up.

We were very glad to get your letter on Thursday and to hear of all your activities, especially Michael's sartorial splash, which as you say should liven up the holiday transparencies. So far this tour I have taken very few colour photos indeed and you have seen all the black and white ones. Glad to hear that Auntie Florence's arm is mending well and Father's shoulder getting better. As a family we seem to be having our ups and downs!

Needless to say we are in suspense over the house between Teddington and Kingston. Like a serial story in a magazine - the installment finishes - Will they buy the house? - see next week - so we are biding ourselves in patience!

On Monday evening this week the party was held - our turkey being the piece de resistance. I had a little turkey - a few ? hard bits, stuffing etc and the following day some turkey soup - but then the jaundice increased and my appetite went so I declined. However it was a nice bird. The Rowlands arrived on Monday and left on Friday having enjoyed their visit. It was very nice to see them and Ray looked in each day for half an hour or so which made a nice change.

David had arranged a weekend for our senior nurses and our dispensary nurses. They met together for a meal on Friday evening and then a service in the chapel followed by films in the Outpatient department.

Then he arranged for the lorry to take them to Ogbomaso Hosp. for a lecture demonstration of leprosy and look around the leprosarium, which I think they all found most interesting. Then they joined nurses there for a mid-day meal and came back in the evening. Eileen went with them and enjoyed it very much.

Our plans for local leave have changed somewhat as Uncle Fred isn't due into Lagos till a week today (24th). My medical advisors state that I should not go to Lagos, but Margaret and Peter will probably go down to meet Uncle Fred, do a bit of shopping and then return. Then when Uncle Fred has settled in we shall go away for a break - probably up to Louie.

Do hope all is well at home and look forward to hearing from you in due course. Love from us all, and a special da da (his only word) from Peter. David

23.6.57

Another Sunday has come round and finds me in the living room - very much better I'm glad to say - and getting around more! The jaundice is going - practically gone now and I am eating well.

Our arrangements have gone a little awry due to phone calls to Lagos as to Uncle Fred's date of arrival! We were told firstly that it was the 24th, then that it was the 21st. We felt someone ought to meet him and Margaret was the most possible so I persuaded her to go on Thursday with Peter. I was much better and with William, well able to cope here. So on Thursday Margaret and Peter went down to meet Uncle Fred on the Friday only to learn that the boat was not now expected until the Sunday and that is today. By this time he should have landed - plus luggage and on his way to the Marina, Lagos. They will have an early lunch and come up if all is well this afternoon. The one snag is that it is Sunday and Bill Mann isn't very hopeful about getting them off early. If they are very delayed they will come up tomorrow. Margaret rang up last night - both she and Peter are very well and I hope enjoying the change. Margaret has done a lot of shopping - a large box of stores has already come up on the lorry to leave the car empty for Uncle Fred's loads.

Your letter arrived on Friday, sorry to hear that you were outbid on the house - am quite sure that something will turn up. You do seem to have had a hectic outing! I should think that outings are something that can be happily left behind in retirement.

The week for me has been a quiet one - much reading and sleeping, a little accountancy, checking of invoices and so forth. I have got through most of the local books, so have had some sent down from the Training College.

Andrew and David have been very busy I fear, but the coming of Uncle Fred should make it a bit easier. If all is well we hope to get up to Louie this week and stay for a week or perhaps a little more, so we shall not receive your letter before we go and our letter will be late in reaching you.

David has had a visitor the last day or two - the editor of the magazine 'Nigeria'. David is hoping that they will do an article on the work at Imesi - fully illustrated - not only for the present publicity but also I think to be able to use the photographs for a book which he hopes to publish when the scheme is through.

The last week has been cool - I imagine cooler than it has been for you, though probably much moister. The hens have gone off laying a little as they do at this time of year - but the garden is doing quite well - ever hopeful we have seven eggs under a broody hen!

I do hope all is well with you all at home you have often been in my thoughts the last few weeks.

Just had a phone call from Margaret - Uncle Fred safely in Lagos, but because it is Sunday no-one to see to his passport so they cannot come up until tomorrow.

Love to you all   David

Ikole, 30.6.57

Here we are at Ikole. It is now Sunday. We travelled up on Wednesday I found the journey a bit tiring, but am very much better, going for longer walks each day. We haven't received your letter for this week because we left before it could arrive so we have it to look forward to when we return.

Monday afternoon I got dressed for the first time and went to the car to greet Uncle Fred and Margaret and Peter who were well - Uncle Fred looked a bit tired and rather older than I remembered - but then shorts tend to accentuate youth or age! He is living in the Pearson's guest room with bathroom and eating with them until they go - two weeks tomorrow and then Sandy, the Pearson's cook will look after him.

Tuesday was a very busy day for Margaret - getting sorted out from Lagos, shopping and preparing for our holiday here. Uncle Fred began to work and was dismayed at the number of outpatients to be seen!

Wednesday morning the car came and we began to load up but found we could not get Peter's cot in so had to unload again and pack the ambulance. Louie hasn't a cot so we had to bring it.

We had a good journey and arrived here at 1.30 - rather earlier than Louie expected us. We had lunch and then retired for an afternoon rest.

Louie has got rather a bad back at the moment - she makes light of it but is obviously in some pain, though says it is improving. She sends her love to you. She is much the same as usual - very sharp! The days have slipped by - Peter has settled down in his new environment and we have been for a walk each day pushing Peter in the 'go chair' that we have borrowed from the Morleys, going a little further each day. The weather has been delightfully cool and last night we had to have two blankets which was a real treat.

Yesterday evening a large car arrived bringing Mr. and Mrs. Simpson - friends of Louie. He was a District Officer in Ado Ekiti ten years ago and they have kept in touch. They are Scottish, have two children at school in Edinburgh, and he is now Assistant Permanent Secretary to the Minister of Aviation and Communication - a very good job - two to three thousand a year I suppose. We brought food up with us - knowing Louie - and they likewise. As you can imagine it is a bit of a squash - but they are returning in the morning. Margaret met them at the Sunday evening singsong at the Jonahs last Sunday and they said they might come. Margaret said that she thought we might be there so they brought camp beds etc. Louie did not believe they would come! We had a pleasant evening chatting, he knows many of the ministers and so forth.

William has come with us - he was very pleased to do so and is in great form! He pushed Peter out the other day and yesterday, having decided that his first Birthday was in sight took him on a little walking practice! Peter can stand well now without support I don't think it will be very long before he begins to walk. If you remember we brought out some 'Kiddiecraft' Bricks and will give them to him tomorrow! I am quite looking forward to them!

Do hope all is well at home, I fear we shall be rather out of touch till we get back to Ilesha perhaps a week tomorrow or Tuesday.

Love from us all and special baby noise from Peter, David

Ikole, 7.7.57

Another Sunday and since last I wrote (I do hope you have received it - it was taken to Lagos for posting) we have had a quiet week and are all feeling the benefit of our holiday. I am quite better and looking forward to getting down to some work again. We have not heard from Ilesha, and haven't had your letters sent on so we do not know how you have all been faring.

The visitors who were here last Sunday went first thing Monday morning, so we have had a quiet week pottering about. On Monday morning we gave Peter his plastic bricks which he is playing with as I write this! He loves them- though not as yet for building. He is cutting two more teeth- upper molars- big ones so he has been a bit fretful and kept his fingers in his mouth more than usual - but he now has ten teeth! Jean gave him a plastic lorry with which he plays too, but I don't think he recognises it as a lorry yet!

Tuesday afternoon Louie decided we would go to the Ado Clinic 36 miles away to get some stores, cement, paint, kerosene etc. for the hospital. The car battery was flat but Louie stated that once we got going it would be all right. With a big push we were off! We had one minor stop in a village and had to have a push but sixteen miles from Ikole it stopped never to go again! Then I was informed that the fan belt was loose! and sure enough it was practically off Fortunately we had Louie's driver with us and he went off to see if he could get it repaired by a shoemaker. Meanwhile it was sweltering so I begged some chairs and put them under a tree for Margaret and Peter, but the usual crowd gathered 20-30 looking at the 'white baby' which is a relative rarity in these villages. Peter didn't seem to mind at all, but it was a bit uncomfortable. Unfortunately there was no luck with the shoemaker so Louie walked to the Mission House of two RC Fathers who lived in this village. They came in their car took us to their house where we had tea and decided to send the driver for a new fan belt to Ilesha. Then the Fathers brought us back in their car!

Incidentally we got some men to push Louie's car into the RC compound and locked it up. Quite a little adventure Peter was very good throughout!

Thursday evening the driver arrived plus car so on Friday afternoon Louie decided we could make a second attempt! I drove and we arrived safely in Ado did some shopping and then went to the Church Missionary Society Hospital for tea and another good journey home.

Emboldened, on Saturday (yesterday) we set off after coffee for Kabba, which is 40 odd miles NE of Ikole in scrub country where occasionally lion are heard and seen. We had a picnic in a rest house with a magnificent view, then had a rest and then went to the WTC where Louie had a friend and she had a large dog - so big that when it was standing Peter could crawl underneath easily. It was the first dog Peter had really been with and he crawled round at speed uttering shrill hunting cries. The dog was very good and could easily have got out of the way but let Peter catch his legs all he could reach but to our distress having got a firm hold on his back leg - tried to bite it. But the dog appeared supremely indifferent. A good journey home completed a very peasant day. The hospital transport is coming to take us home on Tuesday so next week I should be well installed again, with recent news of the hospital. Do hope all are well at home and we are looking forward to catching up with your letters.

Love from us all, David

PS Just arrived Ilesha. Many thanks cards and letter will write on Sunday.

WGH, 14.7.57

It was very nice indeed, on our arrival home last Tuesday to find two letters and two birthday cards for Peter waiting for us. We read through the letters to find out what you had been doing before starting anything else! There was a letter from Thea and one from Mr. Ingham the next day, so we felt once more to be up with the news having been cut off for two weeks.

Already our time at Ikole seems a long time ago - so much has had to be done since we came home, but we have had a very enjoyable and restful time. At the moment the Pearsons' are in the middle of last minute packing - they go down to Lagos tomorrow - sail on Tuesday and both Margaret and I are trying to pick up the threads of being left in charge, with its resultant increase in responsibility! No doubt we shall pull through, but it is a little overwhelming to begin with.

Some time later - Andrew asked me to go up to the office for last minute handover!

House hunting too seems rather a palaver. We are looking forward to hearing about the Tudor/Queen Anne edifice. Would it not be worth seeing the extent of dry rot at the house and getting an estimate? It might be possible to make an economical buy, would the local authority put anything towards the repairs?

Peter is very well and cheerful, fretful only the first day after our return whilst he got used to being at home again. He is really very good indeed. The plastic lorry which Jean gave him for his birthday, he now pushes along, making loud lorry noises as he has seen the other children do.

When the Pearsons' have gone the Morley children will be very quiet indeed and thrown very much on their own resources. William was quite excited yesterday and said that Peter walked in his playpen - but as yet we haven't seen him - but can stand quite firmly.

Wednesday was a busy day here - I had two emergency operations with a long committee in the evening. Thursday was full. I had two emergency operations - two weeks accounts to ledger and the minutes to cope with. Friday too was full with large outpatients in the morning and a clinic in the afternoon, with the nurses groups meeting all together in the evening, to hear Margaret Woodland speak on Papua.

Yesterday, Saturday was the opening of the new Private Block and Laboratory - both excellent buildings, well equipped. The new King of Ilesha performed the

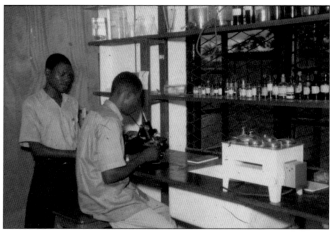

Laboratory

opening and quite a crowd was present. The financial result was not very good - about £30. Last night, Uncle Fred and the Pearsons' came in to chop.

This morning I have been down to Otapete then it was our turn for morning coffee and this evening, after service here all on the compound are coming for coffee to say au revoir to the Pearsons'.

Friday next at 10.30, the Governor is coming to look round (Sir John Rankin) and the following week Erastus Evans is staying with us! And so it goes on. By next Sunday I hope to have got a little more straightened out

We are all very fit - and hope all is well with you all - your holiday is almost upon you! Much love from us all, David

21.7.57

Our passages home are booked on May 25th on the Aureol. This is fortnight later than we are due, because we are expecting a brother or sister for Peter the first week in February. Margaret will be going into the new University College Hospital and will be looked after either by Mr. Lawson or Miss Lister, the two consultant obstetricians there. We very thrilled and glad that Peter will have a playmate! Margaret is keeping well, a little unwell at times but better than last time. The Morleys are expecting a baby too, about a fortnight before ours, so they will be very much of an age.

We were very pleased to receive your letter and to learn all was well at home - It will be a real thrill for Stanley to come home a few days early from school - something that we never did. We do hope you have an enjoyable holiday - we shall look forward to hearing about it on your return - though glad to receive letters from the continent.

We hear from Uncle Fred that Auntie Florence called at Rivercourt one day and that she was going to have tea with you. At the moment Uncle Fred is going to fly home sometime after January 17th when the Pearsons' arrive, but Auntie Florence doesn't like the idea of him coming home suddenly from heat to mid-winter and is threatening to come out and fly with him if he does!

It has been a most eventful week. The Pearsons' went on Monday and left us all feeling a bit flat and depressed, with a lot to be done in preparation for the Governor. Tuesday was busy and Wednesday too. In the evening Margaret and I were invited by Sir John Rankin to a cocktail party in the house at which he was staying - a very pleasant hour with about eight Europeans and 20 Nigerians.

Thursday was the Coronation day of the King of Ilesha. Enid and I did Uncle Fred's work and made it possible for him to attend the ceremony, which was most impressive. In the evening the Owa gave a party and David M and Eileen Searle went down.

Friday was our big day. The Governor arrived at 10.40, met by yours truly who introduced the staff - and then showed him round for an hour, after which invited him for coffee which Margaret and Aileen had arranged. Sir John was most interested in all that he saw and thought that a good job was being done! On the Wednesday he had thanked M and me for looking after Lady Rankin two years ago. Apparently she is in England now and Sir John is going on leave in a week or two. A very pleasant visit but we are glad it is over.

Next Wednesday the Parliamentary Secretary to the Western Minister of Health is coming but it won't nearly be the same sort of do. Wednesday evening was Fellowship, led by Uncle Fred, and Friday evening - nurses classes.

Last night we had chop with the Morleys and then afterwards I had a tracheotomy to do in a small child - successfully I am glad to say!

Our new boiler arrived on Thursday and it weighs 22cwt, so you can imagine that it is proving a bit difficult to set up.

Martin Evans arrives tomorrow for five nights - apparently he is not very well, so we shall have to see how he is. If he is fairly fit we are having dinner parties to get folk in to meet him. It is going to be a very busy week for M. I fear. Our private ward is in use - with two European patients in!

No shortage of news this week. Have a lovely holiday and wish we were with you. Love from us all, David

4.8.57

We were very glad indeed to receive your letter on Friday this week and to hear all your news, especially the preparations for your holiday. By the time this reaches you, you will be well established in Germany and I hope you enjoy your stay in good weather.

We have had a busy week - though mainly with catching up on things not done whilst Mr. Evans was with us. I have not officially been on duty but I have had a number of emergency operations, which I have actually done, or assisted Uncle Fred. Last night I did not get to bed till 2.45am due to operations and had another one at 8.30 this morning. Fortunately David M. took and fetched the nurses so I have had an easier time the latter half of the morning and at the moment am sitting in the house after coffee with Peter in the playpen and Margaret getting Peter's lunch.

Peter is still not walking - though one feels that he could if he wished - but he is saying a few words - he said 'Peter' at breakfast so clearly that anyone could understand it!

Wednesday was pay day - and fortunately it went quite well though I ran out of money. I got over £1000 ready but Elsie asked for £665 for the nurses so I had to leave five till next day! The accounts really are quite a burden.

Last night we had a second showing of 'Nigeria greets the Queen' for the Europeans and serving officers of the town. A year old GB newsreel was shown first and then the Queen film. Margaret and Aileen and Elsie provided coffee and altogether it was a very happy evening, greatly enjoyed by the guests who seemed most appreciative.

Tuesday night Uncle Fred gave a housewarming party - a very nice meal and everyone seemed in good form.

The boiler has taken up quite a lot of my time, but yesterday we got it working and the automatic water feed functioning - but only if the pressure was up around 25 psi - still it worked which is a great thing.

In addition I have had a patient in the Private Ward who needed a Haemorrhoidectomy which I did yesterday morning, all taking time which is most precious.

We had a letter from Andrew yesterday after he arrived in Chasetown. They had a poor journey home Alison having acute otitis media and hardly eating anything and all the children having colds and being fretful. However they got home in good order, Auntie Florence met them and thought they looked not very well.

Andrew's father has obtained a car for them - a Singer 9 for £75. We are wondering - if it serves them well, whether to put in a word for it. It would be very useful for travelling. Also we are wondering about a holiday - whether we should be able to manage it then with children 4/12 and 23 months? We must be thinking about it soon - should be glad of your reaction.

Do hope all is well with you all and looking forward to hearing from you in due course. Love from us all, David

11.8.57

We were thrilled to receive your letter at the end of the week - four very full pages - full of interest- it seems to have been a marvellous place to stay. I hope that the letter I sent to you there arrived - I only sent one and the next, plus Stanley's letter we sent to London, not wanting them to arrive after you had left.

Can just imagine the language palavers. No doubt you are taking some colour photos and we look forward to a session of them when we get home.

At the moment Peter is crawling at speed all over the floor and I am keeping an eye on him. He has just climbed unaided into one of the easy chairs, sat back and held a piece of paper as if he were reading it! Peter is very well though he has had a bit of a cold. Margaret has got a very bad cold indeed, unfortunately, but it should be on the mend quite soon.

We have had rather a hectic week as I had to go down to Lagos for a Standing Committee of Synod. It is concerned with the medical policy of the District and I was asked to go down to it.

I left on Thursday afternoon, taking Eileen to Wesley College, Ibadan because she wanted to have a tooth out, saw the Days, and then went down to the Marina and stayed with the Manns. Michael Mann (KS 2nd year VI - just got a scholarship, is out for the holiday - he is a nice lad and Malcolm Wainwright (also was at Oxford with Michael) and is now at Badagry was also with the Manns. Malcolm does not look well at all - and Badagry is a very lonely spot. He is engaged to a nurse at a Teaching Hospital in London. He has difficulty with his food and the water is very poor - and the area is one of the least developed in Nigeria.

I did a few odds and ends of shopping next morning and attended the committee - nothing very startling, then took the hospital car to the garage to be overhauled. Unfortunately they could not start it until 2.30 so it was not ready until after 5pm too late to start back on the 166 mile journey, so I stayed another night and came up early yesterday morning arriving just before 1pm. I picked up Eileen who had had rather a tottering time at the dentists, and whose face is badly swollen.

On my return, I found Margaret's cold worse, but Peter improving - at the moment he is having yam with peas and chicken - no potato available. I did the accounts in the afternoon and in the evening we were invited to a welcome party for Hon. J. O. Fadahunsi's son who qualified six weeks ago and has just returned - a very noisy affair.

This morning it was our turn for coffee but I went to church and left before the end! The Wednesday before I went to Lagos we had our first Staff committee since Andrew left and fortunately it went well. On the Monday we went out to chop with the Eltons - a very pleasant evening. Margaret wants a little space so I will close - looking forward to hearing more of your adventures.

Love to you all from us all, David.

Dear Mother,
I would like to lend my blue maternity gown to Aileen for her to wear on the boat and until she can get into the shops in England. Her brother-in-law is sailing mid September and calling here in Ilesha, so could bring it. His address is for Mrs. D. C. Morley, c/o Mr. R. L. Morley, Rothwell, Pye Corner, Sandford, near Bristol. I would be very grateful if you could post it to him. It was cleaned before we came away and I hope that you will find it either in the wardrobe or a wardrobe drawer in the bedroom.

With love, Margaret

Sunday, August 18th
We were very pleased indeed to receive your letter yesterday, to learn that you are all well and had a lovely time - and also that our letter arrived.

We were very glad to hear that Uncle E is making good progress and Auntie A is in better form. They will both feel much better after the operation. I'm sure.

You do seem to have had a wonderful time mountain railways, chair lifts -

summits - the lot I can just imagine Stanley - thrilled to bits.

We are all well here - sundry colds and coughs have cleared up - Peter in very good form, crawling all over the place at speed - but not yet taken his first step alone, but with a hand in Margaret's and mine and him between us he walks quite well!

This morning we have been to Elsie's for coffee and he looked very sweet in a blue nylon dress affair and a pair of matching blue shoes plus his very blue eyes. Some words he speaks very plainly - Mummy, Daddy, Peter, Bye Bye, and occasionally others, and he is trying to say many more.

We have had a busy week without any outstanding events. Unfortunately Uncle Fred is in bed with fever - I hope he is soon better. He had a temperature on Friday, worse on Saturday (101) and so is in bed today. The Morleys are well, they went down to Ibadan on Thursday and did not get back until Friday lunch which meant rather a heavy morning.

Tuesday night we went to Elsie's for dinner and played Scrabble afterwards - quite nice, and Wednesday was Margaret's Fellowship. The garden is at last coming into its own. So far, for reasons unknown it is the worst season we have had, but now it is looking up and we have some delicious lettuces ready.

The hens too are not doing at all well. Margaret is looking after Jeans and altogether we are fortunate if we get two eggs per day - from about 20 hens! They are loosing at the moment as you can see! I think that when the rains stop in two months time they will pick up again and with 20 hens we should have sufficient eggs and to spare.

We have a new bank manager on Ilesha (the second since the Albions left) and I was approached the other day to see if our chapel could be used for a wedding, so have written to ask Jonah if we can get it licensed. Apparently his fiancé is flying out early in October and they would like to be married in Ilesha. Mr. Esan, our superintendent Minister would be the minister in charge. Anyway a wedding would cause a bit of excitement among our women folk.

The weather the last few weeks has been wonderfully cool and we have all felt we have had energy to get on with work and so forth - but no doubt as the weeks pass it will be much hotter again. It is five weeks since the Pearsons' left - they are now on holiday in Scotland I believe before going to Selly Oak. Our new Sister Miss Mabel Rowling is having her appendix out and is due to sail in about a month.

Do hope all went well on your return home and you all feel better for your holiday. We are very well Peter sends a sticky kiss; he is trying to feed himself!

Much love, David

25.8.57

We were very glad indeed to receive your letter on Friday and to learn that you are safely home again you seem to have had a wonderful holiday and must have many very happy memories to call on when winter draws on.

Methodism is in its annual upheaval and next year we too will be involved and looking at it from a somewhat different angle.

Very glad that the trip over the channel was accomplished without trouble - you have my unbounded admiration.

Later:- Have just returned from coffee following morning service at Otapete. One has time to commune with ones thoughts! Coffee was Aileen's - very nice - but it is a wet cool day- with showers following one after the other. I am off this afternoon but on night duty this week. Unfortunately a nurse's guardian is coming to sign a bond this afternoon, which will be rather an interruption.

The week has been a good one all round. Uncle Fred is better again and got back to work on Wednesday. Tuesday was rather heavy as David was at Imesi and Uncle Fred in bed but it went very well considering. On Wednesday it was Eileen's turn to take Fellowship - rather slow - not a very easy passage. Tuesday evening we went to the Morleys for chop a pleasant quiet evening - we shall miss them when they go in six weeks - flying home and back, and Margaret will be the only wife on the compound, with Sunday coffee every Sunday and cold store every Friday. It will be about eleven months before we see them again as we shall go just before they are due to come back.

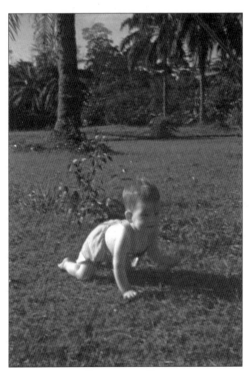

Peter crawling

Last night we had Miss Clarkson and Margaret Grant in to chop with Uncle Fred - a very nice evening, hearing all the news of England - trends in fashion and so forth! We had salmon salad, which was very nice indeed with our lettuce, which are absolutely wonderful. We had some cold for breakfast as a change to eggs and it was delicious it really adds tone to the fridge and with salad from the garden will be something to look forward to for days.

Peter is very well, and at the moment playing happily in his playpen with some rubber bricks from Jean, a donkey from Thea, and a rattle and a plastic parrot. He stands up steadily and bends down to pick toys from the floor, without any support but still has not walked unaided. If Margaret and I take a hand each he walks quite well. His vocabulary remains about the same but he often times imitates what we say and we can hear some words quite clearly.

Margaret is keeping well, though a little unsettled in the earlier part of the day - she is much better than last time. I am keeping well despite a lot of work, which will increase next week when we try to balance the books for our financial year end on Aug 31st.

On Friday a Dr. Bonne of World Health Organisation came to see here and the Imesi scheme - was most interested - a most useful contact. He is Dutch, lives in Geneva and a very charming man. He stayed with the Morleys. Last Monday we had Gwen Davies and Nancy Hall for dinner en route to Ikole.

The hens are still not producing eggs - rather disappointing. Hope all is well and Michael enjoyed the rest of his stay on the continent.

Love to you all from us all, David

1.9.57

Another Sunday is here and I am taking the opportunity of a quiet moment after morning coffee to start this letter.

We were very glad to receive a card from Michael from Germany and your letter yesterday. Although the letter was posted two days late it arrived only a day later than usual. Sorry to hear of Michael's indisposition across the channel - four hours isn't too long though! - the thought of thirteen days is rather worse.

You do seem to have had a hectic time with young people - nine to cope with is rather too much!

Thank you for the thought about the house on the south coast. Could you enquire where it is and if near the sea and so forth.

Stanley will be in France by now, I hope he has good crossings - so that he does not develop a phobia about the sea. They should have a very good time and it should add zest to his learning of French.

This has been an eventful week here. Most important to the family is that Peter has taken his first steps, unaided though encouraged. Just one or two rather unsteady but definite steps on August 27th, between Uncle Fred and myself - a most exciting day. Both he and Margaret are well - as I am. Peter especially looks very well indeed.

On Wednesday I went up to Ikole on trek and as Louie had Miss Davies and Nancy Hall of Shagamu there Margaret and Peter could not come.

Unfortunately I met trouble at Ikole. The Minister of Health was in the district on a tour and visited Ikole where the people presented him with a letter requesting the immediate removal of Louie as both intolerable and intolerant. A most unpleasant letter.

The Minister brought it in to Louie and talked it over in private, but I think that as a result Louie will not return after her furlough. Apparently she had considered it but this letter will be the deciding factor. She is very hurt indeed, though being Louie will not show it. I have had to write letters to Jonah, Bill Mann, Andrew, and Ralph Bolton to explain the situation - and probably we shall, if the government is willing, hand the place over to them. Anyway a decision has to be taken soon because Louie is due to go on leave. We shall have to see what is the best thing to do. The Mission House has never been sympathetically disposed towards Ikole so I don't expect for a moment they will send a replacement. On the whole it was not a very happy visit and it is possible that it is my last with Louie there.

I brought back Gwen and Mary and they are staying with Elsie and Eileen respectively till tomorrow when they return to Shagamu. Incidentally I don't know whether I have told you- but Enid is resigning at the end of this tour so with Elsie only doing one more tour we are going to be a little short. Incidentally don't murmur anything about these troubles yet.

Our new sister Miss Mabel Rowling is due here this month and Elsie is gong on furlough October 7th. Marion is due back at the end of October. Last night we had a party at Uncle Fred's - very nice.

Margaret has heard this week that her father had to have an emergency prostatectomy a week last Thursday. He returned from holiday on Sunday, taken ill and admitted to the Waterloo Hospital on Tuesday, with the operation on Thursday but is apparently going on well. Thea is very busy therefore, because Ernie is in Portugal again for his firm. It is rather worrying, though nice to know that the operation is over. We hope to hear again in a few days time.

Our financial year has ended so I have a frightful lot to do in the office. The hens are looking up - more eggs this week!

Hope all is well with you all - we are in good from. Love from us all, and a coo from Peter, David

8.9.57

I am enclosing a photo of Peter taken last July. It was taken by David M who has given it to us - we think that it is very good and very like him as he is now. It is possible that you might think it worthwhile to get some colour prints to send round the family. I think the minimum number is three and they work out at about 1/6d each, but I should be happy to settle for them and to know that the Aunts, Grandma, Mr. Ingham and Thea had a recent photo of Peter.

Mr. Ingham has ben very ill indeed I fear. Uncle Fred had a letter from Auntie Florence stating that the day after the op. he was very well but delayed shock set in and for three days he was desperately ill but has now picked up again after blood transfusions and continuous drip, and was making good progress. We did

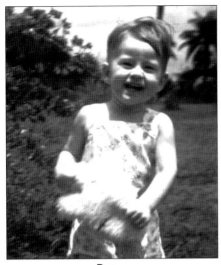

Peter

not know anything of this until it was all over - which is a relief.

Ernie is still in Portugal, so Thea has her hands full. She is bringing a single bed into the front room, so Mr. Ingham can go there after he leaves hospital and so she will be very busy indeed.

We were very glad to receive your letter on Friday - you have had a very busy time with visitors. I hope that this past week has been easier for you. Stanley will have returned from the continent - a really travelled young man! I hope his French has benefited accordingly!

The week here has been a busy one without a great deal to highlight.

Sunday - Uncle Fred's cook has been sick so Uncle Fred has most of his meals with us and a few with the Morleys. Unfortunately he has a bit of fever again and is not very well - I did his night duty for him last night.

We had a good session with the accounts earlier in the week. On my first balance I was £100.10.0 out, but Uncle Fred found the £100. We checked the ledger against the cashbook but could not find the 10/- until the next morning, when casually looking at the cashbook found an error in addition during the time Andrew was doing the accounts when I was in bed - so there we are! Balanced for another year.

Wednesday evening was my turn for fellowship so continued with my study of 1 Corinthians.

Friday our Nurses class - another filmstrip on church history and then last night Uncle Fred, Margaret and I went to chop with Marjorie Clarkson at WTC - a very nice evening though Uncle Fred had a temperature of 101! We had a letter from the Pearsons' - they seem to have had a good time in Scotland - I wonder if perhaps Andrew has been with you for a night - I know that he is due to go up to the Mission House about now, and there is the Medical Committee too.

Elsie and Eileen went up to Ikole during the week for a quarterly nursing committee and Louie has apparently made up her mind to go. Bill Mann is due here tomorrow on his way to see her and with Mrs. Mann and Michael will be staying on Tuesday evening.

During the week we had Rev Bill Wood for a night - there always seems to be someone! This week I must get out a budget for the coming year - no easy task and we shall find money a bit tight.

Garden now doing well - hens not so very well yet I fear. Asian flu has been in Ilesha. Had to visit our King twice - David has had a day off with it!

Do hope all is well with you all - you are always in our thoughts especially on Saturday house meeting days. Peter and Margaret are very well, as I am. Love from us all, David

15.9.57

Sunday afternoon, warmer than it has been previously - I have been in the pool this week and very nice it was too. It has been rather an eventful and worrying time as you will see in due course but I will try to record chronologically.

Monday was made busy by the arrival of the Manns plus their son Michael, who had been held up 90 minutes on the road because of flooding and they had to wait until a lorry dropped some stone chips till they were able to get over. They seemed in good form, had lunch and tea with us and then went on to Akure for the night, and back to Ikole on Tuesday morning. Unfortunately they found Louie had gone to obtain adoption papers of a sort for a girl, Bosede, whom she is going to take home with her. None of us are very happy about it, but Bill Mann talked to her and she has agreed not to decide definitely about returning or not next tour, till she has been home for a while and Jonah has had time to see the people. Unfortunately Miss Sennett of the Mission House is up in arms with Jonah about Eileen going up to relieve and Jonah is very angry about Miss Sennett's letter and so on and so forth. Anyway the situation is not so bad as it was but things are not very happy. I understand that Jonah and Bill are coming up in two weeks time so we shall see what happens

Your letter arrived Wednesday and we were very glad indeed to receive it, to learn all the news and of Stanley's safe arrival home. The house for holidays at Hove sounds as though it would be very nice so we will think about it a little more. Deputation requests have started coming and so we must plan where we shall be when so to speak soon

Wednesday evening was a Committee, which went fairly well - Elsie's last before she goes on furlough on October 5th.

On Tuesday night Uncle Fred had not been very well - up every hour to pass urine and when David and I looked in to see him on Thursday morning he had not been able to pass urine at all so we agreed that he ought to go straight into hospital. We put him in the car and Margaret packed a bag and I drove him straight to University Hospital, Ibadan and he was in bed in a side ward by 12.30 pm having seen the surgeon. We had a message yesterday that he is developing an abscess in the pelvis - rather unusual- but we fear that it will take a good time to clear up. The whole question of his fitness to remain out has been raised and is a question which must be answered fairly soon. I don't know. If it was decided he should return home, whether there would be anyone to give me a hand for the next four months.

Margaret is going down on Tuesday, with Peter - to see how he is and also to see Mr. Lawson the gynaecologist. I saw Mr. Lawson when I took Uncle Fred in and in fact he was most helpful and got him to the surgeon so swiftly and he asked if he could see Margaret this week, so she will go down with a driver and she will have lunch with the Days and return in the evening I expect.

Friday was a very busy day and then yesterday Prof. Emmet Holt of New York and Dr. Collis of UCH Ibadan came to see David about his work and discuss the meeting on nutrition, which is being held next Saturday. I shall be unable to get, as David is playing quite a big part and I shall have to hold the fort because I think it most unlikely that Uncle Fred will be out and even if he is he won't be able to do any work.

Yesterday and this morning were both busy as David was engaged with the two visitors and I had a strangulated hernia to operate upon as well as the accounts in the afternoon. Margaret Woodland brought in a maternity case, who fortunately delivered normally last night.

Margaret and Peter are both very well indeed - since Uncle Fred went to Ibadan his cat has been here - to Peters delight 'ussi' he calls it in a high pitched squeal as near as a meow as he can get! We have not heard from Liverpool this week so presume that Mr. Ingham is making steady progress. The flu is passing over in the town though I have a few aches and pains today and may be the last of those to get it! However it will be better tomorrow. Do hope all is well with you all. Much love from the three of us, David

22nd September 1957

There are a few minutes to spare whilst something is staining in the laboratory, so I thought I would pop up to the office and begin the letter home. We were very glad indeed to receive your letter and also one from Michael with all their respective pieces of news. Glad Grandma is keeping fairly well, that lectures are being prepared, thank you for the Christmas cards which are on their way, they will be here in good time I'm sure. There is a faint note of hope, concerning a house at Godalming in Michael's letter and we wonder if this is the one. We also heard from Thea by the same post that Mr. Ingham is making a slow recovery and has been out of bed, which is good news. A letter also from Andrew they are settled now into their flat at Selly Oak and seem to like it so far, though it sounds a bit of a crush, only two bedrooms for the six of them.

On Friday we received a letter from Dr. Bolton concerning a lady Doctor Dr. Kendrew who is available for nine months from October 16th and asking if we should like her. I am cabling to engage her at once. Unfortunately the news of Uncle Fred is not so good. Jonah, to whom I spoke on the phone last evening, had seen him on Thursday and said he looked terrible and that he felt he should go home. In fact he is writing in this vein to Ralph today I believe. Yesterday there was a big conference in Ibadan, under the BMA, on nutrition and David was one of the several speakers. He with Margaret Woodland went to see Uncle Fred, and they too returned rather worried about him and David says there is no doubt that he will have to go home as soon as he is fit. The Morleys have offered to take him home with them when they fly in three weeks time if he is fit. Apparently he is still having trouble passing urine and he is having to be catheterised. It is possible that he will be coming back here tomorrow - so we shall have our hands full indeed.

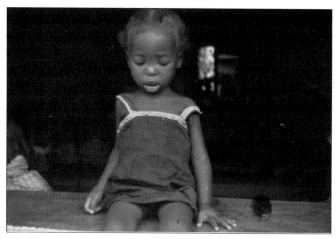

Kwashiokor

It has been a very busy week. Last weekend we had Dr. Collis of UCH Ibadan and Prof. Holt of New York. Margaret and I had dinner with them last Saturday. Each day was busy, especially Tuesday, with David in Imesi, and then on Friday Dr. Cecily Williams, one of the worlds leading nutritional experts, who first described Kwashiorkor in 1933 in Ghana came up to see Imesi, so David was away from the hospital from Friday morning till this morning. Yesterday, whilst they were in Ibadan, I had a strangulated hernia, and a caesarean section in addition to the ordinary work and the accounts! Still we got through all right.

Margaret, Peter and I are all keeping well and Peter's hair is gingery! The colour reproduces hers, then mine, then back to hers again! I hope that it does not fade before we get home and then you can see for yourselves.

The garden has come into production. We are at the moment half way through a large cabbage that is doing us for two meals. The hens too are looking up, though Jeans are doing better than ours - but we had 27 eggs last week, which supplies all our needs.

Elsie is looking forward to getting off now, she will be in Lagos two weeks today, preparing to sail on the Tuesday. Mabel Rowling, the new sister arrives on Friday this week and Marion should be out in about a month's time. Louie should be due to go home next month and is still taking this little Nigerian girl home with her, and Eileen will go up to Ikole. Very glad indeed that you have seen our colleagues to be - we are looking forward to their arrival in January very much indeed as you can imagine.

I have just remembered, Margaret and Peter went to Ibadan on Tuesday. Margaret saw Mr. Lawson, the gynaecologist and all is well but he wants Margaret to live in Ibadan from immediately after Christmas onwards. Uncle Fred had a large ischio-rectal abscess opened on the same day but has not made the improvement anticipated, as I mentioned before.

Peter and the cat are getting on quite well. The latter stands for quite a bit of pulling about. Peter's name for it is Pssi! Do hope you are all keeping well - we are fit and though busy and with some anxiety as you can imagine - very happy. Love to you all, David

29.9.57

We were very glad to receive your letter on Thursday this week and to hear how you all are, and news of Stanley, Grandma and Garth.

Naturally we are most interested in news of the house in Godalming. The Morleys know the village well - apparently St Thomas's Hospital was evacuated there during the war, and they say what a pleasant place it is. Quietness from here sounds delightful! We look forward to further news.

We have had another busy week - Uncle Fred came back on Monday - a little better and since he arrived he has picked up a little but still unable to pass urine so David is having to catheterise him every six hours or so. Uncle Fred has been booked on the same plane as the Morleys and has accepted the fact of going home very well. I think he realises that things cannot go on as they are.

Auntie Florence and their eldest son Dennis (who is in practice very near the London Airport) are going to meet them. I should very much like you to meet the Morleys - could you go to the airport London to see them when they arrive? I will add the time of arrival and date on the end of the letter. They wish, I think to go to the Mission House that day, before going on to Bristol.

Uncle Fred is up and about and remarkably cheerful but he looks very poorly. I wrote Auntie Florence on Thursday to let her know how he was. Because David Morley is looking after Uncle Fred I went up to Ikole - our usual monthly visit - too brief to pack up everything for Peter and so I went alone. Unfortunately I had a strangulated hernia to do so I didn't get off till 4pm. Louie was in good form - as though nothing had happened and she is apparently flying home at the end of October, with Bosede, the five year old Yoruba girl she has more or less adopted

Tomorrow Bill Mann and Jonah are coming up for a board meeting and will be going to see her again and get things fixed up in some way or other.

On Thursday Enid went down to Lagos in the lorry to meet Mabel Rowling who arrived by boat on Friday. I had ordered a load of dressings from the Kingsway Chemists there so they had a big load. They arrived last night - rather late. Miss Rowling has been to Eastern Nigeria with the leprosy service for a number of years and seems a nice person who will fit in well.

Elsie goes this week - Friday or Saturday - Marion arrives about October 20th and we hope that Dr. Kendrew, the lady doctor will arrive about the same time because from October 15th I shall be alone!

This morning I have been down to Otapete - a long service, and at the end we had the introduction of Miss Rowling.

Margaret, Peter and I are all keeping very well, though today the weather is warmer - the first hint of the hot season. Peter has begun to play in a real way, putting things into an old box, putting them on top and pushing it around and so forth. He isn't walking much yet just occasional steps but we think his vocabulary is increasing.

Do hope you are all keeping well. Love from us all, David

PS Morleys and Uncle Fred arrive London Airport at 10.30 am Thursday 17th October

6th October 1957

I am in the office with a moment or two to spare so am starting the letter on the typewriter. We returned from a visit to Afon just before lunchtime and I have had the accounts to do plus letters to Andrew and Ralph Bolton so feel that I have caught up quite well.

Today is your Anniversary Day and once again you have a very good platform - I doubt whether Rivercourt has had such illustrious Anniversary speakers as they have since we came to the church. Do hope it went well and you had a good day from every point of view.

We were very glad to receive your letter during the week and hear about the Godalming house. We had wondered from your description if it wasn't a bit on the large side, so we were not surprised to hear that Rex advised against it on that score, though we can imagine that it is disappointing not to have got settled down, though no doubt the 'right' house will crop up soon. Incidentally we had a young X-ray engineer here the other day whose parents have been in a similar position and they said that in Norfolk and Suffolk you can get a house about half the price as elsewhere. His parents had been to view one, an old rectory, 16 major rooms, two and a half acres, moat, orchard, walled garden. The price £750.

We have had a busy week one way and another, David M. was in Imesi Tuesday, Ibadan Wednesday, and Imesi Thursday, so I had my hands full, but on Friday afternoon we loaded up and went off to Afon in the ambulance on the routine quarterly visit. The Rowlands are well and expecting a third infant on January 21st, the same day as Aileen, so around then the district will increase by three. It is lovely countryside and you can let your eyes relax and look at the horizon about fifteen miles away, a very pleasant experience after being in this forest belt with no views and very heavy foliage all along the roadside. There were but a few patients to see, so we had a restful time.

On Thursday evening we had a party at the Sisters house to welcome Mabel who has settled in very well, and to say farewell to Elsie. Elsie left at 3am on Saturday morning as she wanted to get to the hairdressers at 9.15 on Saturday for a perm. What a character she is. Elsie sails on Tuesday, and the Morleys and Uncle Fred fly on October 16th from Lagos. Dr. Kendrew is coming I am glad to say, but I shall be alone for ten days which will be a heavy stint.

Uncle Fred is better and not having to be catheterised but is having to get up ten times at night still. He has lost two stone in weight, so you can imagine he does not look very fit, though he is in better spirits than previously, but finds time fast on his hands at the moment.

Margaret is keeping very well and Peter is thriving and weighs over 20lbs. He is walking more and will totter across his playpen without assistance quite frequently. He is beginning to play quite constructively too and recognises more people and animals, and is really still incredibly good.

We hear from the Pearsons' that they are settling in at the missionary guesthouse at Selly Oak, but I feel that they must be a bit cramped as they only have two bedrooms and one living room.

I had a letter from Ralph this week confirming that Dr. Kendrew is coming out. She is a Quaker 39, qualified in 1950, the same year as me, married as a student but the marriage has been dissolved. She has a GP assistantship waiting for her in July but is coming out for eight months. She flies on October 22nd so will arrive in Lagos 23rd and probably arrive up here on 24th to start work about the 26th I hope.

The Morleys go down to Lagos on the fifteenth and David will want a few days off before that so I shall have almost a fortnight alone.

Sorry to hear of Father's rash - do hope it settles down soon. Yes, we had heard about John Wrights practice at Nailsea but had not realised that you knew the previous doctor. I understand that they only have a flat over the shop for a year - which does not sound very comfortable.

We hope Margaret and Peter may be able to stay at Wesley College after Christmas perhaps with the Baxters though we haven't asked them yet. Margaret Day is expecting a baby possibly March so would find the extra a bit heavy. As soon as Margaret goes into hospital I shall go down and then bring Peter back - Jean has promised to look after him, with William and me until Margaret returns. Anyway we shall see.

We are well, and hope you all are also. Love from us all, David

13.10.57

Sunday afternoon and the hottest it has been for many months - really very hot and humid. I can hear Peter rattling his cot and telling us it is time he got up from his afternoon rest - incidentally he is getting two more teeth and today had his first taste of ice cream, which he enjoyed very much.

We were very pleased to receive the home letter this week but disappointed to learn that the house plans as drawn was not a possibility! Apart from the price it would appear to be satisfactory - surely the wall between the kitchen and the scullery could be removed to make it a reasonable place.

By the time you receive this you will have seen Uncle Fred if all is well and the Morleys. They are all packed up and ready to go to Lagos on Tuesday, fly on Wednesday and reach London on Thursday.

Uncle Fred has improved considerably this week and is thinking he might almost have carried on but his urine is still quite heavily infected. I do hope that he travels without trouble. David has been very good and he is working until the last minute but in 48 hours they will be gone.

We have had a busy week. On Tuesday I had to go to Ibadan for a committee on the private hospital ordinance - in place of Andrew- a long way for a committee especially as I have to go again in a months time. I have tried too to get a bit of operating in before David went so have had two full operating days, one complicated by having to go to court - a dreadful nuisance. On Wednesday evening Aileen took fellowship and on Friday Uncle Fred took our nurses group - very well indeed.

Yesterday was a full day with a visit from Mr. Lawson who had tea here with us. In the evening Margaret gave a party for Uncle Fred and the Morleys and we had a very good time indeed. It meant a great deal of work but it was a lovely meal and a very happy occasion. We started with chilled tomato juice and 'small chop' (biscuits with savoury things on such as shrimps, pilchards, cheese whilst the folk gathered. There were nine of us, then soup, ground nut stew, followed by lemon whip and American ice, coffee, chocolates, with a cigar for Uncle Fred! We presented Uncle Fred with a tray made by our carpenter, with the names of the hospital staff under glass - so to speak. He may well show it to you on Thursday - he seems very pleased with it.

This morning I went to Otapete service one and three quarter hours and then we had some friends drop in at 12.15 for coffee and then we were due up to the Women's Training College for lunch with Margaret Grant - including Uncle Fred. Very nice but rather hot and just at Peters rest time but he was very good considering. David is at Imesi again so I am taking calls again - no doubt I shall get used to it in the next few weeks. I do hope Dr. Kendrew is a capable sort.

Elsie will be almost half way home by now. Marion flies tomorrow and arrives on the 18th I think. Louie will probably not be returning to Nigeria but Eileen goes up on Thursday so for a day or two we shall be reduced to two sisters and one doctor - the lowest for many years.

We are all very well indeed, Margaret and Peter especially. Our love to you all, David

20.10.57

A very hot and sultry Sunday afternoon. Peter has had his tea and is playing in his playpen - I have just lit the primus to boil the kettle - it is Williams half day. We are all well and should you have heard that my eyes were inflamed they were quite better in 36 hours and have been no trouble since. Peter has been a little fretful - he is cutting two more teeth - but not overmuch.

The Christmas cards have arrived - thank you very much and the blouse for Margaret with which she is very pleased. If Michael would let me know how much the cards were I will settle with a cheque.

Your letter arrived on Thursday and we were glad to have all the news, though sorry to here the Rev. Hopkins didn't draw a large crowd. It was certainly quite surprising to receive Henrys gift - how very nice indeed.

Interested too in the Medical Meeting. We had a letter from Andrew also, and he confirmed that it was not well attended. Very glad that both he and Roy spoke well, apparently Ilesha came in for more than its fair share of publicity.

Henry seems to be in as big a muddle as ever with Mary and Iris. I hope that he gets matters sorted out one day.

As you can imagine we have had a full week. Monday, David worked until mid-day and then helped Aileen with the last minute packing. On Tuesday we all had breakfast together here and then Margaret and Peter went down to Ibadan to see Dr. Lawson. All is well I am glad to say. They experienced a torrential downpour on the way back.

Meanwhile Uncle Fred, David and Aileen and the children left at 9.30am for Ibadan and Lagos and we hear, had a good run down and got off with no hitches. I hope Uncle Fred travelled well - I have dropped a note to him today.

The medical work has been heavy, but not nearly as bad as it might have been. Enid has rallied very well, and has helped in outpatients, so that we have got through in reasonable time. I am keeping the wards as quiet as I can until the new doctor comes next week. However we have had two caesarians, a forceps delivery and a manual removal, so we have not been idle in the surgical realm. On Wednesday evening Margaret took our fellowship and on Friday I took the nurses group. On Saturday Marion came up by train as the transport arrangement fell through. She arrived at Oshogbo at 11.45pm and arrived here about half an hour later. She is in very good form, full of energy. She sees a very big change in Peter, and like others thinks he is a grand little fellow.

Yesterday we had the Clappertons in to tea - a new family with a boy of six.

We had a pleasant time. David Morleys brother, Roger, and his new wife, came for the night. They arrived from leave and are on their way to Kano by road where he is a District Officer. A very nice couple indeed.

Louie and Eileen are here this evening en route for England I think probably for the last time. She is rather cast down. Margaret and I are going in for coffee this evening and we shall finish with family prayers.

Mabel Rowling has settled very well and brings a very placid approach to problems. Margaret had seven chicks hatch (eight eggs) last Monday - we are very thrilled especially Peter, but the hens are not laying at all at the moment which is disappointing.

Do hope all is well at home and we do look forward to hearing from you week by week - you are constantly in our thoughts. We are all very well and though busy, not too busy! Love from the three of us, David

                                                                                    27.10.57

Another Sunday is here, with many visitors so am trying to snatch a moment before our evening service. It has been a busy week but it has seen the arrival of Dr. Kendrew and although she has not done much yet, she will settle down I think and in time be most useful. The weeks seem to be slipping quickly too and it will not be so long before Andrew is out here again.

We were very glad to receive your letter but very sorry indeed to hear of the trouble with meeting the travellers. Glad to hear that Uncle Fred travelled well I hear he is now in Liverpool. Margaret's father is now out of hospital this week.

We are all keeping well but we seem to be busy with odd things. Dr. K arrived on Wednesday in Lagos and came up Thursday afternoon. In Lagos, at the time, were Eileen and Louie. Apparently Louie got away with Bosede and should be in England this night. I think she may well call in to see you. Apparently I have heard - though not from Jonah, that the Ikole people will not have her back at all, so it is most unlikely she will return.

Last Sunday evening Enid fell in chapel and sprained her ankle. It was not better by Monday so we sent her to Ibadan and she has cracked her fibula and it is in plaster now and she is on crutches so we are a little short on the nursing side as well!

Eileen returned on Wednesday and went up to Ikole and on Thursday Dr. K arrived looking tired and all her 38 years. Apparently she was a dietitian at the Middlesex Hospital in the war and then took up medicine after the war. I think she will manage quite well though at the moment is understandably a bit lost.

Last Monday we received a letter from Dr. Ross. He was a student at the London, junior to me. He, with his brother, asked if they could stay two nights. One is working in the Quae Ibo mission and the other in the Leprosy service. They turned up at 3am on Saturday morning and we were not expecting them until

Saturday evening, so we had to get up and make up beds and so forth. However it has been very nice having them, and to be able to talk of friends and so forth. They have been most interested in the hospital, comparing it with their own. On Saturday they went down to Ibadan and took in two patients, which was the point of the journey.

On Saturday afternoon there was a phone call from the Owa saying he was coming up to look round in five minutes. He arrived with the Owa of Ife- Sir Adege Adeoni - a very important leader in Nigeria - and 40 chiefs. However, they did not stay long. Later in the day our lawyer came about the lawsuit we are bringing against one of our nurses and the case will be coming up in November, here in Ilesha. I am not looking forward to it one little bit.

Peter is in very good form and walking quite a lot now - Margaret is well, though this entertaining is really very heavy for her. On Thursday Basil Nicholson is coming for the day and night - the Leprosy advisor for the West, and so it goes on. By the end of this week Dr. Kendrew should have found her feet and work should be easier, which will be a relief, though am longing for January!

Do hope all is well at home. Love to you all from the three of us, David

2.11.57

Saturday evening and both Margaret and I are tired after a busy and rather hectic week. Margaret is doing her housekeeping accounts and I am just writing one or two letters.

We were very glad to receive your letter, which arrived on Thursday even though written and dispatched later than usual. I can just imagine Auntie Alice's enthusiasm for house hunting, and am so pleased that Uncle Edward is better. No. 1 certainly seems to be a home from home for many people.

Last Sunday we had the two Dr. Ross brothers and the Matron and I didn't seem to get much done at all. They left on Monday morning and though we were glad to have them it was nice to have the house to ourselves again for a bit. On Tuesday though Dr. Basil Nicholson came and he took up quite a bit of my time with a visit to the leprosy village and so forth - he stayed Tuesday night so we had Mabel and Dr. Kendrew in to chop.

Wednesday evening was committee, fortunately a very short one because we had a triplet delivery, which I had to help with.

Thursday we had operations, another busy day and then more on Friday. In addition I had to lead our group on animism!

Then today has been a very heavy one with the wedding in our hospital chapel. We have had to get it registered and so forth, but it was a very nice occasion. The bride was in a lovely white dress and groom in a black suit. There were 80 guests, mixed European and African. The chapel was full. I said to Margaret that I wished there was a collection as we had the four wealthiest

Nigerians in Ilesha there!

We left Peter in his playpen with the Sisters but they let him out and then put him back in, to which he objected very strongly, so Margaret had to forgo the reception. I attended but came away as soon as I could, fortunately, as I had to operate in maternity. It has been a sweltering day, one of the hottest this year.

The hospital is becoming much busier again, but Dr. Kendrew (Elizabeth) is finding her feet and she will gradually be of much more help. Now she is settling down she is much less reserved than at first.

Peter is walking much more now and he realises that he can move about more quickly on his feet than on hands and knees.

Now Sunday morning - got sleepy last night so we went to bed and had a good night even though I was on call. This morning I have taken the nurses and Marion and Elizabeth to Otapete and have returned to give a hand with coffee but with so few, a maximum of six, it is not such hard work.

We have heard that Dr. Roy Goonewardene and Beryl will be coming straight through to Nigeria and so arrive in Lagos on Christmas Day. It does mean he will be here earlier than expected, and Margaret will be able to get them settled in before she goes down to Ibadan.

The chickens are three weeks old today and seem to be doing well. As we are in loco parentis to all the fowl in the compound we have enough eggs to sell to the sisters, but it is quite a lot extra for Margaret as well as looking after their gardens. All told it must be three acres at least. The weather has warmed up considerably the last week or two and the pool is coming into its own again. Do hope all is well - we are very fit. Love to you all from the three of us, David

10.11.57

It is Sunday morning. The wards, which I have just been round, are quiet, so there are a few moments, in which to write a few lines.

We have had a busy week but not frantically so - and have all kept well. Peter is really walking now and walked all the way to the Morleys house and began playing on the back verandah and several times he has been down as far as the orchard. He is very pleased with himself and laughs away as he walks. He seems to be developing a love of roses because he makes a beeline for the rose bushes and pulls off all the petals! At the moment he seems to have gone off tea - he starts very well and then suddenly decides he does not want any more.

Sorry to hear that Father is still in the hands of the physicians and hope the matter has been sorted out by this time.

Last Sunday evening I went to our hospital chapel service - quite a good one, Margaret staying in with Peter. With all the houses round about being empty there are no listeners for babies!

Monday was busy and on Tuesday I had to go to Ibadan again for the second

Committee for revising the Hospital Ordinance.

Wednesday evening Elizabeth came in to dinner and then Marion led a fellowship. Thursday was library for Margaret and on Friday evening we had some films for the nurses. They were from the United States Information services - one on Woodrow Wilson and the other on Washington. The first interesting but difficult to follow and I don't think the nurses understood it at all

Yesterday was a quiet day - I got the accounts finished in good time and a quiet evening. Elizabeth has survived her first week of night duty and does very well I think. It is a great relief to have someone else to share the work.

The garden continues but the poultry are a bit disappointing about eggs - only just paying their way at the moment. The chicks are thriving - just four weeks old but this morning there was a hawk around.

I had a letter from Dick West again, asking me (with Margaret) to go to Queens Hall, Hull, again - what do you think? The only reason I shall go would be for Dick's sake, but I must make it clear that it is the last time. We might fit it in with a visit to Yorkshire but two children will add to the complications!

Do hope you are all well. We are expecting the Crossleys for an 11 day stay, tomorrow. Love to you all, David

17.11.57

Another Sunday morning and quite a busy one, so I am snatching a moment to get this letter started. We haven't received yours this week - but expect it will be here in a day or two.

We have had a busy week entertaining the Crossleys. She is young and decorative but has not given Margaret any help, which is a bit odd I think. She is so different to John who is intelligent. However it has been pleasant having them - they go tomorrow to Lagos for some meetings or other I gather.

Margaret went to Ibadan to see Mr. Lawson and all continues to be well with Margaret and with the new baby I am glad to say - but she does have a lot on at the moment, with dispensing, stores and keeping an eye on the compound and so forth as well as having Peter to keep an eye on. He is now walking much more and in a matter of seconds disappears - and there are such vast spaces he might wander in sometimes it is not easy to find him.

On Wednesday afternoon I had to go to

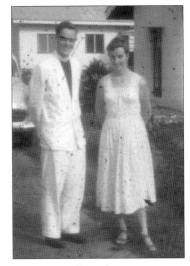

Crossleys

305

Ikole on our monthly visit. Eileen was well but finding it lonely and rather worrying. She is used to having a doctor around who takes responsibility. They were not over busy fortunately, and finding it easier going than at Ilesha. She is coming in tomorrow ready for our entrance examinations that are on Tuesday and Wednesday next week.

Friday was a busy day - made more so by the visit of the new Matron (a Miss

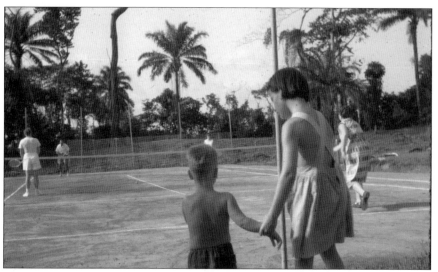

Tennis

Johnson) of the new University College Hospital, Ibadan. She was most gracious and thought what a nice place it was, but she had only been in the country two weeks so hasn't much to compare it with.

Yesterday was busy with operations in the morning but in the afternoon we were determined to get a game of tennis. The Sisters also have two visitors (teachers from United Mission College Ibadan) and five of us went up to play on the Women's Training College court. Marion and Elizabeth are obviously good players so if we could find a fourth on the staff we could have a good foursome.

This morning is our coffee morning, I have taken the nurses to chapel and have given Margaret a hand with making the coffee and so on, but am now waiting a summons to the theatre for an emergency operation.

Our Hospital Management Committee is fixed for Saturday December 7th so I must get out the notices and so forth for it. The chickens are thriving though we were wakened by the night watchman at 5am to say that the ants were in the Morleys chicken run so Margaret got up and put on Wellington boots to go and rescue them - what a business it is!

Do hope you are all well - looking forward to receiving your letter in due course. Love from us all, David

23.11.57

We have been very well off for letters this week - three, but sorry to hear that Grandma is not well. It certainly seems as though her span is near the end, and expect and hope she will slip quietly away. I will write to her this weekend

We were most interested in Michael's letter concerning the house. I think that it is a good thing to look in the higher price range - it is an investment. How long we shall remain here I don't really know. When we get home I am going to suggest a further two tours to Ralph Bolton and see how he reacts. I shall then have done ten years on the field and Peter will be six when he should be at proper school. I shall be 35 and it will be as late as one can reasonably leave it to get into practice in England and still have a pension at the end. If we were to stay on, Peter could go to Kingswood School for very little though.

We are thinking of you very much at this time and realise how trying it is for you all. I have no doubt though that something will turn up quite soon.

About the car - we have decided to obtain a second hand one if we can. With two children it will be a necessity especially as we would like to get around our honoured relatives in various parts of the country. Reliability is the most important factor, plus economy of running petrol at 4/6d a gallon I believe, and here it is 3/4d. An eight or ten horsepower car, which is not too expensive. I don't know how we shall be placed when we get home and I am not sure of the price of a car? I certainly should be most grateful if you could locate something. Incidentally whilst I remember, Bill Mann has told us we may be coming home on a boat arriving at Tilbury about the middle of April (15th) but will let you know more definitely when I know. Also my deputation this furlough is in London N.W district, but quite where I have not heard yet.

This week has been very busy - our Nurses entrance exam on Tuesday, then on Wednesday I went to Ibadan for 5pm being invited to the Official opening of the new hospital by the Princess Royal.

Unfortunately it was a very difficult time of day for Peter, so Margaret could not come. I saw the Princess Royal very well, about four yards away, the Governor General and the other notables. Then on Friday I had to go to Oyo for a committee at the Maternity Home. Today, I am writing this on Saturday night, Margaret, Peter, Elizabeth and I have been for a picnic to the Women's Training College.

Just broke off for chop when a young couple looked in and asked if they could be put up for the night. They have got stuck on the way to Akure.

Peter is getting much steadier on his feet now, and his hair is growing much more. We were looking at earlier photos of him and are surprised at how much he has changed! When he is out now, he shouts 'car car' every time he sees a vehicle and jigs up and down in the seat.

Tomorrow is harvest festival at Otapete so we shall go there for a while I expect. It will be a very noisy occasion.

Margaret is keeping fit except for two holes in her leg - pecked by Clarence the cock. Much love from us all, David

1.12.57

Once again, Sunday morning. Coffee is over and we had two folk up from the town with medical problems so we had rather more to coffee than anticipated. Peter is playing in the room and on the front verandah, so concentration is not easy. Margaret has gone round to give the three lots of fowl their midday corn.

We have had a busy week but unfortunately Margaret has had a septic leg from the bite of Clarence the cock. It was all right for a few days and then seemed to become inflamed. However with poulticing and penicillin it is settling down and it is not so painful to walk as it was.

Peter has been well and gained this month so that he is now over 20lbs. - not very much considering his age - but he is rather a twee little boy and looks well covered!

Last Monday I had to go to Ibadan for the Medical Advisory Board. Unfortunately fifteen miles out of Ibadan the lower water hose began to leak, the car got over heated and almost seized up. I had to wait until it cooled off, and then fill with some water from a stream. I tried to patch it without success, and we had to stop and fill the radiator six times before reaching reasonable habitation where I wound insulating tape round and got to the secretariat one and a half hours late for the Board. However I was there for half of it.

I had not intended to stay in Ibadan but went and had my picnic with the Days and then went to the garage to get a new hose. It took one and a half hours to fix it and I could have done it in 20 minutes at the outside. I got home about 6.30pm and found an obstetric problem waiting and had to do a hysterectomy immediately and I have rarely felt so tired as I did that night! However a good nights rest was all that was needed to feel restored.

The hospital has been busy through the week, then on Friday I had to pay the staff. Unfortunately their income tax is also due, so I had to decide to whom to lend a little money to be tided over this month - a rather exhausting afternoon. However it is settled, the books balanced and ready to start another month. One more payday to cope with and then Andrew will be back again.

We now hear that Beryl (the new surgeon's wife) will arrive in Lagos on the 24th and Roy will come on later from Accra where he is attending a conference, so it is possible that she will be here for Christmas.

Our court case against the nurse is to be heard on January 14th in Ilesha, so we shall get Christmas and the New Year over first. I suppose there is still a chance that she will settle out of court - I sincerely hope so.

At 2am on Saturday morning we were awakened by the night watchman who said the ants were getting at the Morleys baby chicks. Margaret got up to look and didn't return. I got worried and went to look and found her attempting to get the ants off the chicks, one by one. It took an hour and out of seven chicks only four are still alive and they are very poorly - rearing hens is a most hazardous business.

Next week will be a busy one, with our Hospital Management Committee on Saturday. We are expecting the Manns and Jonah up- perhaps to stay on Friday night, which will make a lot of work for Margaret. It will be a good thing when she goes to Ibadan and has a rest, though we are not looking forward to the separation.

Hope all is well with you at home and house hunting is progressing

Much love from Margaret Peter and me, David

7.12.57

Saturday evening after an exhausting day dominated by our Management Committee, of which in Andrew's absence, I am secretary. However it is now over for another six months!

First of all I must let you know that the Christmas decorations have arrived without any trouble and will do very well indeed on our Christmas tree. Thank you very much. It will be a real thrill this Christmas with Peter, (he is now running) because he will appreciate the decorations and so forth! Also a book has arrived from Michael, thank you too for that. I have not seen it - Margaret has popped it away until Christmas.

However we are glad to receive last weeks letter, though sorry to hear of the trouble at Abbots Langley - it will be a merciful release when Aunt Ruth slips away I feel.

The week here has been a full one, fortunately with a minimum of emergencies, so the medical rounds have not been too heavy.

Our twelve nurses who are taking their finals went down on Monday, but their papers have been postponed for ten days - there was a leak of the test questions so the tests have to be reset!

On Tuesday we expected Mr. Lawson of Ibadan to come through but he failed to turn up after we waited until 2.15 for lunch! However he turned up at 2.15 on Wednesday - as M and I were resting! He examined Margaret and found all well and then I took him to see a girl in the ward. He decided she needed an immediate operation and did it forthwith! He was most affable and friendly and was going on holiday, leaving his wife and 6/52 old son in Ibadan!

On Thursday we went out to tea with the Clappertons and had an enjoyable hour. Peter was very good indeed - a perfect pet! Took his tea ever so well and captured all the hearts present. They have a boy aged seven who played very well indeed with Peter.

Friday was again busy. I had a very full antenatal clinic in the afternoon and in the evening Jonah and Bill Mann arrived for the Committee. We had a quick meal - Elizabeth was also with us and then Jonah spoke to the nurses in the chapel and then we all came back here for coffee and a chat - a very pleasant evening.

This morning I got through the wards and so forth and we began the Committee meeting at 10.15am after Margaret had provided coffee and biscuits and we finished soon after 12.00 - the business having gone through quite well.

Jonah and Bill had a quick lunch afterwards. Unfortunately I had to sign a Bond with a nurse and so got held up and they left at 1.10 to return to Lagos. However on Monday Jonah and Mrs. Jones and Mr. Beetham, from the Mission House, London, will be here for lunch. It is possible that on Tuesday I have to go up to Ikole for a committee.

In addition on Wednesday, Thursday and Friday mornings I had to attend court to give evidence in four cases.

We are all keeping well I am glad to say, our cat is expecting kittens, the garden is doing well still.

David Morley is thinking of accepting a lectureship at University College Hospital, Ibadan next tour! which means we shall see less of him. Roy Goonewardene has failed his FRCS again.

Do hope all is well with you all. Love from Margaret, Peter and David.

15.12.57

A lull in a rather busy Sunday morning so I thought I would get this letter started anyway! We were very glad to receive your letter on the usual day this week.

We have had a very hectic week what with one thing and another. Last Sunday night Peter suddenly shot a temperature of about 102 and was so fretful Margaret went into his room to sleep and he was unwell for two full days with a cold and sore throat. However he is much better now apart from the occasional cough and is his usual happy self. On Sunday night, in addition to being worried about Peter I had nine hospital calls so you can imagine I did not feel very ready for work next day!

On Monday the Jonahs and Mr. Beetham came for lunch and stayed several hours. I showed the latter over the Hospital and he seemed quite impressed. He will be here for the Africa conference (Ibadan) in January so we may see him again.

Tuesday Peter improved, and on Wednesday the x-ray technician whom we had asked to come to look at our machine arrived late in the afternoon, so we had no alternative but to ask him to stay the night, which he did - not a very exciting guest!

On Thursday Mr. Lawson, in very good form, looked in after his holiday to see the patient upon whom he had operated. He stayed to coffee in the morning. That day we had a telegram from Mr. Mellanby saying he was arriving Friday and sure enough he arrived - much as usual and is going on to Benin tomorrow - then back here on Wednesday and up to Zaria on Thursday and then back to us possibly just after Christmas. Thus he is going to be around for a bit, though on the whole he is an unobtrusive guest.

Yesterday (Sat) we received a Dr. and Mrs. Taylor and two children – one four years old and the other seventeen months for the weekend. They have only been out two months and I met them at the Official Opening of UCH and in the way one does, asked them up to the hospital sometime and they quickly took me up. They are a very nice family. He was at University College Hospital, London, much the same time as Winston. We have had a very pleasant weekend and I am sure it is good for these folk to see what it is like in the smaller hospitals.

What it has meant though it has been a very busy week for Margaret who really does need a rest. This coming week should not be too busy, though we know of four people who are coming but it is the unexpected people that make the work.

In addition I have had a very busy week of night duty with major surgical operations five nights out of seven and last night did not get to sleep until 4am so we shall try to get to bed in good time tonight. In addition I have had five police post mortems to do!

Despite the work we are all well and looking forward to Christmas. We shall be thinking of you next weekend wishing we were with you

With love from the three of us, and best wishes for a very happy Christmas to you all, David, Margaret and Peter.

22.12.57

Christmas is about upon us here and when this arrives you will be anticipating the New Year, which will be a busy one all round I feel. Do hope you have had a very happy Christmas and perhaps you have found a suitable house— and that would be a good piece of news.

It is Sunday morning and I have taken the nurses and Elizabeth to church, our guests are busy packing up gifts for the hospital staff - a very useful job they are doing. Margaret is busy with the accounts and Peter is asleep. He has been very well this week so we felt we ought to give his TAB injection - he should have it when he is about a year old. Unfortunately, as with all of us, he had quite a severe reaction and Margaret and I were awake with him until about 3am when he dropped off and we likewise were able to drop off. This morning his arm is sore but he had a good breakfast and is making up for his lost sleep.

Margaret's cold and cough are much better, but preparations for Christmas are making heavy demands and yesterday we had nine visitors, some expected and some unexpected! The Boltons who are here now, are a young Methodist couple who work for Esso petrol in Lagos and are on their way to the East for Christmas. They asked if they could stay here for two nights to break the journey and to see the hospital about which they had heard.

One of the Sister's visitors has arrived from Ibadan, but Malcolm Wainwright (Oxford with Michael) our guest will not be here till Christmas Eve and we are having Margaret Woodland as well.

During the week we had a letter from David Morley telling us that Andrew - their youngest boy fell out of an upstairs window on to concrete and has broken both arms, one collar bone and his skull - but they think he will be alright - an awful shock for them it must have been. We have not heard from them since.

Have you heard that Mr. Barnes, late of Kingswood School, is now in Lagos? He has gone to the Boys High School there for a year in the first instance but seems to be enjoying it very much indeed - I hope he will be able to come up to Ilesha some time, it would be quite something to have him stay with us.

The other day I saw an advert for a new Riley car (one point five) - Michael could you investigate? I have been wondering if we would not be wise to buy a new car! If we brought it back here with us we should not have to pay purchase tax on it, but we should have the cost of shipping and also import duty- but they are less than purchase tax and a new car would be more reliable than a second hand one. What do you think!.? Anyway it is worth thinking over but I have not actually seen a model yet though I hear there are some in the country.

A little later, Peter has perked up and is playing with John (Williams son) on the front verandah.

Do hope all is well with you all. A very happy New Year, and much love from Margaret, Peter and David

29th Dec 1957

How did Christmas go? We have had a lovely time - Peter has had some lovely gifts, but the one that he likes best, is the one you sent - The Barking Dog Car! It really is fascinating and he has played with it for hours. Thank you very much too for our gifts - the manicure sets are most welcome. Neither Margaret nor I have one, and the bath salts and powder are Margaret's favourites.

Sorry to hear that Grandma was not so well and that you had to go over by train and bus - I hope the car is out of dock soon.

We have had a busy time but not so busy as on previous occasions and I seem to have spent more time at home, which has been most enjoyable.

Last Sunday night the Carol service went very well - and was greatly appreciated by many folk - the collection was over six pounds and the Owa of Ijeshaland came - so we were very, thrilled.

Monday was a very busy day with many outpatients and then on Tuesday,

Christmas Eve we again seemed to be very busy.

Our two guests, Margaret Woodland and Malcolm Wainwright both arrived and after the evening meal of hot duck, pear - a delicious meal - most went carol singing around the town. Elizabeth went and I stayed in and decorated the tree, with Margaret and finished preparing parcels. Then there was the fun of distributing to other houses and receiving numbers of parcels for Peter.

After supper we filled Peter's pillowcase, left many round the tree and went to bed. Unfortunately I was up from 3-4am amputating a finger! At 6.30 Malcolm took Communion service and then we returned and helped Peter unpack his presents - he was most excited. After breakfast we opened our other presents.

There was hospital work to do, then services on the wards. Enid and I went to the leprosy colony and had a happy time with them, distributing gifts.

Then coffee in our home followed by preparation for lunch, which we had altogether under a bamboo and palm shelter with the nurses - chicken and rice.

In the afternoon we managed to have a rest, but I had to take the nurses who were doing their nativity play to the leprosy patients who enjoyed the little play immensely.

Tea was in Elizabeth's house and then we enjoyed a large swimming party - wonderful fun and then in the evening thirteen of us for Christmas Dinner at the Sisters. I had to carve the turkey - a lovely meal.

Boxing day was relatively quiet, most going up to Imesi for a picnic and then Friday it was the nurses party which needed a great deal of energy but went well and the nurses seemed happy.

Saturday I had quite a lot of operating to do all morning and part of the evening. Malcolm tried to get a local bus or lorry down to Lagos but had no luck and had to leave at 5am this morning. Margaret Woodland left after coffee. On Friday evening Beryl Goonewardene arrived and she seems a most capable person and will fit in well. Roy comes on January 10th.

Margaret is busy packing up - she and Peter are off to Ibadan tomorrow. Mr. Mellanby arrived today

We are all very well - Peter Margaret and myself. Our love to you all, and a chuckle from Peter, David

5.1.58

Another Sunday is here and I am starting this in the office in a lull as it seems to be going to be a busy day.

I was glad to receive two letters this week, one written just after Grandma's funeral and one after Christmas. Despite the rather depressing start you seem to have had quite a good time - I should love to have heard Freddie on keeping fowl in the Philippines. I have not got your letters beside me as I have sent them on to Margaret, whose address incidentally is care of Mrs. Day, Wesley College,

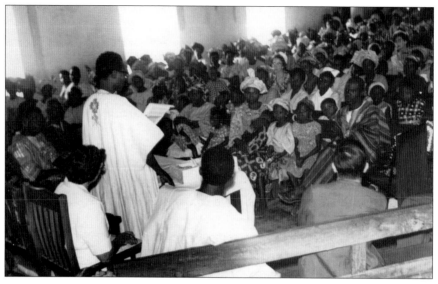

Imesi

Ibadan. As you may imagine I am feeling more than a little bereft. The house is very quiet without Margaret and Peter. I seem to have none to talk over the current hospital problems with - however another two weeks and Andrew will be here and I shall be able to get down to Ibadan for a little while - I need a break!!

The week has been a busy one, Margaret and Peter got off first thing last Monday morning and had a good run down to Ibadan. Peter has been a little unsettled, meals at slightly different times and that sort of thing and a long gap between first and second courses as their household does not seem to tick quite like our and apparently Peter gets very impatient for his custard!

Hospital work has been busy and unfortunately Elizabeth has had a bad cold, Marion lost her voice and Enid is still in plaster. On Wednesday night at fellowship we all felt very low indeed, but we seem to pick up towards the end of the week.

Yesterday was the first anniversary of the WACMR Imesi scheme and Margaret W had arranged an anniversary celebration and had asked me to speak at the public meeting. The Sisters suggested that Beryl came out to see the place and we took a nurse and her sister out too.

It went quite well, finishing with a traditional dance through the village from the Town Hall to the dispensary. Afterwards we returned home to Margaret Woodlands and had a very nice evening meal including roast duck and then back here by 9.30pm. Fortunately the hospital had been quiet but I really enjoyed getting out of the place for a few hours.

Mr. Mellanby was with me till Friday mid-day completing the lagging of the boiler. He has made a good job of it and I am sure it will be easier to keep the steam up and save on fuel. He charged the hospital £10 which I felt a bit steep.

Although it is quieter than ever I am pleased he has moved on to his next stopping place.

On Friday next Beryl is going down to meet Roy and they are returning on the Saturday. I have asked them in to dinner that night. It will be very nice to have another man around the place!

In a few minutes I am expecting Charles Day who is coming up to take our Covenant Service, which will be a pleasant interlude. Only two weeks till Andrew comes - and only about twelve till we sail! Much love to you all, David

12.1.58

Sunday morning and a few spare minutes so I am starting this letter. I was very glad to receive yours on Friday - it came quickly so perhaps the mail is back to normal.

Here, at home, it is terribly quiet without Margaret and Peter and I do feel at a loss — no one to talk problems over with and that sort of thing - but the days are slipping past and it should not be long now before I can get down if only passing through to Synod and then after Synod to stay for some days.

It has been a very busy week here - Thursday being one of the heaviest surgical days I remember. In the morning I did two hernia operations and a D&C and one other and then the emergencies began coming in and I had to do five major surgical emergencies in the afternoon. Coupled with a heavy week of night duty it was rather tiring.

The big event of the week was Roy's arrival on Friday evening, plus a Ceylonese friend a Rev. de Silva who had also been attending the conference at Accra - a very nice man indeed. Roy is a very self assured fellow, and Beryl does not seem to get much of a look in at the moment, but no doubt things will settle down. I wonder what place they have in Ceylonese life? He will be starting in the Male ward tomorrow and will be a great help in a few days when he has settled down.

The other event has been the arrest of one of our staff - the theatre orderly. He had his leave just before Christmas and apparently whilst at his home (150 miles away) posed as a Doctor and gave injections. Enquiries were made to the police here, who visited his house, found drugs, syringes etc. (obviously stolen from WGH) and will be charging him. He has incriminated another man who has also been arrested- so where it will stop I do not know! The theatre orderly was a man we all liked and trusted - it is a blow when this sort of thing occurs - one begins to wonder about the worthwhileness - but looking on it overall - it is only an occasional incident.

It would have been nice to have a new car to travel in but not a practical proposition. Space has gone. Often think of you all and wonder just what you are doing.

Hope worries soon resolve - I am sure they will. Love to you all, David

Wesley College Ibadan, 15.1.58

Here in Ibadan all is peaceful. Peter is having his mid-morning sleep and I am enjoying the relaxation, which is only possible whilst he is in his cot.

David will be keeping you informed of events at Ilesha, but I'd just like to let you know that all is well with us here, and to add my thanks to those already sent by David for the Christmas gifts. Peter's car is still a favourite and in spite of some hard knocks is still as good as new, which speaks much for its strength.

Apart from a weekly visit to the clinic, where I continue to get a good report, we don't go out very much. It is a leisurely life, but I can make use of any amount of time for sewing and knitting. Peter's wardrobe is more adequate again now, and the baby's is complete. Few additions were needed there, as more than one layer of clothing is inadvisable in this heat and Peter's baby clothes can all be used again.

This morning the Hospital lorry called in on its way to Lagos for repairs and to bring up the Pearsons' at the weekend. I was very glad to have up to date news of David, as the post between Ilesha and Ibadan takes three or four days and the phone is out of order here.

David has kept remarkably well amidst the strain of long hours of work and responsibility and already things will have taken a turn for the better with Roy's arrival. When Andrew is back and Synod over David will need to get away for a while and then we hope to see him here, but I don't know when or for how long that will be.

Peter has settled down very well here. It was rather difficult for him at first, with a completely new routine and surroundings, but his rest times and 12 hours sleep at night have remained undisturbed. Once up, he is on the go all the time and moves very fast - this morning he caught a chicken, which is quite an achievement - he flashes from room to room, up the stairs, round the corners and off across the compound, full of the joys of life. I get plenty of exercise!

With love, Margaret

18.1.58

Saturday evening, and a few minutes in hand so I thought I would start this letter. It has been a most interesting day - I have entertained Mr. Beetham, Miss Sennett and eight others to tea. They are delegates to the All Africa Conference in Ibadan, and came up to see what the hospital was like. They all seemed most interested and I think impressed.

It was thrilling news to hear that your house has been obtained. I'm sure that as the weeks pass it will become more and more settled in mind and after all - one can be happy in any kind of house almost. I am sorry Margaret wasn't here to share the news when I opened the letter but I will send details down to her. How far is it to Worcester Park from Rivercourt ? I imagine there will be quite a lot of tripping to and fro to be done. Peter I fear will be at the crayon and mural stage so we shall have to watch him!

Margaret and Peter are keeping well in Ibadan, but I think Margaret is getting rather low in spirits so I am hoping to get down to see her next week - perhaps to and from Synod, and then the week after go down and stay down for a bit.

Andrew and family are due back tonight. Unfortunately the boat is a day late - but as the people they were going to stay with are away tonight they are going to have to come up - so I fear they will be very late? - about 10.00 pm - and the children will be very tired.

The week has been a busy one - but Roy is settling down - though he does not get through many outpatients yet and he operates slowly. However I have no doubt he will speed up in time. I have had five inquests to attend this week - but the lawsuit against the nurse is not until March 4th - but I wish it were over.

Miss Sennett said that Louie Trott was returning to Ilesha but where she got the news from I do not know. We have not heard that news yet! Whether Jonah is just thinking wishfully or not I don't know.

The work here is increasing with the dry season - it is very hot and dry now - and the nights are relatively cool. I have been on afternoons this week- but go onto nights this coming week with Roy on afternoons. Elizabeth has the week relatively free, though the children's ward is a colossal task.

Office work is up to date I'm glad to say - there is little to be done there for Andrew so it should be a fairly straight forward change over. Do hope you are all well - with Andrew's imminent return my spirits are high though rather tired in body. Shall be glad when Synod is over and I can have a rest.

Love to you all, David,

Wesley College Ibadan, Jan 22nd '58

Thank you for you letter which was very welcome. I had just written to you before I received it, and now another week is over, during which we have seen David again.

I could not be sure that he would be able to get away for Synod, but was delighted when he called in yesterday afternoon on his way to Lagos. To our surprise there were five people in the Ilesha contingent, so Margaret Day and I had good company for tea and we were a very happy crowd. David was in good form, Andrew was with him and Jean too. You will have heard that they travelled straight up from the boat on Saturday and so they had no time for shopping. They left the children with Beryl yesterday and Jean is having a mornings shopping and returning today. David is coming through on his way back tomorrow, but hopes to return to spend the weekend with us.

Unfortunately Peter was not at his brightest because we had both just developed colds with runny noses and Peter had just woken from a hot and heavy sleep. He is more himself today and we hope to be quite better when David comes again. My report from the clinic on Tuesday was quite satisfactory and this leisurely life is suiting me. I feel a lot less weary now than I did over Christmas.

No doubt you have heard that Daisy Rowlands baby has arrived - another boy. A cable was received at Ilesha with the news of another arrival. Aileen Morleys baby, a girl, to be called Ruth, both are well.

I was very interested indeed to hear of the house at Worcester Park, and to see Michael's plan and read the description. I am sure that as soon as you come to accept it as your own and to see your furniture in it, you will forget all other dream houses and even the few disadvantages of this one and be delighted with its very many good points. It would appear to be in good condition and although a great deal of money, there should not be as much to spend on it as there might have been on a cheaper house. Looking forward to hearing more about it.

With love, Margaret

1/2/58

Saturday evening, and a few minutes to spare before going to the Pearsons' for chop, so I thought that I would get the letter started.

Margaret is well and no signs yet of anything happening - the Rowlands came up today and brought news that she was well and Peter also and tomorrow I hope to go down in the afternoon and stay there until the baby comes - it is due on Tuesday.

Things are more or less handed over to Andrew and I have got the accounts done and the WACMR account completed for January, so can leave everything tidy with a clear conscience.

Glad to have your letter this week with the excellent news of Ken Parker. We must keep the date free so that we can slip in at the back of the chapel. I am so pleased that it is at Rivercourt - I wonder if Ralph Butler will be invited?

Sorry to hear the house palaver is not yet settled - perhaps your minds will become adjusted to it in time despite the smaller rooms. If it isn't settled by the time we get home I shall be able to join in the hunt.

Ibadan was very hot indeed - most depressingly so, but a letter from Margaret tells me that it has got a bit cooler - I am so glad because it really was most trying and the Day's house is the wrong way round for the prevailing breeze, which makes it worse.

On Monday we went shopping and bought a number of things - but most significant material for new curtains and cushion covers and a new colour scheme. The ones I got in 1953 are finished - material doesn't last long out here - so we bought this stuff in order to enter it in our last years house account which is in a healthy state, but we shall not make up curtains or cushion covers until our next tour. On Monday night we went out to dinner with the Boshiers and had a nice evening, though we were all very tired.

I gave Peter his second TAB injection on Sunday evening and he woke at 2.30am and didn't get back to sleep again - a bad night. However he picked up and was quite a lot better by Tuesday, the Boshiers also had a bad night on Sunday. Their baby, David, is teething and they were up most of the night and so we didn't stay long on Monday evening and all turned in early.

On Tuesday morning I went with Margaret to the clinic, saw Dr. Lawson and all was well and in the afternoon returned here to find all well. I had kept busy the last few days, largely office work and not ward and am thinking now of things to pack for Ibadan tomorrow. Margaret wants her button box and one or two other things, which I must gather together and this time I must not forget my toilet things as I did last time.

Peter has a few more words and is very fast on his feet and climbs with agility! He still remains quite small bless him. I have missed them but if all is well we shall be together again soon

Hope all is well with you, love from us both, David

PS The Morleys would like you to let them know when the baby comes, 36 Mill Road, E Denton, Newcastle on Tyne

Wesley College, Ibadan, 9.2.58

Another Sunday is here - and we are still in status quo! Margaret is keeping very well, but we shall be glad when something begins to happen. Peter is in fine fettle - very lively and we are able to distinguish new words in his vocabulary almost every day. When he wants a second helping he says 'please' and points to what he would like - he really is most engaging. He goes off when we are not looking, for long walks around this compound. The other day we followed him at a distance unbeknown to him and he did not seem at all fearful, trotting along. Whether he intended to return to the house or not we don't know because he saw us at the point he should have made tracks back to the house.

Christopher, the Day's eldest sometimes attempts to take it out on Peter, but by and large it has been a happy week. Charles and Margaret are in good form though Charles feels a bit left out of things at the moment. There is now United Methodist and Anglican theological training but it is at Melville Hall the Anglican college and as Charles lives here he feels a bit out of touch also. However it is not very long before they go home and at the moment they are wondering where they will be. They have had a number of invitations but nothing that 'rang a bell', so it looks as though stationing committee will place them somewhere.

I arrived in Ibadan last Sunday evening and then Margaret and I went to the college chapel here for the evening service. Monday morning we did some shopping and then Tuesday went to see Mr. Lawson who was quite satisfied with things.

On Thursday evening we drove out with Margaret Day and Christopher to the University Botanical Gardens. They are most interesting though not very extensive, with many tropical shrubs, rather than flowers. Perhaps next tour we shall call and get some cuttings to put in because they are happy to supply them at 6d each.

Enid turned up here on Friday, she has come for the weekend to stay with a Sister Tutor friend of hers at University College Hospital and brought down mail including Michael's letter to me. Hilda Porter also looked in to see us, she seems to have had a very good time at Ilesha. She has had a talk with Enid, who is now again undecided whether to return or not. I am sorry that it has all been raked up again - much better to have left it as it was I feel, though our chances of getting another Sister Tutor are remote.

The other day we mapped out our furlough time roughly It is not easy to do at this distance, but May meetings occur as soon as we are home almost. We are booked to sail on March 27th on the 'Winnebar' due in at Tilbury or Dover on 11th April. We would send you a cable or you could enquire at Elder Dempster's London Office.

We should spend about a week at Rivercourt, then to Liverpool, returning to Rivercourt for the May meetings about the end of April I expect. Then comes my deputation 10-19th May. Ken's wedding 24th May, and Layman's Swanwick 29th May to 2nd June.

Then in June or so we thought we would travel north beginning with Layman's Swanwick, calling at Matlock then up to Yorkshire for a while possibly Hull then over to Liverpool and stay there some weeks, returning to London in August to be present to assist in the big move and having helped with shelves flooring to which I am much looking forward.

Incidentally to return to the secondhand car - is there not a scheme whereby a reputable firm will buy it back after six months and what about an examination by the AA? I think also we should be wise to become temporary members of the AA I think it is 10/6 for overseas visitors. Well time and space gone.

We look forward immensely to your letters and to hear how you all are.

Love to you all, David

Wesley College, Ibadan, 13.2.58

Thursday evening - the baby arrived about 4.30pm. I don't know the exact time. I will send a cable in the morning, which should reach you before this does.

We have had rather a worrying time since the infant was due (4th) as each day late seemed to make it more like last time and then on Tuesday this week there were signs that things were happening so I took Margaret in about 9pm. However after a sedative she seemed to settle too much and Mr. Lawson said she could go home on Wednesday afternoon - so I went and fetched her at that time yesterday.

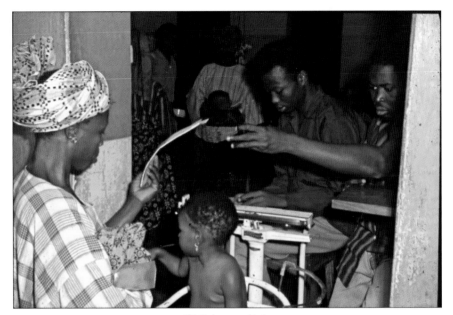

Childrens clinic

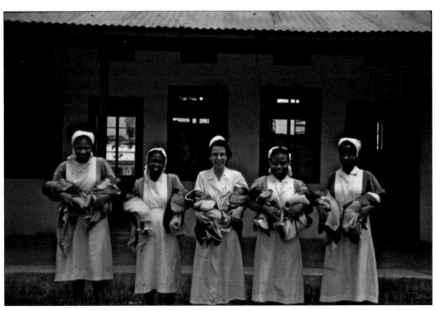

Sister Marion Lethbridge with Midwives

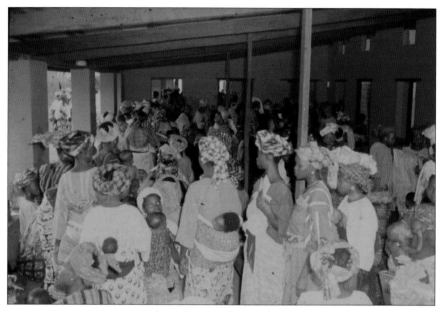

Imesi under fives clinic

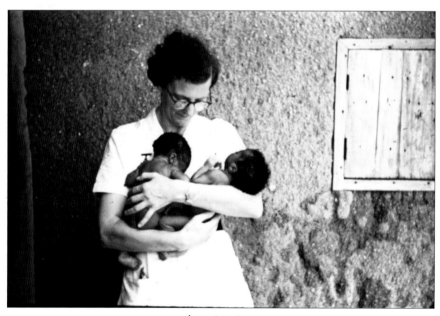

Imesi twins

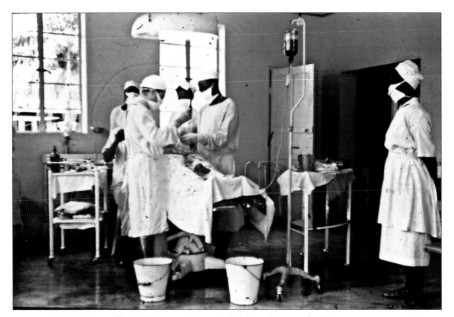

David operating with blood transfusion

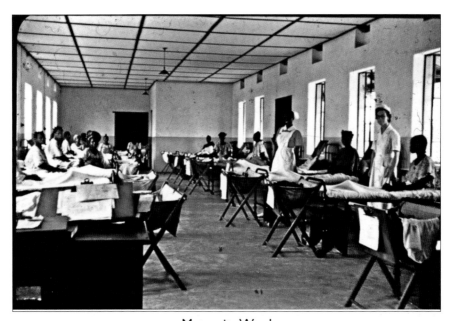

Maternity Ward

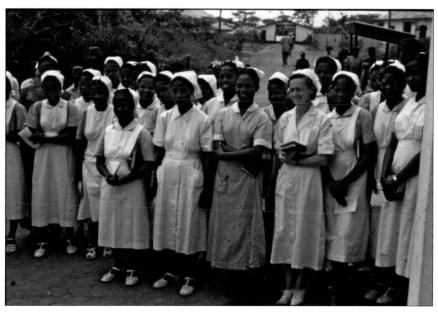

Sister Blake with nurses

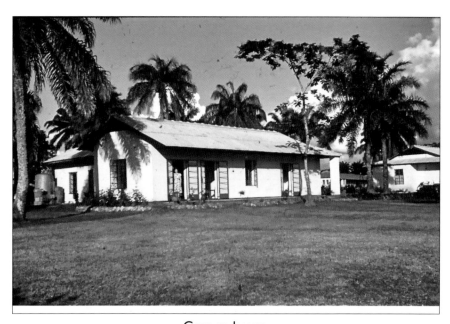

Cannon house

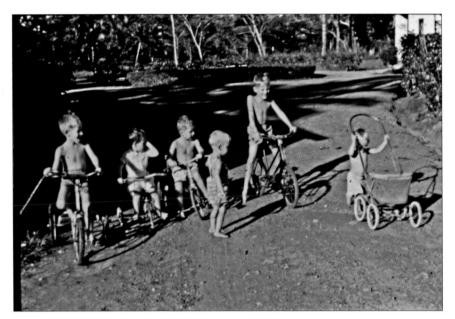

The doctors children

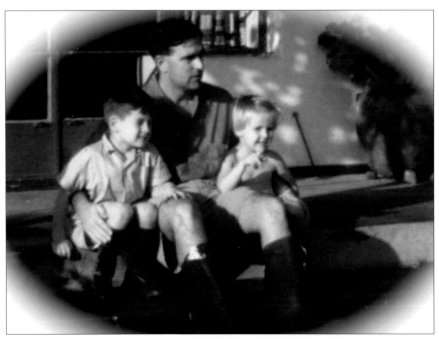

David, Peter and Elizabeth (must be wet season note the boots!)

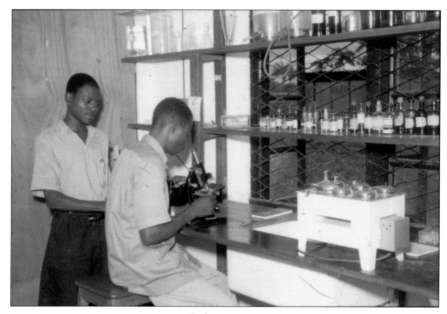

Laboratory

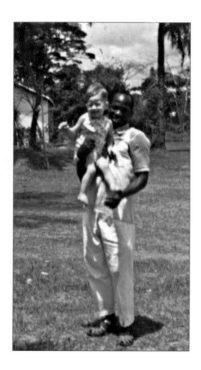

William with Peter

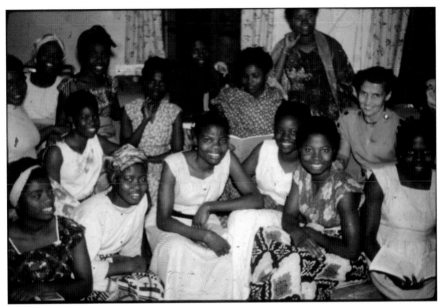

Nurses Friday group with Jean Pearson

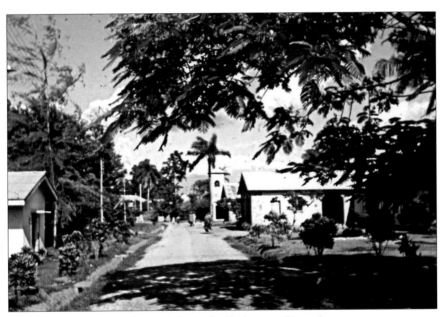

Hospital drive Stella Leony Chapel

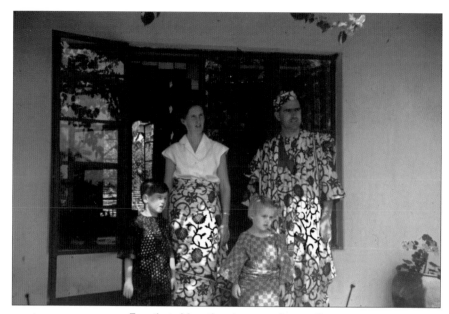

Family in Yoruiba dress at farewell

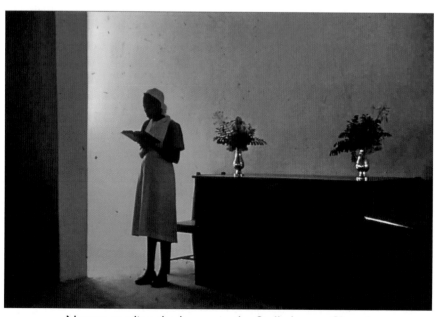

Nurses reading the lesson in the Stella Leony Chapel

However at 4.30am this morning painful contractions occurred again so we crept out of the house and went over to the hospital. I rang at 11 this morning to enquire and they said she was in labour, so I planned to go at visiting time this evening.

However Mr. Lawson himself rang about 4.30am and said I had a baby daughter and she had red hair like Peter!

She had almost normal delivery with a little help at the end in order not to endanger the scar from the caesarean she had with Peter. I rather think if they had not been quick she would have got the baby out first!

I went round this evening. Margaret was still in the delivery room, so I put on a mask and shoes and went in to see her. She is very well indeed and very, very happy - though being a bit sick with the injection, which they gave her. However it will wear off before tomorrow.

Elizabeth Margaret Cannon looked well too - gingery hair and seemed very similar to Peter to me, though I didn't see much of her 7lbs 6oz unwashed but as pink as pink. I didn't stay long- and will go back again tomorrow evening at visiting time.

I must get the cables off first thing in the morning and then set about getting a birth certificate and put on Margaret's passport.

Whilst writing this I put a call through to Ilesha to let them know, they all seemed very pleased. With Ruth Morley that makes three girls on the compound and six boys. They all seem to be well there and in no hurry to have me back, which is very nice. I think Margaret will be in for about eight days as a minimum so we shall have to see and then it is only six weeks today before we sail and so we have quite a bit to get through yet! Love to you all from the four of us

With love from us all, David

Saturday evening, 15.2.1958

All is quiet, so I have decided to try to finish this tonight, whilst Peter is asleep! The day seems so full I cannot get anything done.

By the time I am writing this you should have received the cable I sent off yesterday morning. Sometimes I fear there is a bit of a delay before they are telegraphed from this end. I was in again this evening, Margaret is really very well and Elizabeth seems to be a contented baby so far, very little crying and feeding well and really rather bonny! Her hair is black - not ginger as previously mentioned!

Margaret is in a ward, about fourteen altogether all the others being Nigerian and one or two quite ill. Every thing is beautifully appointed and of the most modern design - there can be few hospitals in the world to compare.

Mr. Lawson has been most kind and attentive and all the staff very pleasant. They have not had many European patients in this department I think because

321

Mr. Lawson only takes in those with some unusual condition.

Both Margaret and I are very thrilled to have a daughter. Although we didn't really mind and I have always appreciated a brother. A little girl is quite an innovation in a family in which boys predominate! We are very pleased indeed, Margaret especially wanted a little girl.

I have just sent off a letter to the Methodist Recorder with the notice of Elizabeth's arrival- with the proviso that they have not already received one- there is no point in having it in twice.

In six weeks we shall be on our way home - it seems almost too good to be true. It will be rather a hectic trip I fear Peter is up to no end of mischief and I have my hands full at the moment and certainly will have on the boat.

He is off like a shot, trotting along, climbing through the large rain gutters we have, running down to see the Boshiers and then over to the College. Every vehicle is looked at and cars and lorries so named. Today whilst in the town shopping we saw an engine and tender which elicited 'coo' it is the first one he has ever seen.

William is here and he is doing the daily wash and iron of Peter's things and mine but the rest falls to me. Peter is eating more now than he has recently and I am sure he is putting on weight. He misses Margaret and occasionally a bit fretful. I am trying to introduce the idea of baby to him. I hope he accepts her without difficulty, I think he is young enough to do so. One thing has occurred to me and that is fireguards. Peter has no experience of fires at all and I wondered if something could be perhaps borrowed to put round the fireplace in the front room.

We are very glad to have your letter sent on from Ilesha with all its news. Have had a letter from Auntie Ruth asking me to speak at her Garden Party - so will probably fix up an early Saturday in June and we could combine it with a family visit. Looking forward so much to being home again. Love to you all from us all, David

Ibadan, 22.2.568

Sunday evening and Peter has just gone to bed, Margaret is bathing and Elizabeth is sleeping though due for a feed in a few minutes time. I shall go over to the College service in a few minutes also.

Well once again we are a family - now four! Margaret came out of hospital on Friday morning, and has remained well, though naturally finds the stairs a bit much so I am hoping that I shall be able to give quite a bit of time at home to give a hand - nappies seem to be very thick on the field at the moment. Elizabeth has had a good day today and an excellent night last night, though yesterday she was very unsettled. However today she has been as good as gold. Peter also has been good, and loves to look at 'baby' but he seems to poke rather hard with his finger! He seems to have accepted Elizabeth quite well though he has been a bit more 'clingy' than usual.

Tomorrow we hope to get back to Ilesha and when we are once more in our own home we should get settled down into a regular routine. Charles and Margaret Day have been very kind and hospitable.

We are a bit out of touch with Ilesha - no communication of any sort for ten days or so, so we shall have to see how they are faring on our return. We were a bit worried about Peter's cot. It is too long to fit in the Morleys car and only the hospital ambulance, or the lorry is long enough. However a friend of the Days was travelling through today and has taken it up plus two of our cases so we shall manage quite well as far as luggage goes tomorrow.

We were very pleased to have your letters this week ,yours to me was forwarded from Ilesha and glad to hear of your delight over Elizabeth's arrival. It won't be long now before we are packing to come home - four weeks on Friday I think it is, then two weeks voyage to arrive on 11th April.

Do hope Stanley's finger is healing up.

The Days are wondering where they will be going to on their return to England. They fully expect to be placed by the stationing committee. So far Charles has been in the southwest, apart from the Seaman's Mission in the East End of London I think.

It is now after service - Frank Longley was preaching. Supper is complete - Margaret has got ready for bed and given Elizabeth her 10pm feed (last night she slept from 10-6). Long may it continue! Love to you all from us all, David

PS Does Gladys know about Elizabeth's arrival?

2.3.58

Sunday evening. Margaret has just gone along to chapel. I am baby sitting for both our and the Pearson's family. Peter is asleep - Elizabeth woke a few minutes ago, but having been changed she seems to have dropped off again. It has been a sweltering day 95F in the shade this afternoon and at 6.30 as I put Peter to bed it was still 90F and with a high humidity. We are all feeling a bit played out. As we rested this afternoon we were perspiring so much we had to cover the pillows with towels. However three weeks more and we shall be virtually packed up if all is well, ready for our boat on the 27th. We were glad to receive your letter on Wednesday and to learn that all was well. I had one from Auntie Florence too earlier in the week so feel to be fully informed. Margaret has had a number of letters and some wee gifts for Elizabeth that are most acceptable.

We left Ibadan on Monday morning last and had a good journey up here with only one stop to give Peter a drink - Elizabeth slept in the carrycot all the way.

Everyone seemed glad to see us and gave us an excellent welcome - the nurses especially seemed very pleased to think we had a daughter. We had lunch with the Pearsons' and then after a rest settled back into our own home again. It was two months since Margaret left!

Margaret is getting stronger each day I'm glad to say - and we have managed to get a girl to come in for an hour each morning to wash through, boil and put things through the wringer, the nappies and Peter's clothes, which is a great help. William knows her mother and although she does not speak or understand English she is quick on the uptake and does very well indeed. It saves Margaret standing for hours, which is a good thing. She will help until we go home I expect. Next tour Margaret will be unable to leave the house to help with the dispensing and so is thinking about doing our own cooking and hiring an electric cooker such as the Days have. William has not been very satisfactory of late and it may be that he is wanting a change. Many factors are involved such as whether the hospital goes onto the town electricity supply and so on.

On Thursday Elizabeth was two weeks old so we had a weighing session and she was just 8 lbs. having put on 10oz in the week since leaving hospital. Peter on the other hand has only gained 3oz in two months. Apparently Bryan Pearson was the same at his age. The heat takes away appetite completely. Peter is very active and very well and is beginning to understand quite a lot. He is being difficult about his midday meal though and eats very little of it which is most distressing - I expect it is just a phase and when he gets in the colder weather his appetite will improve.

We shall be bringing our pram home I expect, crated up. Shall be glad to take the Rivercourt Missionary Supper, but must make it the last time. Spent one morning this week taking photos for deputation! I hope they satisfactory.

Wonder how the decoration is getting on! I trust Peter doesn't attempt any murals! Hope you are all well. We are all very fit if a trifle hot!

Much love to you all from the four of us. David

8.3.58

Saturday evening and a few minutes peace so I thought I would start this letter. We were very pleased to receive yours on Wednesday. By now the decorators will have finished and order will have been restored once again and no doubt Stanley will be coming home. Incidentally - a question to Michael - should I bring some of my tools home for the flooring and the roof or will there be enough at home? Would it be worthwhile lagging tanks and the roof whilst we are at it to prevent paternal excursions into the loft? Are there any open parks around the new house - what type of shops?

We have had quite a good week however and Elizabeth does very well and sleeps until the next feed is due, usually though she still needs one at 2am.

Margaret is stronger now and well on with the sorting of drawers as a prelude to packing, which we shall start in a few days. There will not be any need to pack everything away as last time so it is not such a task. Linen and so forth must all be washed and dried thoroughly before being put in airtight trunks to be kept here.

Peter is up to mischief the whole time - and 'helps' with the drawers taking everything out and scattering them over the whole house. He is keeping well but still not eating very much. It is not that he doesn't like the food, but he seems to be in a sort of a negative phase. We hope it will soon pass as meal times tend to be a bit noisy. I think that when he can talk more and explain himself, he will settle down.

I have had an interesting week catching up with the malaria slides and working out the results for our second paper. I think that I shall have shown that the giving of anti-malarials to women in pregnancy will give them bigger babies - more able to survive the neonatal period. Numbers at the moment are small but in the next few months should increase.

Next week I have to go to Ibadan for the court case against a nurse who has broken her Bond - I am not looking forward to it in the slightest and shall be very glad when it is over. After next week there is only one full week before we sail on the 27th. We shall travel to Lagos on the 25th as there are one or two purchases to be made before our journey.

The Rowlands are still with us but hope to go soon. A letter from the Wrights at Nailsea - they are expecting a fourth baby on August 4th!

Looking forward to being with you before very long - love from us all, David

16.3.58

Sunday again and no doubt you are writing your last letter to us for some while. A week today we shall be in the throes of packing - sorting is now complete and tomorrow we shall get out the trunks.

It has been our coffee morning and folk have come and gone, leaving the clearing up which is also complete. Margaret and Peter are going down to feed the hens, leaving me a minute or two to start the letter. The colour film is back - most of the transparencies are good - one or two good ones of Peter and Margaret with a glimpse of Elizabeth and some quite good ones of the hospital for deputation.

I have had a note about my conference deputation. I am in St. Albans, Bedford, High Wycombe, Berkhamstead, and Dunstable in the ten days! Rather too far to return home after evening meetings I fear. I have not had the programme of meetings yet but there can't be much overlapping.

This week has been a busy one - Margaret is finding the clearing out tiring - Elizabeth is now 8lbs. 12oz. having gained 8oz in the week and she looks well. Peter is very well and eating much better than previously. At coffee this morning there were seven children, and Peter insisted on sitting at the picnic table with them and ate two biscuits and drank his squash with the minimum of attention.

Last Sunday evening I went to chapel where Ray was preaching - an excellent service and then I have been on night duty this week- fortunately a good week, with two nights completely free of calls. On Monday afternoon I motored down to Ibadan, staying with the Days, for this court case. Unfortunately very little happened, I did not have to appear but have to go down again this coming Friday for Court on Saturday. It is an awkward time - just three days before we go down to Lagos.

The weather had been very hot indeed - temperatures over 90 in the shade every afternoon- though we had one shower which cooled it down one day.

It drops to 80 in the shade we are grateful! No doubt in a few weeks we shall be wishing we had brought a little of the warmth with us.

We are seriously thinking of having an electric cooker next tour. Having chopped up some logs to burn on our stove to heat the coffee has given me even more thoughts on the matter. It would be so much more convenient just to turn the knobs and get the heat! Our wood-burning stove is in a very poor way. It must have been on the go for a number of years and the grating is broken where the fire goes, and the top is cracked so that smoke fills the kitchen which is therefore quite a depressing place to keep clean.

Peter is getting a great deal of pleasure from the car you sent him for Christmas with the toy dog that barks. I have had to repair it twice, but it is still going strong. Cars are his passion at the moment, he parks them and un-parks them and makes many noises appropriate to such manoeuvres

The Rowlands are still in the Morleys house, waiting to hear of a passage - very unsettling for them. They are going to Peterborough next September.

Hope you are all well and looking forward to seeing you soon —four weeks today we shall be with you! Love from us all, David

                                                                    24.3.58
Our postal strike now being over letters have come through - Father's, your's with Michael's notes. I have returned from the court case - my evidence was taken at last, so my mind is free from that concern

Car - If you think it a good idea to go to Boston for one it sounds an excellent idea to me. Our first week home is likely to be a very busy one - land Friday, then Sat and Sunday - followed by visit to the Mission House - must get a suit - welfare foods and so on, and to fit in a visit to Boston might be difficult.

If Michael and father are able to get up before our arrival I shall be very happy to leave the choice to you - a countryman type certainly would seem to be a good idea.

If you think that I ought to go with you we will try to fit it into the first week - A car that will sell well would be an excellent thing too! If I have to put down

£400 I shall want to pick it up again!

As I mentioned in yesterday's letter we shall be landed at St. Pancras Station and shall not require meeting at Tilbury but time and station would have to be ascertained from Elder Dempster's.

Our light luggage will consist of, we hope, two suitcases, two holdalls, two children and one dispatch case!

Packing is practically complete - just our overnight things to put in tomorrow morning and then we hope to get off about 10.30 to arrive Ibadan about 1pm for lunch and Elizabeth's feed and then to Lagos about 5.30pm

On Wednesday we have a bit of shopping to do I have a yellow fever inj. to get and one or two people to see and then to the boat for 8am on Thursday morning. Two stops only Takoradi and Freetown and then Tilbury.

Elizabeth is well, though watchful at the moment. Peter found a pot of baby cream and plastered his face thickly with it - he must have seen Margaret putting some on at some time! It was very difficult to get off.

I have sent off a colour film addressed to me at home and it has some of Peter if you care to open it when it arrives.

Love to you all from us all - It won't be very long now before we are together. Love from us all, David

TSS Winnipeg, 27.3.58

We are safely aboard - about one day out from Lagos and nearing Takoradi where I hope to post this.

We had no trouble with customs and were almost the first on board. The cabin is small and incredibly hot. There is an electric fan, which we keep on constantly but despite the noise we all slept well.

There is a very fresh breeze and a good deal on movement on the boat. We have managed to keep going so far, we have to, with Peter to look after!

He is beginning to settle down and he has done very well so far and Elizabeth seems to enjoy the movement of the boat. It is a friendly boat - with only 100 passengers altogether so we should get to know them fairly well in time.

The Jonahs, both very tired are on board, the Hale's, with two children are coming home for the last time, the Edmonds returning from Oran - the first time. She is expecting a baby in about eight weeks I should say, they don't look very fit, either of them, and Gladys Clarke, a senior missionary from the Rural Training College, Asabar.

One snag is that children have separate mealtimes from the adults 7.30 - 12.00 - 5.30 and ours are 8.30 - 1.00 - 7.30 so far I have taken Peter down and have seemed to spend most of my time in the dining saloon. The food is good as usual with a wide selection and one feels that if the boat would stay still for a while one could enjoy it more.

With washing, ironing, feeding Margaret is kept very busy, but at the moment having a rest after the 10am feed and as Peter is also resting I have an opportunity to write this. The boat is rolling pretty heavily and a strong wind keeps flapping the paper up.

Looking forward to seeing you all on the 11th - I think we arrive in the morning. Our love to you all from us all, David

RRS John Biscoe, 4th March 1958

Dear Auntie and Uncle,

Thank you very much for your letter. I wish that there was time to write long letters to everyone, and especially to Mother and Dad and to you, but there does not seem to be. But I have asked them at home to pass on all the news to you. The main part of it is in diaries, which I have sent to Iris and asked her to send home later. It seems the best way because it avoids forgetting things. The only fault is that I could not avoid writing it to somebody and that makes them sometimes rather personal!

I do hope that the new baby has arrived alright. I've heard nothing to the contrary so I assume it has. I wonder how little Peter is. If he is as fit and bouncy as Dr Pearson's children there won't be much to worry about. I am very sorry to hear that David is having such a worrying time in Ilesha. What a great man Dr. Craddock must be to go out as he did. The MMS must be most concerned over it all. The whole thing is a thorn in my conscience anyway. Here, life is interesting and new, tough and varied, but there is nobody to love and to help. The other fellows seem to be such a well-adjusted and self sufficient lot.

I am glad that you had such a good holiday last year. As you say Stanley is a very well travelled young man by now. I hope there'll be time to write him, but I am much afraid there won't (last minute rush as usual). Anyway I send him my love and I very much look forward to meeting him again and going over the years. The natural history of this place will interest him enormously - there are whales swimming round and under the ship often when we are at anchor and seals and birds in abundance.

Thank you for news of Michael and his work. He would be very interested in problems of man sledging rations and of their packing, and I look forward to discussing it. I think I have at last got through my emotional torment and am hooked and landed well ahead of Micky! I wonder how he is managing. He is the only surviving mysogonist - though none of the others proved very sincere anyway.

Both you and Mother and Dad seem to be in the midst of housing problems. I gather you are staying in the home counties, which I suppose will be closer to family and friends - though you must have friends all over the country having left in so many parts. I do hope you find somewhere soon, and I do look forward to seeing it. There is so much about coming home that I look forward to - I shall be very, very glad to see it again. One thing is, of course getting married and I don't think I shall delay long. Thank you for having Iris over, and for looking after her.

About the money to the Anniversary - as I told uncle before I left I did arrange it with the bank but I did not really want people to know about it. It takes all the merit out of giving somehow. It was only because I was coming to prize money so much (the old false gods but how true that is) and I am afraid I still do, but at least it is a gesture to give some of it away. I spend so much more than that on myself anyway and I save so much too. It is really only a years collection in a lump.

When I read back I don't seem to have told you much of what life is like, and of what we do, but as I said earlier its all in the diaries. Because they tend to be written to Iris and a little personal I have told her to vet them and pass them on if they are OK!

I am sorry that grandma is having more trouble from her complaint. Please give her my love. And I send my love to you all and to David and Margaret, Stanley and Michael.

I so often think of the very happy times I had with you all and look forward very much to coming home.

With much love, Henry

FOURTH TOUR, 1958-60

2.10.58

Just a note, to let you know that we have arrived, and safely in Ilesha. All appears to be good order.

Monday in Lagos we spent shopping with a visit to the beach in the afternoon. Andrew arrived about 10.30 and did some hospital shopping. He seemed in very good form and in the evening Margaret and I and Andrew had dinner with Mr. Barnes, my old house master during which, he called me Cannon!

On the Tuesday we were delayed in starting as Andrew. who had a broadcast to take, and then more shopping so we did not leave until 1.15 and called at WACMR on the way out seeing the Gosslings and Dr. Macnamarra.

A good journey then to Ibadan, where we called and had tea with Beryl awaiting her baby and so on to Ilesha about 5.15. We were warmly welcomed, supper for the children in the Pearsons' and to bed. We had dinner and a talk, the Morleys coming in to coffee also at the Pearsons'.

Wednesday and today we have spent unpacking - everything has arrived safely - the record player working though again a little troublesome to start.

The children have been very good, Peter has slept through both nights a record! They are each in their own cots in their own room now

Peter too has begun to feed himself again, though his appetite is not yet back to its full strength.

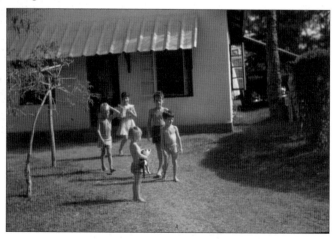

Peter and Elizabeth

A phone call this morning from Roy in Ibadan informed us that Beryl had had a baby boy - but no details - the girls on the compound are still at a premium.

It is raining again, it has been very wet since we arrived, but apparently it has been a dry wet season on the whole so far. All here are well, Elsie and Marion back at work again. Our love to you all, David

PS - Michael - I left the electric fittings for Peter's garage on the garage shelf. Could you send them please?

5.10.58

Sunday is here and we have been in our Ilesha home about five days and are once more settling down.

It is almost lunchtime and Peter has climbed up into his high chair (one we have borrowed), Elizabeth sounds too as if she is ready and Margaret is just putting the finishing touches to the meal. William is in good form - if anything a little over helpful I gave washman the trousers of my grey palm-beach suit to wash as they were marked. Unbeknownst to me he gave them to William who boiled them with Omo! They are now dappled. The only solution is to dye the suit so we wonder if you can get a dye in a tin - grey and post it out to us. I should be most grateful.

Peter and Elizabeth have settled down very well and Peter is still sleeping through the night in his own cot - a great relief to us as you can imagine and is once again feeding himself. Last night David M. gave a children's film show. Michael P called for Peter, who in pyjamas and red slippers went hand in hand. M said he looked very sweet indeed. Apparently he was very good indeed and enjoyed the films immensely, calling out with great gusto when he saw a horse or other recognisable animal. Later in the evening we went to chop with the Morleys and had a very pleasant evening.

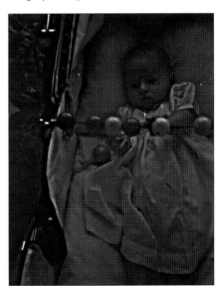

Elizabeth in pram

Today I have begun work and have taken over the female and maternity wards and am on duty this afternoon. I have been trying to get the hospital accounts settled up - but they are not yet balanced- I will continue this afternoon if all is well Roy is in Ibadan and Beryl still in UCH we have not heard anything from them at all yet, so do not know how big the baby is.

This morning we had a call to say the ambulance had broken down in the town, so Andrew and I had to go out in the lorry and tow it back which we managed without mishap.

Our vegetable garden is in good form - Jean must have given quite a lot of time to it. We have lettuce, radish, cauliflower, beans and onions ready now. The hens are a bit disappointing so M is killing off the older ones for the pressure cooker. We had one today which was quite nice, and we intend to get six pullets from the University farm in about three weeks time.

The weather is very warm- apparently it is just getting warm again after the cool season, but we have had one or two very heavy storms since we arrived.

Time and space are gone. We look forward to hearing from you and how you got on at Scarborough and Hull and how the garden goes.

We are all very well indeed and send our love to you all, David

12.10.58

Actually it is Saturday night - almost 10pm. Margaret is tidying up her sewing box - I have been reading some obstetrics - the children are fast asleep so an excellent opportunity to start this letter. Tomorrow morning I hope to get to Otapete and the rest of the time I am about, Peter will no doubt be keeping me employed!

We received two letters this week from you - one on Monday and the second last Friday, so we are well up to date with your news. We note that Stoneleigh has become your choice - by inference if not by direct note! Glad to hear of light fittings, has the new piano stool come yet? Have you managed to dispose of any of the furniture that you had in mind?

By this time you will have got well tidied up and got the kitchen cupboards settled to your liking.

Your note re the Ludlows and the dispensary van put up my blood pressure for a bit but it settled down again in due course! We are all very well. Peter and Elizabeth are sleeping much better and when they wake up in the morning are content to lie in their cots until M goes in. We are up well before seven so it is not much of a wait usually though. We are profoundly relieved that Peter is sleeping through. We have had better nights than we have had for months!

Margaret is keeping very well and beginning to feel that the house is getting tidier - it does take a while to get through all the drawers and cupboards.

With the new electricity supply we are able to use our electric kettle and toaster and we have had a shelf and electric plug put in the kitchen to accommodate them. It makes things much easier. Unfortunately William broke our water filter a few days ago by putting in boiling water, so we have had to get a new one (aluminum) which has cost our house allowance £5.5.0. However it is virtually indestructible which is a great point.

Roy, Beryl and the baby arrived back from Ibadan yesterday. They all seem well the baby apparently very like Roy.

In the hospital we have been very busy and I seem to have had numbers of operations in the afternoon. In addition a lorry accident and a tree which fell on a house during a storm produced twelve post mortem examinations to be carried out which took a lot of time. However I have got last years accounts sorted and have completed the weeks accounts today so am fairly straight there.

Peter is settling down well and often 'plays with boys' usually in the role of spectator at the moment - he looks very small compared with Michael and Roger. However he has taken to Andrew and Jean, David and Aileen and will go off with them if they ask him - say to the town in the car which he enjoys very much. He is still rather difficult over food, but is eating more.

Elizabeth, bless her, eats anything - is absolutely colossal and tried to crawl today for the first time.

Do hope all is well with you. We are all very fit and have settled down once again. Love to you all from us all, David

18.10.58

Saturday night, children are asleep, Margaret is checking the house inventory and there are no urgent calls to do at the Hospital so I thought it a good plan to start this letter.

Yours arrived on Friday and we were very glad indeed to receive it and learn how you all are. Before I forget - did the photos I took the last few days come out? If so should be pleased to see one or two of them in time.

We were very glad to hear of the garden and shall be interested to hear what Mr. Pearson has to say about the fruit trees. It must be quite thrilling to be thinking about stocking the pool too, it should be ready about now, does it still hold water? Most interested to hear that Mr. Sackett is retiring. There has been talk for a long time but this is the first real news. I wonder if Bill Spry will be his successor.

This week has been a very busy one. I have been on nights (tonight is my last night) and Andrew and family went on local leave on Thursday so I have had the administration to do too.

Last Tuesday we had a 'Tramps supper' on the lawn of the Morley house. We all turned up as tramps. Margaret and I looked a very odd couple. I made a beard to wear - cotton wool dyed in blue/black ink - but it was more blue than black! Elsie was much the best and looked a real character!

A nice supper sitting round a camp-fire and then films - a selection from various film libraries in the country - a very happy evening. Wednesday night was my turn for fellowship, rather spoilt by two urgent admissions.

Friday night was fellowship - but we listened to the wireless talk by Dr. Collins

- head of Children' Dept. UCH Ibadan who was with David Morley at the time! I had an operation to do on a 3/12 old baby afterwards and Dr. Collins asked if he could assist - which he did - not often one is assisted by a professor - and an MD FRCP. He seemed quite pleased to do so.

Today he and David have gone to Ado to see Dr. Hare and are returning tomorrow evening - so we are down to Roy and myself at the moment. Roy spent all morning and half the afternoon operating so I have had a busy time.

Since I began writing a nurse has been to tell me two more patients are waiting - which makes five to see, so I had better go up and have a look and do the night round.

Now, Sunday evening. Last night it took a long time to get round the patients then straight to bed. An easy day today at home most of the day, and a walk with Peter as usual this evening.

Peter is developing rapidly and beginning to use quite long sentences with association of ideas. He is also learning to play with others and to take a few knocks, and a little to give some back. Elizabeth is still a very good baby though today she has not wanted her food and was sick after tea, though she appears well, it must be something she has sucked I expect. Apart from this they are both well and thriving. Peter seems very happy and sleeps all through, as Elizabeth has done the last few nights. So apart from hospital calls the nights have been better and this and next week there should be no hospital calls either.

We often think of you all and the garden and should love to be able to see you all. Love from us all, David

26.10.58

Friday was a very good day - two letters from home and the two dyes all by the same post. What an awful blow for the Parton family and Graham - I am sorry for them. I wonder what the trouble was?

Glad you had a good time at Stoneleigh - the ice seems to have been broken- but rather a trying operation for you.!

We were very glad to hear that a table has been bought - it sounds nice and we look forward to seeing it in due course. Shall be interested to hear how the copper beech came down.

About Marley tiles - the amount was £13.7.6 sent 9th August. Unfortunately the cheque was from a cheque book I have left at home, just where I don't know. I am sorry not to be more helpful. Incidentally have you seen Ilesha in the KO for October.

We have had a busy week. Andrew is still away but is due back on Wednesday back to work on Thursday, which will be good. They are travelling to Ibadan tomorrow I think, and will stay there two days before coming up.

Last Wednesday we went up on trek to Ikole - a very good trip each way Louie was very well and in good form. I had to do an operation for her on the Thursday morning, which was a pleasant break in routine. The children were very good indeed - we did both journeys without a break. We took William with us because Louie has two girls in the house, neither of whom is very good! It made a pleasant but busy break. On Thursday Mabel went down in the lorry to meet Sister Grant (Lilly) she did not arrive until Friday and they came up last night after a good journey. She has been almost a month at sea and is glad to have arrived on terra firma.

As it happened David M had managed a film show - Nigeria meets the Queen and there were quite a number of people present I am quite sure I am on the film - back view!

This morning I went to the service at Otapete and on arrival back was called to operate on one of our senior nurses - all went well however. Roy gave the anaesthetic. This afternoon was busy (I am on afternoons this week) and I was only home for half an hour for tea between 2.15 and 7.30pm!

Tonight we have both been to our chapel.

Peter is well and eating better than he was. Elizabeth thrives and makes Rohan look a very small baby though he has gained 12oz. this week and is now 9lbs. Margaret and I are both very well.

Our internal phone system is well under way, another two weeks should see it completed and another month for the nurses dining hall. Do hope all well at home.

Love from us all   David

2.11.58

Sunday afternoon and I have had a long rest and read - Margaret not so fortunate and at the moment she is getting tea ready. Peter is already sitting in his high chair waiting, baby is in the play pen playing with some 'toys' which Peter has given her - largely the less lethal kitchen implements!

We were very glad to receive your letter yesterday - so not late really even though posted on the Tuesday. We read with great interest of all your activities especially your getting into tow with Mr. Pearson and the Rotary luncheon for Father. Hope the clay disposal system works. Have you tiled the front of the lounge window? Shall be glad to see the photographs in due course. I am just finishing off the colour film I had in for our journey - I must get it in for processing very soon or it will not be very good.

We have had a quiet week in some ways. Andrew and family got back last Wednesday evening having had a very nice holiday. Unfortunately a suitcase with all the clothes for their second part of the holiday got sent up by mistake with Lilly Grant, so their few days at the University were somewhat marred by lack of suitable raiment! Apart from that they had a good time. It is very nice to have Andrew back to administer.

On Tuesday evening we had Lilly in to an evening meal - she comes from Sunderland- though her home now is in Houghton-le-Springs, and she went to school at Bede School - which strikes a cord, though rather a dim one. She knows St. Bedes Park very well, including the Manse as she did her midwifery at a Nursing Home very near there and looked after a minister's wife in that capacity. I think she will fit in very well and be less temperamental and upset than Mabel, who is in bed again this weekend with tummy upset.

Margaret took Fellowship on Wednesday very well. Thursday and Friday I coped with accounts and got the month completed in the books and the WACMR account off.

Yesterday was an easier day - in the afternoon after an emergency operation I took Elsie down to the Eltons (Peter came with us) to get her hair permed. It is the first time she has had a home perm and it seems to have turned out very well. In the evening we went out to dinner with Dorothea Taylor of the African Girls School. We had a nice time but the evening was brought to a conclusion by the house being struck by lightening - and a colossal explosion via the telephone which was shattered into remnants and all the lights went out! We were worried about the children so left and came back - they were both fast asleep.

The other big item is the completion of our phone system with 18 extensions in the hospital. This means I can ring up M and so forth and saves David running along with messages etc. Our telephone is in the bedroom beside the bed and we hope that it will save some excursions in the night. I am on night duty this week so we shall see.

We are all very well Peter is very active and is playing more with the other children. Elizabeth is eating well and although not putting on much weight seems very well, (18lbs 5oz). She is cutting another tooth, which will bring her total to five but she is still very contented and much the nicest baby on the compound!

Tomorrow is a welcome party for Lilly at the Sisters, which should be good fun if Mabel is better

Our love to Auntie Pop, Pop and Uncle Michael and Uncle Twink who Peter referred to last week, David

9.11.58

At the moment Peter is standing by my knee saying 'Auntie Pop', Pop, Auntie Pop, Pop as I told him to whom I am writing and he seems very pleased with himself. He has been to Sunday School (Jean's) for the first time and brought home a picture he has coloured. I fear there is no sign of budding artistic ability. Margaret has always kept those he has strictly under supervision, but one day this week he must have obtained a blue pencil from another house and when M came in, all round the play pen and on the wall are squiggles in blue crayon. When asked what he was doing he said 'showing baby' which was virtually unanswerable!

Both Peter and Elizabeth are in good form, Peter eating more and Elizabeth eating all that is put before her, and Margaret and I are well.

We are very glad indeed to get your letter on Friday - glad you had a good time at Tooting and had the day with the Pearsons' - a most interesting fact.

How did Thursday go? How was the Duchess of Gloucester? We are looking forward very much to hearing how things went in church, the PRESENTATION!

Is the beech tree completely down now? or has it only been trimmed? It will be exciting seeing the garden again in 1960 - and see what changes there are. The vegetables seem to have done very well on the whole. Is the motor mower still functioning or has the grass stopped growing?

The week has not been very special except for the dying of my trousers with the dye you sent out. The two tins (½ lb dry weight clothing each) only did the trousers but we shall also have to do the jacket - another two Dylon No. 54 please, will be required! Could you send them out? Sea mail will be adequate, airmail I feel is rather expensive. The trousers have done very well indeed, a grey similar to my Terylene trousers. We are very pleased indeed with them.

On Thursday evening the Sisters gave a party to welcome Lilly - quite nice - with a little music and dancing after dinner. Last night we had Roy and Beryl and Marion in to dinner in the evening. After the meal we played Table Croquet - and had a most enjoyable time with much noise and laughter.

Today has been easy as I am not on either afternoon or night duty - a pleasant break, though I had an excellent week last week on nights - the telephone is most useful and I do not have to get out of bed at all.

This morning Andrew introduced Lilly at Otapete so it is my turn to go next week again. This evening after service we are having hymn singing in the sisters house a most interesting revival of an old custom!

Next week looks like being a busy one centred round Thursday. Margaret Woodland arrives in Lagos and is being met by Aileen who is going down to do some Christmas shopping. It is our medical meeting here and we are having the Orthopedic surgeon from UCH Ibadan to speak and we shall have to entertain several Doctors from other hospitals. In addition Joan Ryeland is coming to Ilesha on her job and is staying with the Pearsons' on the Sunday. Incidentally Janis is coming up for Christmas when she will be staying with the Sisters I believe.

We are trying in a gentle way to brew some ginger beer, starting with BCL, dried yeast. The plant has been on the go almost two weeks but does not look very active. Unfortunately I have forgotten the brewing recipe, and wonder if you would forward it in the next letter please. The rainy season is almost over now and it is already getting very hot in the afternoons

Do hope all is well with you all. Love from Margaret, Peter, Elizabeth and me

23.11.58

The oddest thing happened with your letter this week - the second one, addressed by Michael arrived on Wednesday - and the first addressed by you arrived on Saturday. Actually I have just noticed that his was posted last Sunday and the other on Monday, so the Monday one must just have missed a plane.

We were very glad to hear all the news- and to hear of gardening progress - the front must look very much cleared - have you done anything to the acacia trees and hedges on the very front?

The 'Friendship House' must have been a bit dampening and run at a loss judging by the supper!

We have made a note of the Wyatt's new address, and the same week we had received Margaret's uncle Harold's new address- so bungalows seem to be quite popular - they must have got on quite quickly with the Wyatts, it will be very interesting to hear how they settle down. Any news of Henry's return? I saw that the relief boat had sailed and wondered if Henry would be returning with it.

We have tried the GB recipe from memory without much success - absolutely flat with a film of growth in the bottle - no doubt a secondary culture. We tasted it but it was quite unpalatable. However the plant continues and looks much like the one at home, so hope with the correct formula for a better result.

Very thrilled to hear of the clarinet I look forward to a recital when the theory is completed!

The week has been busy but quite ordinary apart from yesterday. Margaret has started on the curtains for the house and we hope to get them finished before very long but the new cushion cases will take a bit longer. I have started reconstructing the garage for Peter from Father Christmas, which is quite fun and I hope to get the roof made from a piece of five or three ply which has recently become available here.

Yesterday was our November Medical committee in Ibadan. Elsie, Andrew and I were up early (breakfast at six) and away by 6.30 arriving at Wesley College about 8.40. It seems quite different there without the Days- the Todds are in their house.

We had quite a good Committee, Jonah and Bill Mann were there. The unusual feature was that - after the committee Jonah asked Andrew and me to see him and he told us that the Church Missionary Society has asked if we would take over the Ado Ekiti hospital about 80 miles away. It was a bolt from the blue. I don't think we should have anything to do with it - but Andrew is not so definite.

After the Committee we went to the shops, Elsie buying 150 yards of sheeting! So home about 3.40 having a picnic lunch en route. At 5.30 we set out for Imesi where a party to welcome Margaret and to mark the first electricity in the village was held. A very noisy do. I left about 7.40 to bring back the two Pearsons' and the two Morley boys who had gone to see the bonfire.

Last night for the first time Peter said his prayers - 'Gosh Mummy, Gosh Daddy, Gosh baby, Gosh Peter, happy Day Amen'!

Tonight Roy and Beryl are having Rohan Christened at Otapete, much excitement. Tomorrow is our Hospital Management Committee so we have our hands full. I have got to get a stencil cut yet for it.

We are all very well. Christmas will be here very soon!

Love to you all from all   David

30.11.58

A very hot and stuffy afternoon, the children are still resting, though Elizabeth is making 'waking up' noises, so it won't be long before they are about again.

We were very pleased indeed to receive your letter and to learn all your news, yesterday. I should think that having a Sunday morning at church in the West End did more to assure your selves of less responsibility than anything else! It seems to have been a very pleasant trip. It does sound thrilling to hear of lots of apples and pears. Are they keeping well and how have you managed to store them?

Is the roof loft used much or not? There will not be the need at the moment.

I wonder who is to be the new Head Master at Kingswood School? I know that Bill Storey was going to apply for the headship, but if a scientist has got the job it can't be him I think.

We are all well here - Peter though has had some unpleasant bites on his legs which have made him a bit off colour, but he is really quite well.

Elizabeth too is flourishing - still looks very much as she did as a baby - but is now able to crawl after a fashion - more pulling herself along with her arms. She seems to get much dirtier than Peter used to. Margaret and I are very well - have had rather a hectic week - I have been on afternoon duty and last night went on night duty.

Andrew went up to Afon on Friday returning Saturday, taking Joan Ryland who is still with us - they had a good but tiring trip. David M went to Ibadan on Tuesday and up to Kaduma on Wednesday and back here on Friday so we have had his work to do also.

Margaret Woodland is settled in, but does not seem very happy - feeling that the job is too much for her. She will need very careful managing to get through the tour satisfactorily - it is a bit early to feel under the weather!

Betty Simms has gone - flying from Ibadan last Friday. She is going to stay in Rome for some days on the way home.

We are considering an electric cooker very seriously - but the running costs we expect to be rather high and it is a problem whether to get another wood burning stove or to have a Baby Belling cooker. The latter is cheaper to purchase but more expensive to run, somehow one would like to combine the best of both methods.

Robin Morley has had tooth ache for some days so they have to go to Akure tonight at 6pm to have it seen to - 50 miles away.

The children are now practically up! Unfortunately I have a little work to do in the office, so perhaps Peter will come with me. Do hope all well at home with you all, All our love, David

6.12.58

We have had an eventful time recently and the reason that I am typing this is to demonstrate my new typewriter and to try to get used to it. Behind this lies quite a long story, see later.

We were very glad to receive your letter this week a most interesting one full of you activities, especially in the garden. The progress should be a real show by 1960 when we hove too again, already we are looking forward to seeing them. The glass house too seems to be having a new look and the paving in front of the lounge should be very nice indeed.

About three weeks ago I woke up one morning to find that during the night a burglar had been in the bedroom and taken a complete drawer from Margaret's dressing table. We were not a little mystified. I went up to take prayers, and when I returned Margaret had found the drawer in the orchard, its contents strewn about, but nothing stolen. Since then the carpenters have been busy and have fitted wire mesh to the windows and doors in the two bedrooms and we now lock our doors at night. It is unlikely to be repeated. However about two weeks ago Marion Lethbridge had a record player and a sewing machine stolen from the Sister's house. Then just one week ago our hospital office was broken into by the burglar getting into the roof through another room after making a hole in the ceiling and then coming down into our office by making another hole into the ceiling of that room. The only things they removed were two typewriters, one mine and the other the hospitals. The police have 'investigated' but nothing discovered except that it is the work of a professional burglar, and not a member of our staff. That being so, on the strength of getting back the value of mine on the personal insurance scheme, I have bought another machine, another Remington, a slightly different model as the other one I don't think they make nowadays. All quite exciting and we have another night watchman.

On Thursday a representative of one of the firms came round with the model of the adding machine I was enquiring about in England. Andrew liked the model very much indeed so we bought it on the spot and it has already made a wonderful difference to the accounts.

Last Sunday evening we had the visitors from Eastern Nigeria on their way home. Our Guest was Alan Worall, a minister completing his first tour, landing on December 15th and getting married on January 1st- all a bit of a rush we felt. He was very excited indeed and could not eat any breakfast on the Monday morning!

On Wednesday we had Tony Wilson as our guest for the night. Michael will remember him from Kingswood in School House, one year junior to him I think. He is now a representative of the drug house Parke-Davis and also a conservative candidate for parliament, hoping to get a seat in the next House. We had quite an interesting evening, though unfortunately we had a hospital committee. However we heard a great deal of his adventures travelling to every hospital in Nigeria, some of them in most inaccessible places. He talks a great deal, and is rather a smooth character as befits a salesman.

Somehow I seem to have got this air letter somewhat torn!

On the Monday evening, incidentally we went out to dinner with the Morleys and had a very nice evening. They have gone over to the east to the Church Missionary Society Hospital at Ieanu to advise about welfare, quite a nice trip for them. They went on Wednesday morning and return on Monday next,

Tomorrow we are getting two Birmingham medical students who are on a terms exchange at UCH Ibadan, and the Professor of Medicine there thought they ought to get to Ilesha to see what work in the country hospital is like - next week I shall be able to report how successful the experiment has been.

Peter and Elizabeth are very well. Both are eating well. Peter was most amusing yesterday, for the first time feeding Elizabeth with small pieces of cake, As Peter put the piece into her mouth, his own mouth opened wide in sympathy, and his thumb came into use to push the morsel home! Elizabeth has just begun to stand, holding onto a chair or table and she will stand beside the washbasin and hold on whilst having her face washed. Peter is talking much more and making quite good sentences, and expressing his ideas. Most evenings last week he and I have been in for a swim, he enjoys it greatly and will now jump in from the side into my arms. When in the water he seems quite buoyant and has begun to splash around with his arms and legs, though it will be a little while before he can swim.

Christmas will soon be here, I am pressing on with the garage and hope to start painting it tonight. It is beginning to look quite like what it is supposed to be. Margaret is making arrangements for food, some from cold store. We have been tempted to buy a goose, but feel it would be rather much for us at the moment

Do hope that you are all well - we are all in very good form, Love from us all and a wet kiss from the children, David

13.12.58

Dear All,

By the time this letter reaches you there will be a real house full of you and I know that you will have a very happy Christmas together. Auntie will have inspected all the improvements made to the property, including the patterned terrace. A very Happy Christmas to you all, from Elizabeth, Peter, Margaret and me. At the moment it is Saturday night and Elizabeth is sitting on Margaret's knee here in the living room. She has awakened and we have found her rather hot, so have given her some medicine and are waiting for her to get a little sleepy again before putting her back in her cot. She has been very well today and is cooing at the moment and not showing any signs of somnolence.

Peter is in excellent form just now, is talking much more and his swimming is progressing slowly. This afternoon I took him into the pool, but every time he got his face wet he clambered out and dried his face thoroughly and then came back and jumped in, only to repeat the process - it was most amusing. Thank you very much Michael and Uncle Twink for the book for Peter, which arrived today, without any damage - we will save it until Christmas Day and perhaps put it on the tree.

Margaret and I are very well. The former is busy with Christmas preparations, the cake is made and looking delicious. We have ordered a few specialties through cold store, which we hope will arrive two days before Christmas. The cushion covers are coming on - five out of the eight are now completed. Christmas cards and calendars are beginning to arrive and we have them arranged around the wireless in the corner of the room. Another piece of news is the arrival in Nigeria of the fridges. As you know the Mission has not so far provided fridges, but recently they agreed that they are really essential to life in the tropics, and we are going to have an electric one. This means that our present one (kerosene run) will be extra so we shall try to sell it, but the second hand value of such fridges is not very great. Bill Mann has written to say that he will be coming up for Christmas, arriving on Christmas Eve about tea time and staying to the following Monday. We shall be very pleased to have him, to repay some of the hospitality we have enjoyed with him.

During this last week we seem to have had a number of visitors. The two Birmingham medical students have been here for a week, and seem to have enjoyed their week with us. We had them in to dinner last night, with Lily Grant, and had a very pleasant evening.

The Northern Region of Nigeria asked us if a Health Visitor on their staff could come up for a week to see what was going on here, so she has been around and is coming in for lunch tomorrow. Last Monday evening John Lawson, the gynaecologist from Ibadan rang me up and asked me if we could entertain and show round Prof. Bull of Belfast University. His is a name well known in the medical world for his work on diseases, so it is a real honour to have him. He arrived about 12.45 on Tuesday. I showed him around here, and then we had lunch together and then he set off for Imesi. Unfortunately he was delayed on his return by a tree, which had fallen across the road. This prevented him from calling on his way back as he had promised. However we had a very nice letter from him thanking us for our hospitality. He was a very nice man indeed , and a very able Professor of Medicine I should think.

We have had some more bad luck with the hens. For two weeks Margaret has been complaining that we were not getting any eggs, and then one day in the orchard, found a nest containing eighteen eggs and a hen sitting on them. William looked at the eggs and took out those that were fresh, leaving the hen on thirteen eggs. All went well for a week and we almost began counting our chickens, when one day the hen could not be found and there were only nine eggs in the nest. William said 'a big snake'. Margaret had then to come back to put Peter to bed and when she went back half an hour later there were only five eggs so William said 'snake very close'. As it was pitch dark, and there was only one torch a hasty retreat was beaten! Next morning all the eggs had gone. The garden boy found a hole nearby amongst the roots of a dead tree, where they said the snake was, so they built a big fire and wafted the smoke down it, which they claimed would either drive it out or kill it. It has not been seen since. However Dorothea Taylor of the Anglican School is bringing us half a dozen pullets at 15/- each, seven months of age and about to lay. So again we hope for the best.

Once again a "Very Happy Christmas" to you all, with all our love, David

20.12.58

Saturday evening. Peter is with me in the office, but I am expecting Margaret to appear at any minute to take him for his bath.. I have been doing some typing, and I thought he was rather quiet, I had sat him on Andrews desk, and when I came to look he had located the office glue and was busy spreading it, fortunately only on blotting paper, but he was about to put one of Andrews plans on top, which I feel would not have pleased him! In addition he seems to have found the ink pad and has got a lot of it around his mouth, so what M. will say when she tries to get it off in the bath I do not know.

By the time you receive this Christmas will be over, but only just. At the moment you will all be busy as we are, in preparation. We were very glad to receive your letter today and to learn of the efforts of the firm of contractors, Bert, Sid and T-toes and that some work is still proceeding in the absence of the technical advisor! We look forward, very much, to seeing all the improvements. I trust that being in a higher form hasn't sapped the energy of Twink.

Thank you very much for your Christmas present to M and me. We were just considering a subscription to the World Book Club, which is we think the best of all the book clubs, and we look forward to a years happy reading - thank you very much.

The parcel for Peter and Elizabeth has come and I am sure they will each like their presents. Margaret and I wound up Peter's doggie and roared with laughter - it is absolutely wonderful and will give real pleasure not only to Peter but to all who see it! I have finished the garage for Father Christmas, complete with electric light and it looks quite well.

It really has been an exciting week here. We have got a new cooker which runs on Calor gas. It is a tremendous change to the wood stove. How economical it will be we do not yet know we shall have to wait until we finish the first bottle of gas which costs about £2 to refill - we hope that it will last us a month. It has been used for bread and cakes and has done very well, and is tonight being used for meat for the first time - we have Dorothea Taylor of the Anglican Girls School coming in for chop, so we are a little anxious. Like all new cookers it takes a little getting used to.

In addition, yesterday we got our new hens - six which are just about to lay , in fact we got one egg from them today, which is very good considering they travelled 100 miles the day before. In addition our old hens have gone into lay and this week we have had one and a half dozen from four of them. In addition a patient who wished to show gratitude gave us four dozen eggs so we are well away. Fortunately both children are keen to eat them at the moment.

Last Wednesday we had the 'Messiah' on records instead of fellowship, a very pleasant change. Mabel has been unwell this week, starting last Sunday, when the other two went out for a ride without her (she was on duty and could not have gone anyway). She goes on furlough on the Monday after Christmas and I think it is unlikely that she will return - at the moment she is psychologically unbalanced, and really in need of treatment at home. The work here is stressful, we each carry much responsibility

Peter is very well, and now swims with the aid of an air ring in the big pool quite without fear, though for several evenings we have had much spluttering as he does not seem able to keep his mouth shut. He loves it, and I should like to think that it will not be very long before he can swim without the ring.

Elizabeth is developing fast. She crawls at speed and makes a beeline for the kitchen, and all the dirt she can find. She stands up herself in the play pen, by pulling on the sides and I don't think it will be long before she is walking. She will eat anything that is put before her. Last Thursday, I had a choir practice and M had the nurses library, so we asked Aileen to sit in. E was awake, very bright and would not sleep, so Aileen put her in our bed with the mosquito net tucked in round her and the light on and some toys to play with. When I returned M and Aileen were telling me that she was quiet and just dropping off, when there was a chuckle and round the door came Elizabeth, having got off the bed, out of the net and crawled to the door. Peter all this time was fast asleep.

Elsie and Louie have returned from their holiday in the Cameroon, Louie has not been very well, and it is possible that she will spend Christmas here and her guests also. If so we shall be 28 to sit down for Christmas Dinner! There has been much planning to get the food cooked, because we all have tiny ovens, only one of which will take a turkey of any size. We shall be thinking of you all this coming week.

A very Happy New year to you all. Love from Margaret, David, Peter and Elizabeth.

28.12.58

Sunday morning and just a few minutes before lunch. Peter is as active as ever, Elizabeth playing placidly in her playpen. Christmas is almost over and we have so much to be grateful for. Peter is thrilled with his toy and it has proved a source of amusement to all our visitors and now when the bunny is clapping, Peter claps too.

We were very glad to receive the photos too - some of them are excellent aren't they. The typewriter ribbons and the dyes also arrived on Christmas Eve - thank you very much for them. Peter says 'Tank you' to Uncle Michael and Twink for his book and Elizabeth too.

We have had a very busy time - and are still having but tomorrow most visitors will have gone and we shall settle down into routine again.

Last Sunday evening was our Carol service and I numbered among the male members- amongst the bases except for one carol where I was the sole tenor!

Monday was a very busy day we seemed to have hundreds of patients - I have been on afternoon duty. Tuesday was a day of preparation. Shopping to be done and the first of the guests arrived. Louie at Ikole had invited two teachers from the School at Gabu - but sent a message to say she was too ill to have them and would be coming down herself. So we had to put up two extra in the Sisters house. Louie came later and she has got infective hepatitis and is as yellow as a canary, similar to my illness eighteen months ago. David Morleys brother and his wife from Kano, arrived too, so already, we began to get a full compound. On Tuesday I had two difficult maternity patients and I have a private patient delivered so Marion and I had to go out to see her. I was offered a bottle of whiskey as a present! Wednesday was another hectic day. Bill Mann arrived and Olive Osborne who wanted to stay, Jean Ryland and Gwen Davies from Shagamu and John and Nancy Gill with the three children from Lagos and then Margaret Woodland from Imesi! What a crowd!

On Christmas Eve at 7pm we began caroling at first around the houses and then round the wards. The wards were decorated rather better than previously (more people about) and looked very nice. I fitted up a light in the model of a church in the female ward. Then we went to the leprosy village to sing, and then down into the town, first to the Owa then to the senior members of the Methodist Church in Ilesha and finally to Mr. Fadahunsi - the local chairman of the town council and so back to the compound for ham sandwiches, mince pies and coffee.

Unfortunately the children were most wakeful and Elizabeth was cutting a tooth and didn't get off until 1.45am so we had a very short night - Communion was at 6.15 to which I went but Margaret stayed in, in case the children woke. I will leave room for a note from Margaret. Letter is continued in Auntie A's letter.

Dear Mother, Thank you very much for the beautiful gift. It was a lovely surprise to receive it on Christmas Eve. Elizabeth would say thank you too for her doll, she takes great interest in it. We've had a busy but happy time and have thought of you all very often.

Love from us all, and to you all, David and M

4.1.59

It was a very pleasant to receive your letter earlier this week and to hear of your happy Christmas. I hope that our letter has arrived. Already we are in the new year and time does pass quickly doesn't it? Last Monday all our guests returned to their various homes, having had a very happy time I think The week has been easier all round, though I have been on night duty which is a bit disturbing.

Last Wednesday evening John Gill showed some movie pictures of the Cameroons, quite a different world from Nigeria, and yet adjacent territory, rolling countryside, with scattered villages - different due to its height and different climate although it is nearer to the equator than we are.

In the evening a Watchnight Service, taken by the senior nurse. I attended, with Andrew and David but the others had gone to bed. We had a few days of harmattan, with cold nights and we are very glad to get to bed at 12.20am.

New Years Day was an easy day. It means much more to the Nigerians than Christmas and they have much more in the way of celebrations - drumming, dancing and fireworks, so New Years Day is given to merrymaking rather than coming to hospital. In the evening we went round to the Pearsons as did Marion and Lily and had quite a pleasant evening, though the game we played -a form of patience - was a bit slow!

Friday was a full day as I had to go to Afon. I left after lunch and got there around 5pm. I took my gun, but did not see any bush fowl! They were burning the grass all round which doesn't not encourage the birds!

I saw the patients the next morning and returned in the afternoon, good uneventful journeys both ways and found all well here on my return. We expected Frank Morton to stay and he did not come until 8.30pm so we had to get a meal for him at that time. Fortunately William was still here, because two other folk had come with him!

Today I have been busy in Maternity Department, but it is my easy week, so I have the afternoon and evening to get on with other jobs.

We have all had colds, quite severe ones with running noses etc. However we are all improving I am glad to say and by the end of this week we should all be better.

We were most interested in your Christmas and shall be eagerly awaiting our next letter to hear how you spent the week after Christmas. We often talk of the garden and picture the modifications you are making, concrete paths and so on and are looking forward even now to seeing it all again. Is the lawn in good shape and the mower working well? How does the willow tree look? Does the fountain stay primed?

Peter is chuckling a great deal - he is called Mr. Sharp by some of the clerks here! Elizabeth is getting more agile on her feet though as yet has no sense of walking.

Louie is still here, not very well yet, Mabel Rowling has gone on furlough, possibly not to return. Eileen arriving on Tuesday.

Our Covenant service this evening led by Frank Morton, the purpose of his visit. Hope you are all keeping well, Love from us all, David

17.1.59

Your letter with the enclosed cartoon from Twink arrived today and both were greatly appreciated. Peter is certainly developing quickly and even Elizabeth now scorns her play pen.

Peter this morning was out 'with the boys' when he came back for his boots, as he wanted to see some cows which we allow to graze on our grass. Margaret finished her elevenses, no sign of Peter. Shortly after, Peter appeared as Margaret was coping with Elizabeth, with his boots in one hand. M. said 'drinks are ready'. Peter replied 'Oh sankou' and disappeared into the dining room, climbed onto his chair and had his elevenses! The last few days he has followed 'the boys' around a great deal though it is a case of following in their wake, but he does seem to be growing up. He has out grown his pyjamas and Margaret is at the moment making him some more, but as she said, he will never look as sweet as he did in his first ones.

Elizabeth also is developing quickly - eight teeth, and standing quite firmly, though not yet walking. She has a mind of her own and if she doesn't want an article of diet, she lets it be known!

You seem to have had some very good outings one way and another and there seems to be a real hive of activity over the orchidarium if that is not a mixed metaphor. Where is this thing being erected? and how large is it? Will it do for keeping the children warm next furlough? Should appreciate the odd constructional drawing.

It sounds very cold indeed two feet ice on the pond - I hope it does not affect its water holding properties. Perhaps when it is covered with water lilies next year it will not freeze over!

We are having a busy time here. Andrew, Roy and Elsie are all in Lagos, they went last Thursday. David too was in Ibadan Thursday and Imesi today so I have had a busy time.

Elsie and Louie (who is better) set out at 8 am on Thursday but unfortunately the car broke down and Andrew and Roy picked them up by the roadside at 5.30pm, so they must have been tired out with just waiting. I think it was the coil that burned out.

David has been appointed a part time lecturer at UCH Ibadan. I am pleased for his sake, but feel that he has rather a lot of commitments to take on the extra work. It seems that we shall be having students here, three of them for three weeks at a time. As yet we have no accommodation so David is suggesting using the private block which is not very satisfactory. However we shall see what pans out. Unfortunately our government bill has not been paid in full for the last quarter, as they have run out of money so we are having to postpone building plans, including the ante-natal block until the financial situation improves.

Next week looks like a busy week. I am on night duty and David will be away Tuesday and Thursday, however it is surprising how one gets through if one takes one thing at a time.

The nurses had netball this afternoon, we have just taken in twelve new girls in the Preliminary Training School and some are very good. Peter continues to enjoy his swimming and potters about in his air ring, but still unfortunately keeps his mouth open and tongue out. If there is a bit of a wave he has what he calls a 'big cough' which really means a choke! We are all very well and hope you are all well despite the cold.

 Love to you all from us all, David

7.2.59

A few minutes to spare in the office, so I thought that I would start this letter to you. We were very glad to receive your letter yesterday and to know that my letter had caught up. There has been strike in the Airways Corporation here so that may account for the delay though you do seem to have ben having some fog at the other end.

How exciting that there are bulbs coming up already - it will be most exciting to see this part of the year in the garden, with the daffodils etc. coming up. Will the roses flower this year?

 I can see that you hanker after one of the trees that produces three types of apple! Have you still got fruit left in store?

I should not care to be an orchid at the moment, with a faulty thermostat - the fact that some of the leaves have dropped off does not sound good to me.

This week has not been over busy for me, as I have not been on either nights or afternoons - I start the latter today though I had to do night duty last night, including a caesarean section, as my colleagues all seemed to disappear! Andrew went to Afon, Roy to Akure for the weekend and David who had had a tooth out had to retire to bed. Today has not yet been so busy as it might have been considering the lack of Doctors, though Andrew will be back tonight.

The highlight of the week has been the visit of Monica and Bob Cundall and their three children. They are staying with the Pearsons', though at the moment they are in Ibadan having gone down yesterday morning to see the new hospital there. They are coming back tonight and going back to Ituk Mbang on Monday morning. They are in good form, thinking of settling down in Harrogate, setting up home. It is very nice indeed to see them, and they seem very pleased to be here. Ituk Mbang has only just got a hospital car, so they have never been able to travel at all previously. Harry Haigh had his own car and has felt that that was sufficient for the compound!

They came to dinner on Tuesday evening and we had a good talk about our contemporaries and the folk at Rivercourt in his day and so forth. They send their regards to the Pattersons and to Mrs. Ranger.

At the moment of typing this Peter is beside me with the adding machine, a wonderful machine for a small boy, as there are 72 keys to press, and they stay down when pressed or occasionally push others up. Both he and Elizabeth are very well indeed Elizabeth is standing on her own without help and any day now will take her first step. She walks if you hold one of her hands, but it is fascinating to see her standing by herself away from all furniture, teetering back and forward, and then suddenly sit down.

One afternoon I made a wooden seat of Peters size to fit on the toilet seat, in order that he can manage himself. He seemed very pleased with it at first, but the novelty has worn off. Another job on hand is the painting of the old refrigerator in an effort to sell it. At the moment it stands on our verandah, not being used at all. Today we are just finishing laying a water pipe down to the vegetable garden. Although Margaret has managed to grow some vegetables all through the dry season, it is far from easy, so we have bought 200 feet of half inch plastic cold water pipe and run it down to the garden- I am hoping that it will be finished today. It will make watering so very much easier.

This evening we are having coffee with Elsie who is expecting a lady Doctor from Uzuakoli for two nights. She does not know her so it is all rather a surprise parcel!

Last Monday Andrew, Jean, Bryan, Peter and I went down to the Grammar School to see a football match for a few minutes. It is their 25th anniversary and are having a week of celebrations. They have got an English couple to teach chemistry. Actually, he is the teacher, she was a nurse till they married I suspect only a short while ago. They seem a very young couple or else I am beginning to feel a little ancient.

This week I have to go to Ikole. Unfortunately Margaret and the children cannot come with me because Louie has Beryl House living with her and she can hardly give up her room; as it is I shall have to sleep in the sitting room.

Sunday night: A busy weekend with a caesarean this morning, then to church at Otapete, an afternoon on duty, and chapel again this evening. Unfortunately all our lights have just gone out due to the terrific storm we are having - quite unexpected, but at least it will make the air cooler - it has been stifling today. David off to Imesi in the morning and the Cundall's starting back to Ituk Mbang. Roy is back from his weekend off. Elsie's visitor never arrived!!

Do hope you are all well. Love from us all, David

1/3/59

Your letter arrived on Thursday, and we once again we devoured it eagerly to learn how you all were, how the garden grows, how Stoneleigh is being penetrated and so on. You all seem to have ben having a very busy time what with one thing and another. Your speaking seems to be increasing again and no doubt when the circuit wakes up to the full potential of No. 12, invitations will begin to flow in. You will now be at the MMS Conference at Haywards Heath - quite a new experience for you, and we shall look forward to hearing all about it.

We were very sorry to hear about Dorothy - by implication rather than what you said. Is she not well then? From what you wrote I gather she needs nursing care so presume she is quite ill. What is Rex doing?

We were very glad to receive your Birthday card for Elizabeth - a very smart one - this week and she is delighted with it and has celebrated by walking five steps and remaining on her feet, so at last we can say she is walking and before long she will be trotting off.

Peter sometimes comes all the way up to the hospital and once or twice after examining a patient I have turned to see Peter regarding me gravely and saying 'has the patient got a sore Daddy' to the delight of those around. Frequently he comes to the office to 'help' and I can get little done until he has trotted home again.

At the moment of writing it is Sunday evening, Margaret is at chapel and the children are just dropping off - occasional sleepy murmurs from Peter only. It marks the end of a busy week. David has been away, I have been on night duty and then Andrew and family have been away today and yesterday. Andrew was preaching in Ibadan so I have had his work to do also. However they are back now and I should have a quiet night. David and family returned from Jos on Friday evening having had rather a hectic time. All three children were unwell - Ruth so much so that David got one of the delegates from the conference, a Prof. Walters, to travel out to see her. However they are safely home again, Ruth better, but Andrew not very well today.

Yesterday I was on duty unfortunately but Margaret and the children went to the Ilesha Women's Training College to the annual sports meeting, which made quite a pleasant outing . I have struggled with a trial balance and am 19/6 out in £26,820 odd over six months. It isn't very much but it must be found somewhere!

Last night we had the Morleys and Elsie in to chop and had quite a pleasant evening, except that I had an operation from 7.30 to 8.45 which took rather a large slice out of the evening. This morning I took the nurses down to chapel at Otapete - a one and three quarter hours service and really very hot indeed. Meanwhile it was Margaret's coffee morning, so we have had a very busy day but Peter and Elizabeth have both been good children. We had a very sharp storm two nights ago which put out the lights in a third of the hospital and blew down most of our garden fence - so that is to repair. The hens however are doing quite well still between two or three dozen eggs a week, very welcome indeed. Do hope all well with you all. We should be home by this time next year I think

Love from us all and a hug each from Peter and Elizabeth, David.

11.4.59

Saturday evening and at last there is a cool breeze, It has been a very hot day indeed and what breeze there was seemed as hot as the day, and was no relief but it does seem a bit cooler now though still well in the 80s and it is 10pm.

Jonah and Rowena arrived this evening. (Mrs Jones had a stroke and came up to stay with Elsie. The Mission House flew their daughter out to help.) None of us have seen them and Elsie has very thoughtfully vacated her house so that they are there together this evening. Rowena's plane had to turn back to Tripoli with engine trouble but came on by the next plane - spent one day resting in Lagos and came up here today. It is quite an experience for her, as neither she nor Allan have ever been to Africa. They will now have to decide what they are going to do, whether Mrs. Jones returns to England or they return to Lagos where Rowena takes over the housekeeping etc. - quite a task for her. Mrs. Jones has been a bit of a worry but is making steady progress, though still has not got fine movement in her right hand.

We were very pleased to receive your letter with its news of the garden - the top right hand corner would seem to be very nice and with a greenhouse, would supply seedlings to perfection! One can foresee vegetables all year round, and some of the more exotic fruits! Has anything been done about the grass in the orchard and does the fountain still work?

You seem to have had some very nice outings, we can picture you all setting off etc and wish we could be with you, though we should add to the transport problem.

We have had a good week and we are all well. We have had the two American men from the Pocket Testament League to lunch every day and next week are having them to high tea instead, really quite a lot of extra work. Next Friday they move on to their next town, having 'done' Ilesha. They are distributing copies of St Johns Gospel to as many people as they can. Their aim is five million copies in Africa. They have been to east and south - over four million to date so

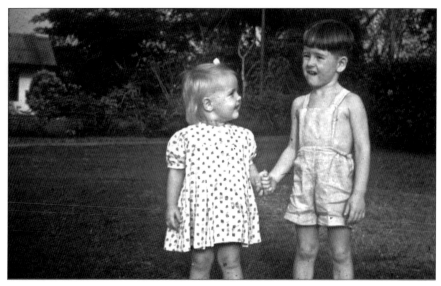

Elizabeth and Peter

it looks as if they will reach their target.

They have two beautifully fitted vans with three amplifiers in each, two projectors and electricity producing machines. They do not seem to be short of money!

Peter and Elizabeth are very well. The latter walking more and the former seems a little put out with her progress at times - but they play together very well indeed. Peter is talking much more and putting together quite complicated sentences.

Our hen is still sitting and has now completed two weeks so that there is another week to go and in that time I have got to get a chicken run made! At the moment I have only made about a quarter of it so shall have to get a move on.

Last Sunday we were late getting down to Otapete and as I searched for a seat sat down in a row in which we do not usually sit but noticed that just behind was a strange English lady. As I took stock I realised I was sitting amongst several rows of girls but did not give it a thought until the notices when it was announced that the new Girls Life Brigade Company was led by Dr. Cannon and Miss Fletcher! The steward seeing me sitting there had jumped to the wrong conclusion!

The garden is struggling or rather Margaret is struggling with it. She has been sowing beans weekly since February and has only just got a complete row. We think that it is ants which come and bite them through at night which is rather distressing.

Have just been to a concert given by the nurses Student Christian Movement branch in order to raise money. It is going very well but won't last less than three hours! Our love to you all from Margaret, David, Peter and Elizabeth.

2.5.59

This will - or rather may arrive on Michael's birthday - Many Happy Returns old chap and welcome to the 30s - sagacity etc. will now rest upon you in full measure no doubt! Though, I must say, as the years roll on each seems better than the last, so although 40 sounds quite advanced no doubt it will be quite acceptable when it comes. But away with philosophy - we do all hope you have a happy day though no doubt it will be a work day.

Glad to hear Mother's disc is settling down and no doubt you will soon be pottering around the garden. The pond sounds to be coming on apace and we look forward to hearing the weekly bulletin of plant life. When are the fish added? I suppose it is when the plants have taken hold and are doing their stuff with producing oxygen etc. I hope sundry birds don't take them out again. Does the fountain still function? Have you had it going for visitors yet.?

Sorry to hear of Twink's mishap with the chisel. He will have had his staple out by the time this arrives no doubt. I am glad you had got into tow with a local Doctor who copes with such things. Interesting that Twink is having dancing lessons - we are still very keen to try and pick up something here.

We have had a steady sort of week. The children are both very well again and full of beans. Elizabeth is trotting all over the place and was brought back from the nurses home to which she had walked unaided. Unfortunately she is also able to climb up onto Margaret's desk - today she scattered lecture notes all over the floor!

With Maria at home and Mabel not returning to us, Lily is staying here as a permanent member of staff. She is a good ward sister, but not cut out for teaching, so Margaret, Aileen and Beryl are all giving lectures in the afternoons. This means that the nurses are receiving lectures from ten different lecturers, quite an achievement in a Mission Hospital. It means that the mothers take it in turns to keep an eye on the children and as far as ours go, Auntie Beryl is much the most popular.

Last Monday we had the McGraths with their new baby (2/52 old) up to tea. She is finding it difficult to feed it so we encouraged her. This morning Margaret and Jean went to see the Woods and their baby (ten days old) and she has got it on the bottle already - but she is American! Our great excitement of the week was the visit of Sir James Robertson, the Governor General.

I was invited to the reception in the Town Hall with Andrew and Elsie. It passed off very well and then we hurried back to the hospital and welcomed him there. Andrew, of course did the introductions and led him around and on the whole the visit was satisfactory, but we all feel that Andrew didn't shine! He never took him to the maternity unit or to the school as arranged as they were short of time but wasted quite a lot of time demonstrating the organ! However we have some photos for the album which we shall bring home.

This evening Peter and I have been making a car. Recently Margaret has had a half share in a carton of packets of cornflakes (20 packets for 28/3) made by Quakers and each one has a car to cut out and stick together on the back. It really is most fiddly and Peter lost interest half way through but no doubt he will enjoy the car tomorrow when it is dry.

Next week is quite busy one way and the other. Andrew has a committee in Ibadan on Friday, Roy to Ikole on Wednesday, Medical Meeting here on Thursday and I am speaking at a Scripture Union boys camp in Akure on Saturday and to cap it all there is a Ministers retreat in Ilesha (40 men) from Tuesday to Friday.

Space gone, love to you all from us all here, David

9.5.59

I had expected to be in Akure this evening - but a letter arrived at mid-day today to say that they did not have electricity as they expected so there was no point in me bringing the filmstrip, and so here I am. Margaret is at the moment bathing, the children are, I hope getting sleepy and soon we shall be going round to the Pearsons' to chop.

We were very pleased to receive your letter and to gather that the back is much better and judging from the activities - very much better! We are all well here, the children and M and I in good form. It has been a busy week as expected but the cancellation of the boys camp has made it easier.

Tuesday was a very heavy day, Andrew had to go to Ibadan and David M to Imesi and Roy and I struggled on. However it was the day that the building of the ante-natal block started which was a memorable day. They are due to finish in nine weeks. I have had some cards printed and have worked out a new system which I hope to get into going order quite soon. We are getting about 150 attendances a day so we have to get a bit of organisation into it otherwise some are kept waiting a long time.

Wednesday we had a good number to our evening Fellowship. Nancy Hall from Shagamu is here on holiday with the Sisters, and Jessie Longley was also here as Frank was at the ministers retreat. Mrs. Jones and Rowena were also staying on the compound, so we had a good number of folk about. Mrs. Jones is about the same. I didn't see her myself, but Elsie, with whom she stayed wasn't very forthcoming so I gather there was no great improvement.

Thursday I held the fort alone for most of the morning, quite a task nowadays, as Roy had to go up to Ikole on trek. Yesterday was busy and today a little but not too much so, fortunately.

Most afternoons Peter and I have been swimming and he prefers to be without his air ring which is a little alarming, he cannot swim yet but one feels that if he would learn to keep his mouth shut and swim a bit lower in the water he would manage.

We have had (or at least Andrew has) a letter from Dr. Bolton who is a little alarmed (as I am) at the outside influence there will be if we build the students hostel with Glaxo money and Dr. Collis of UCH has a say in the students who come and the appointment of a House Physician. It will all have to be discussed fully at the Hospital Management Committee next month, but whether that will be much help or not I do not know. It is a very big decision to take.

Our local leave will be coming next month. We hope to go up to Ikole for a few days with the next trek and then to stay with some friends (the Hands) at University Hospital, Ibadan. Then if all is well we are going to spend a few days in Lagos to do some shopping but we are not yet sure where we shall stay.

At this moment Elizabeth is 'creating.' She has seen Margaret go past the window to the bedroom and wants her to come in! Peter is telling her to stop crying - with no effect whatsoever!

The Sisters have gone away for the weekend and the Morleys have a pediatrician and his wife staying with them for the weekend. Do hope all is well with you at home, with love from us all, David

16.5.59

Saturday evening, a few minutes in which to start this letter. I am on night duty, so may be called away before I can finish it. We were very glad indeed to receive your letter by midday on Friday - which was very speedy indeed considering when it was posted!

You do seem to be having a busy time with orchids! Stanley does seem to be keen on them at the moment. Perhaps he ought to read for a B. Hort. if there is one! Have you sent to Ireland for the necessary factor which seems to be missing? and what do you spray the roots with?

Today you will have been to the suppliers for the fish if your plans worked out. How many and what varieties are there? Does the water stay clear? I must say it is all most thrilling.

Now Sunday morning - I was called away twice during the above to see patients so gave up and went to bed. The second call was to a private maternity patient who had a normal delivery, quite quickly so I was not late to bed.

This morning has been very busy. I was called up to the hospital before breakfast to see a woman who was injured in a motor accident. However I got her stitched up and was about to set out for chapel with the nurses when a lorry brought in nine patients from another road accident which kept Roy and Andrew busy all morning, and then a short while ago another patient was brought in following a third accident! I am off this afternoon, but have a ward service as well as two minor ops so it looks as if it is going to be a rather busy day, as I am on duty again at 7pm.

The week has been much as usual. Last Monday we had the Pearsons' in to chop and then went to the pictures. Andrew and Jean had never been and so were most interested in the place. There was a short cartoon film - very good, and then the main picture which was about wrestling. Not what we would chose to see but it wasn't bad really and we all enjoyed it. The same day Margaret and the children went out to tea with the McGraths and apparently they behaved beautifully. It only goes to show that Peter can do well if he wants to!

They are both very well, eating much more readily and more food. The quantity that Elizabeth is able to eat is quite extraordinary! Anyway they are both very well indeed, as are Margaret and I.

It is now Sunday afternoon! I have had a ward service to take and two small operations, but those are completed and I am home for tea and a couple of hours before service tonight.

The Pearsons' have the Dodds staying with them at the moment. They are new teachers at Shagamu.

Yesterday we were visited by Prof. Daley, who is Professor of Surgery at UCH. He has only been appointed six months. He is a keen Moral Rearmament man apparently and we found him most approachable and sympathetic.

Next Sunday, Mr. Lawson is bringing up two Obstetricians who are visiting UCH, so we shall be busy then.

Do hope all is well with you all - sorry this is such a scrappy letter. Love from us all, David

The Methodist Manse
PO Box 19, Savanna-la Mar,
Jamaica BWI
from my father's twin brother

My dear Arthur and Jessie,

It is a long time since we wrote you. The extra work devolving on us through the repair work (Earthquake repairs and consequent additions) has kept us so occupied that we have had little time to write personal letters. However here we are.

First of all, we are so glad to hear of the proposals for Stanley - he wrote us and I answered the letter this week. What an opportunity the lad has had because of both tragic and happy circumstances - tragic in the loss of his mother and happy that you gave him a home with such principles and training. Anyhow, you can feel if he continues in this way, that your love and service have not been in vain. We rejoice. I wonder if you can enter into our feelings in it all - being thousands of miles away with only the possibility of communication through correspondence - and seeing the lad develop so beautifully with promise of taking a useful place in life! We are grateful to you and to God. I say we because Theda loves him as if he were her own. We are praying that he makes the grade and enters Peterhouse Cambridge.

Then we are overjoyed to learn that he was received into membership at Easter. He is old enough to understand what it all means. Accepting Jesus as his Saviour and taking his stand for Him will put him on the right track for life. We do thank God for the way He is leading the laddie.

Then, your house is rapidly becoming a home in every sense of the word, with comforts and conveniences and increasingly beautiful surroundings. We are just longing to see it and to see you all enjoying it.

Apparently, Arthur, you are kept busy which is a good thing. Don't over strain, old boy, with the pastoral charge you have. Of course you are free from a superintendency, which is a great weight off your shoulders. With the pastoral charge and the house and the garden you are kept busy. There is no doubt that if, when we retire we really 'sit down' we soon go to seed - or to dust! Am glad Jessie keeps active in her Women's department. We only heard the other day from the Blackburns how you Jessie, gave a gracious and warm welcome back to Mrs. Quibell. What a gracious and wise woman she is! We did enjoy associating with her.

Our Chairman is in England - the Revd Hugh B Sherlock OBE the son of a minister and brother of the Vice Principal of the University College of the West Indies. He is a man of character and with all his gifts and position is both humble and approachable, I gave him your address and if he has time he will contact you. His schedule is very full and after Conference he is to go to the United States for a month to speak on our plans for the bi-centenary of Methodism in the West Indies. He spent seventeen years in charge of Boys Town in Kingston and put that institution on its feet. He is a great cricketer - trained Collie Smith. You can contact him at the Mission House.

We have finished our Savanna-la-Mar church repairs and additions. We have added vestries both Choir and Ministers, and a delightful children's chapel to the building. It is a dream of years come true. The children's chapel is most effective. Over the Communion Table there hangs a large picture of the Head of Christ. Theda saved and saved and procured it from America for the chapel. There are other pictures of Jesus and there is a small lectern. I am holding my candidates preparation class in it and I find the atmosphere helpful - very helpful. We are grateful that we have been privileged to execute this job - I think I should say 'task'. I have two more churches to tackle and a Mission House to build. We pray for strength to carry on until it is all accomplished, if the Lord will it so.

I gave notice of retirement at Synod - to take effect from 1st September 1960. Pressure is being placed on us to continue a wee bit longer - until a pipe organ is installed in the church - but I feel we ought to retire at the date mentioned. Like you I want to be an active supernumerary, able to supply here and there where there is need. We have no active supernumerary now- indeed we have only one who got up three years ago after being on his back for nine years (or practically on his back) with a bad heart! I'm sorry, I have misinformed you - forgot the latest Supernumerary - Revd Claude Cousins, the father of Revd Caleb Cousins, who came to see us from Richmond. He is more or less active, but not very strong having passed through two serious operations. To have a man on whom the chairman can call in an emergency is helpful to the District generally. I should like to be that man and serve as needed.

The Missionary Committee has also very generously granted us furlough. I have asked however that it be postponed for a time. It will be our last regular furlough and I want to have it before me for a while and not behind.

Theda has been in Kingston for a few days - returns tomorrow night. She would probably have added a line if she had been here. We both keep fairly well but get tired more quickly than we used to do. Such is life! Her father has been very ill - had to send for the brother - but he is improving at 91. We sympathise, Jessie, with your sisters in the loss of their husbands and we pray that your dear husband may be spared to you for many years - indeed that you may be spared to each other for a long time.

Please give our love to Michael and tell him we are glad he is enjoying his work so well - we hope he has had further opportunity for exercising his musical talent in public worship. Rosemary - our adopted daughter has passed grade two in violin. Much love, Stanley

23.5.59

Your letter arrived on Friday this week and we were very glad indeed to receive it. You all seem to be very busy indeed with all your activities. Naturally we were very glad indeed to hear about the garden - it would sound to be very nice indeed at the moment, and now that there are fish in the pool an added interest. I wonder if they will multiply! We look forward to further bulletins.

Mr. Thompson, the successor to Mr. Clutterbuck, is in the compound this weekend. I believe he is now living in Birtwhistle's old house in Worcester Park and that Mrs. Thompson knows you! Does she worship at Stoneleigh? I should be interested to learn if you know them well. He seems very much alert to what is going on around the medical world, and we naturally informed him of our problems! Unfortunately he is not well. He has been around East Africa and is now within ten days of the end of his tour. He has had a tummy upset which has left him feeling as though he had cotton wool inside him! However he seems better this evening. He has just returned from Ikole where he has been looking into Louie Trott situation.

Also on the compound we have Dr. Frank and Mrs. Davy from Uzuakoli who are on their way to Ibadan where he is lecturing to UCH on leprosy. They arrived yesterday afternoon and are staying on until tomorrow when they go on to Ibadan.

Today has been a hectic one for us. Mr. Lawson, the obstetrician who is at UCH rang up and asked if he could bring two visitors - two senior British obstetricians who are inspecting UCH to see if it is acceptable to offer candidates for the MRCOG. They arrived for lunch at 1.30 and we had a lovely meal - ground nut stew, American ice, coffee, followed by a look around the hospital and they seemed quite pleased and interested in all they saw. We returned for tea and a talk and they returned to Ibadan at 5.15. It was quite a strain having them but very much worth while.

In a few moments we are going over to the Pearsons' for coffee and a snack followed by hymn singing. Both the Daveys apparently are very musical so it should be a good evening.

Last night (Saturday) we had the Morleys in to chop and afterwards played Cludo - a very good game indeed which we enjoy. Again we had a very nice meal - lamb chops from cold store - a special treat.

Both Peter and Elizabeth have had an attack of fever and have been rather out of sorts and fretful but are picking up again now. Peter is getting to the stage of asking Why? What? which makes Father's life a little more interesting!! Last Monday we went to Dorothea Taylor's for dinner and had a quiet but pleasant evening. She is on holiday at the moment - these teachers are certainly in the right job.

The other major event was the arrival of the stove for the nurses dining hall so at last we shall be able to get it into use. The antenatal block is growing and is beginning to show its outlines.

Do hope you are all well at home, I do wish we could see you and you, the children. Much love from us all, David

31/5/59

We were very glad indeed to receive your letter towards the end of the week and to receive also the photos and Michael's letter last Monday. The photos are excellent and show the garden well and you all looking very well indeed. We showed them to Peter and he picked out all except Auntie A who he does not know so well. I don't know whether he recognised the garden or not.

The story of wild duck and the pool is a very good one, has gone the rounds here with much amusement - but I am very glad to hear that the fish have so far escaped the ravages. You all seem to be blossoming forth in new clothes in preparation for holidays - when exactly is it that you are going?

We are most interested in the photo of the orchidarium which is much larger than we had imagined - it is almost a small greenhouse! I feel we ought to read some book such as 'Teach yourself orchid growing' before coming home in order to keep up with the family on the subject and to be able to understand Stanley when he discourses about them!

We have had a busy week again here. Last Sunday as I wrote last week we had the obstetrician who left us feeling rather weak! but we had a nice letter of thanks from Mr. Lawson during the week. On Monday evening we all gathered at the Morleys and showed recent colour photographs which we had each taken, not withholding the poor ones, so it was a pleasant and amusing evening.

Wednesday was Fellowship. We are going through Hebrews with the help of Barclays commentary, which is rather heavy going and I think we shall all be glad when we finish it - next year sometime!

On Thursday it was the Doctors medical meeting in Shaki which is 170 miles from here towards the French border. Andrew decided to take his family, quite a complication as it meant by taking a second car to Ogbomosho, going on with them to Shaki and I had to get a lift back with some Americans returning to Ogbomosho, staying the night and coming back to Ilesha early the next morning as the Pearsons' were staying at Ifaki a little longer and then going up to Afon on trek.

It worked as per plan except that no-one was returning from Shaki that night and I had to spend the night there,

Fortunately Dr. Edwards and his family were returning early the next morning, but it meant I had to be up at 4.45am, have breakfast etc. We left at 5.40am and I was in Ilesha 170 miles away at 10am but feeling as though I had done a days work and not feeling like tackling a full days work, and a pay day without Andrew. However we got through somehow though I was very tired and shall give Shaki a miss unless I can spend the night there. Yesterday was again busy and Andrew did not return until last night.

Last night we had Eileen and Lilly and Dorothea Taylor round and played table croquet afterwards. Peter and Elizabeth are both very well and eating well and Margaret and I are both fit.

Next Sunday's letter may be a little late as we are starting our local leave on Wednesday and going up to Louie Trott on trek and staying on, but I have to be back here next Monday for our committee,

Do hope all is well with you all and that Auntie is enjoying her stay in Switzerland. The antenatal block is coming on quite well   Love from us all David

Ibadan, 14.6.59

At the moment it is 9.05am. Elizabeth is playing at my feet, Margaret and Peter have gone to Sunday School with Jean Hands, our hostess, and Arthur Hands and I will be going to the University Chapel at 10am, so I am taking this opportunity to start this letter.

It has been a very happy and restful week. Last Sunday (we were still at Ikole) I went to the service in the evening and early the next morning we set off back to Ilesha and had a good trouble free run.

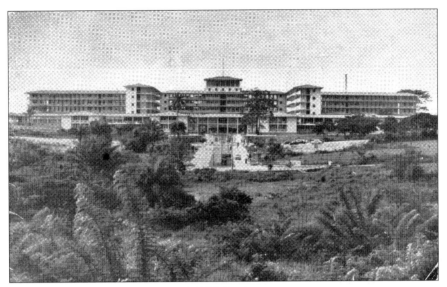

UCH Ibadan

On Monday afternoon we had the Management Committee, without any very startling business except that Marion was appointed deputy Matron, although Eileen was the senior. I do not know how things have settled out since the committee, and hope Eileen is not too upset.

When we arrived back in Ilesha we found your letter waiting. How thrilling that the orchids have bloomed! and Henry will now be in England, or very nearly, with all his emotional problems still to face! He must also feel very out of touch medically, we shall be most interested to have further bulletins.

On Tuesday we had a quiet day after the party the night before! It was a most successful party and the treasure hunt and games went very well indeed. The treasure hunt was a tin of Nescafe and was won by David Morley and his partner.

On the Wednesday we travelled down here in the morning and received a warm welcome from the Hands. He is a lecturer in the Classics Department, of the University. It has been most interesting to live in the University for a few days and to hear how things are done and so forth.

On the Thursday I spent the day at UCH with Mr. Lawson, first in the clinic, then in the wards and finally in the theatre - a long day. On Friday I went in the morning again to UCH and saw the people in the blood bank and was given some pieces of equipment for the hospital. Unfortunately it was rather wet so we had to stay in during the morning and in the afternoon I went again to UCH, where Mr. Lawson had invited me to assist at an operation. It is only the 15th of the type of operation in seven years so it was quite a privilege. It took two and a half hours and was really quite exhausting. It was very nice indeed to work in a theatre with air conditioning and with every conceivable instrument.

It all passed off very well and I returned home. That evening we baby sat for the Hands who had to go to a farewell party for a member of staff. Yesterday, Saturday we started our shopping in Ibadan and had quite a good day, but it is a bit tiring with the children - so hot and busy. In the afternoon, after tea we went to the 'Zoo', run by the Zoology Department here. It is in the University Campus and consists of animals caught locally. Some birds, rats, squirrels, monkeys (many) chimpanzees, terrapins, python, crocodiles, and Peter was thrilled with them, especially the monkeys! It is the first time we have been to a zoo - we must go again next year, perhaps to Chessington.

Last evening we went round to the Lawsons for coffee. He had a service dinner and came about 10.15pm. I had three cups of black coffee and when I got home I could not sleep a wink!!! It was very nice of them to ask us over and we quite enjoyed it. They have a vast living room - 20 feet wide and 40 feet long!!

This afternoon we are travelling down to Lagos and then back on Thursday next week. With moving around we seem to be having a nice long local leave.

Do hope all is well with you all at home. Your holidays can't be far away now. Love from us all, David

June 21st 1959

Here we are settled in at Ilesha again, and already our holiday is a happy memory disappearing into the past. It has been the best holiday we have had here, and we have all enjoyed it, especially the children, who did not seem disturbed by the travelling at all.

We were glad to receive your letter on our return and to learn that you are all well, but very sorry indeed to hear about the fire at Manor House, and hope that the insurance will come through without any trouble.

Activities in the garden seem to continue with the erection of green house and side gate. It will all look quite different when we come home, I have no doubt, we are looking forward to seeing it all.

We had a good journey from Ibadan to Lagos last Sunday. I went to the University chapel in the morning and heard Professor Ferguson preach on 'and your joy shall be full'. In the evening I went to Timinu church in Lagos and heard Jonah on the same text.

We stayed in Lagos at the Church Missionary Society guest house on the Marina, only five minutes away from our mission. A Miss Hines runs it as a guest house so one feels one can do more or less as one likes, and as we were the only guests we had a really good time. The children were very good indeed.

On the Monday we went shopping - rather a hectic business with the children - but we managed to get most things we needed one way or another. In the afternoon we went to the Gills for tea and had a pleasant time though one of their children wasn't very well so we did not stay long.

Tuesday we shopped again and in addition I got Elizabeth's Yellow Fever injection from the health office, so that is another ticked off the list. After tea we all went down to the beach - most pleasant and the children enjoyed very much playing around.

Wednesday was a Muslim festival and so a public holiday. All the shops were closed so we went for a walk in the morning and visited the museum which was interesting. In the afternoon we took Miss Hine to the beach where we had a picnic tea and played in the sand.

Thursday we got off about 9am and stopped first at Shagamu where we had squash with Joan Ryeland. She had just moved into her new house and very nice it is indeed. She and Pauline Webb are going to spend Christmas with us.

We then came on up to Ibadan where we had lunch at Wesley College and then decided to travel from Ibadan to Ilesha by a new road, 20 miles of it are not tarred and have a poor surface, but it is a much more interesting ride, through quite interesting countryside - not so thickly wooded as the other road.

We found all well here on our return. William had tea ready and we went to the Pearsons' for chop.

Friday and Saturday back at work again but this weekend we have John Dean staying with us. He is travelling secretary for the Scripture Union, we came out on the boat with him.

Next week will be spent catching up with everything - the office is very much behind hand. Our love to you all   David

28.6.59

We are going to try sending this to your hotel! I don't know whether we shall be able to from your itinerary but we shall try.

We were glad to receive your letter by now you should be well into Switzerland and having a lovely time, and shortly to enter Italy. How wonderful to see Venice, we certainly envy you this trip. Do hope Auntie A had a good journey to London and is well - give our love to her. We look forward to hearing all the details in due course. Are you taking any photographs?

Most interested in the news of Henry - husky dogs! What a lad he is! It almost sounds as if he was reluctant to pick up medicine again. Most interested also to hear that Mary is not forgotten.

We received the prints of the black and white film I sent home - some of them are quite good don't you think?

Here we have had a usual sort of week. I have been on second night call for surgery and one night had four operations beginning at 10.00pm and two other evenings have been busy, but the rest fairly normal. This week I am on afternoons which I feel is the most trying spell of duty!

We are all very well, though have had colds and Peter one day had quite a high temperature but it was quite normal the next day and he has been as frisky as ever since then. Elizabeth has some charming little mannerisms, she now nods her head up and down when asked a question to which she wants to reply in the affirmative. A very weighty ponderous nod! - most amusing. They are both eating quite well and playing together more, but Peter is also being accepted more as a playmate for the older children.

Unfortunately the Morleys will be off on July 9th and the Pearsons' ten days later. The first flying home the second by boat, so we shall then be reduced from our present five Doctors to three and Peters playmates all disappear which means he will be about the house more and short of things to fill his time with.

The garden under Margaret's green fingers is thriving and we are well away to salads again. Cucumbers especially have done well although they do not grow as large as at home, we often have three in the fridge waiting consumption and the English tomatoes are very nice indeed. Cauliflowers are just about ready but the cabbage has not done very well at all carrots and beetroot also haven't thrived due we think to the rather long dry spell which we have had over the past three weeks, not nearly so much rain as usual for this time of year.

Last evening we went round to the Morleys for chop and Kay MacWilliam was there. We had a very nice meal indeed and played 'pick up sticks' afterwards.

On Tuesday this coming week we are having the official opening of the Nurses Dining Hall at long last. The Owa is going to open it and in the evening Elsie is giving a party for the nurses as eight are leaving this month having completed their bond. We are really going to be rather short of staff nurses for some months until more qualify. Once again we do hope you are having a lovely time. Our love to you all, from Margaret Peter Elizabeth and David.

5.7.59

By the time you receive this you will be back at home and I hope have had a very good holiday. At the time of writing you should be at the Hotel Belvedere at Hedgesville if we have interpreted your itinerary correctly and I hope have received last Sundays letter which was addressed there.

We were very glad indeed to receive your letter written just before you set out, and with Auntie's note enclosed telling us she had given us 50 pounds - it certainly came as a most pleasant surprise. Auntie really is most generous. As Margaret said we shall remember this when we are on furlough and perhaps get down to the seaside somewhere for a week or two where the children can enjoy the beach.

We are having a busy time at the moment. David and Aileen leave here at 6am on Thursday morning and they will be in their own house in Newcastle on Friday night! it is incredible isn't it?

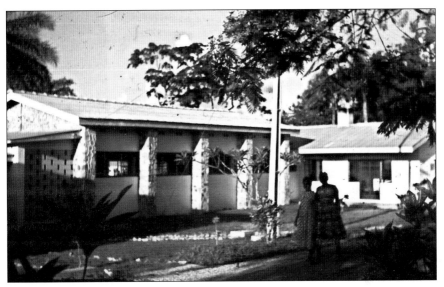

Nurses outside dining room

They are all looking forward to it very much indeed, though David is off to Canada and the States within a few days of their landing and will be away a month, so Aileen will have her hands full as she will not have any help in the house at all and it will be all to open up and air etc.

The major event of the week however was Peter's birthday last Wednesday. He received a number of cards and presents. Michael's and your cards arrived very promptly and Peter immediately annexed them and took them to bed with him each time he went down!

We gave him the Kiddicraft barrels. Which he can manage quite well. Unfortunately they are the type of plastic which breaks, especially with our thin rush mats and concrete floors! Rohan gave him some hankies and other families Dinkie toys, which are a permanent favourite with all the children.

Margaret made a boat out of sponge cake. It had two decks and two funnels and three candles and iced over it and looked very much like a boat and tasted as well as it looked. After tea the elder children went into the bedroom and played with the Dinkies of which between them they have a very big fleet, and the garage I made for Peter which is still in favour and still complete.

This week however has been tinged with sadness as it is the last time all the children will be together. The older Pearsons' go on the 16th and will not be returning to Ilesha, but staying at Culford. Andrew and Jean hoped that they might be able to join them in Ilesha for the summer holidays but I do not think they will be able to afford it.. They are finding it a bit of a struggle to get them fitted out.

We have been looking forward to Christmas a little and wonder if you could

365

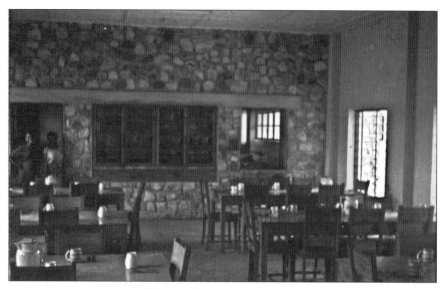

Nurses dining room inside

purchase, on our behalf (for Father Christmas), a doll for Elizabeth. We tried to get one in Lagos and couldn't. We should like one in soft unbreakable plastic and without any elaboration if possible. If you could buy such and send it out by post in due course. I will send a cheque by return on behalf of Father Christmas.

We are all very well, though Elizabeth has a little fever today. Much love to you all, David

11.7.59

As I write this you will be speeding across Europe in a train and I gather not very comfortably! We were very glad indeed to receive your letter during this week, written on two or three occasions and latterly at Herganville which seems a delightful place. I have no doubt that all three of you were ready for a rest after your first week of travelling. It certainly must have been a memorable holiday. The Dolomites we must certainly visit in due course. We gather from your letter that the second week was not part of the tour, but your own holiday which must have been very pleasant. We look forward to hearing all about it in due course.

We have had quite a busy and quite a worrying time. Elizabeth has not been well at all, but at last is picking up. She has walked for the first time for a week today and once again starting to eat.

David Morley saw her and decided it was a virus infection of unknown aetiology! Anyway certain tests were done which were all negative so we just had to wait until she overcame it. She is now more like her old self 'talking' and laughing and playing so it just remains to build her up. Peter has been in very good form. He seems to be growing up quite quickly, and is playing much more

366

imaginatively pretending and playing at shops and so forth.

The Morleys went on Thursday at 6am and have left rather a gap. David was busy up to the last minute as usual and they were here at 6am on Thursday and will be in Newcastle at 6pm on Friday such is the speed of travel! There are now two flights to and from London from Lagos, so if you wished you could leave London at 8am and arrive Lagos 8pm, leave Lagos 10pm (two hours later) and be in London for breakfast!

Mabel Rowling came through on Thursday. She is now appointed to Ituk Mbang and arrived by air in Lagos, travelled here in the hospital car, which took the Morleys to Lagos. She seems in good form and very cheerful. She left by lorry to travel around to the East, not a very comfortable journey I am afraid. I do hope she settles down there - but I gather that Dr. Haigh is not the easiest individual to get on with.

To add to the weeks complications, Andrew has been in Ibadan to examine. He went down on Thursday, very early and only got back this afternoon so we have all been rather busy - but really just as we shall be when the Pearsons' sail on Friday next (17th). They are in the midst of preparations - the boys looking forward very much to going away to school

Louie Trott has been through too. Her car is needing attention, so she is now in Ibadan, having left Bosede here. Lily went up on holiday to her for a few days and has now gone down to Shagamu to stay with Joan Ryeland.

Margaret and I are both keeping very well and just now very busy. The rains have set in in earnest and there is much to do in the compound. In addition we have four separate areas of building to supervise! The ante-natal clinic roof is on and we hope it will be completed by the end of the month. Last night we had Kay in to chop. she seems to be settling down and becoming adjusted to things and tonight we have the Pearsons' in to chop.

Do hope all are well, Love to you all and to Auntie A, David

20.7.59

Sunday morning and a few minutes in which to start this letter. Yours arrived yesterday and we were very glad indeed to receive it and know that you had arrived home safely and that the return journey was not as bad as you had feared. You seem to have had a very good time in the second week and the boat journey seems to have been quite enjoyable! Michael seems to have coped in his usual excellent way with boiled ham and no doubt enjoyed getting things ready. Interested that you heard a Doctor from Wimbledon preach - I suppose he won't need an assistant with a view in 1962? Interested to hear that the greenhouse is now completed, shall be glad to hear what you are going to grow in it first!

I had not heard anything about Twink and the telescope - is this some new adventure? Don't say that orchids are now in decline!

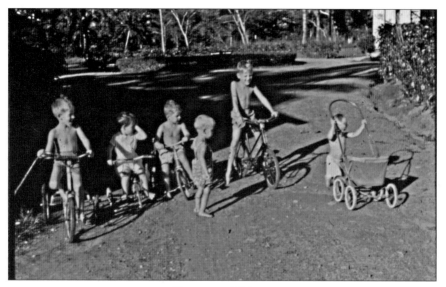

Doctors children

We wonder too, how Michael's term is progressing and when he sets out for foreign parts? Is the college moved over to Weybridge yet and if not when does the big move come.

This week has been a mixed one. We were just getting adjusted to the Morleys departure when the Pearsons' went too and so are feeling very quiet. Fortunately Bosede was here at the time and she, Peter and Elizabeth played together very well indeed. Now Louie has returned from having the car serviced in Ibadan and Bosede has gone. Peter does not appear to miss the children much, but he is now around the house all the time whereas before he would sometimes be away for an hour or two playing with Brian and Andrew Morley. Elizabeth though is growing up quite rapidly - it won't be long before she talks and will soon be able to play more constructively with Peter. They are both very well indeed as are Margaret and I.

Last evening we had Elsie and Kay in to chop, and then I had to chair a debate by the Student Christian Movement that "This house believes a man can be a Christian and a polygamist" the motion was lost 7 to 22.

The Pearsons' left here on Wednesday and sailed on Thursday morning. They arrive London on Thursday 31st July and are going to stay over the weekend at Methodist International House, London. Would you ring them up please to welcome them on the Friday evening? I doubt whether they would be able to get down to Worcester Park unless it was Sunday afternoon. They were all in good form, the boys looking forward to getting to Culford at the beginning of September. Andrew has quite a lot of deputation to do, and will be up for the Valedictory - he may be glad of a bed. Incidentally he will want the Ilesha slides *in the wardrobe of the spare room. If he came over whilst at MIH he could collect them which would save packing them up.*

We are all rather busy, reduced in staff as we are but no doubt we shall manage. Hope you are all well and settled in again. Love to you all and Auntie A, Love, David

26.7.59

Sunday morning. I have just taken the nurses to a special service (SCM) at the Apostolic Teacher Training College , and have time in which to start this letter before returning to pick them up again.

We were very glad indeed to have your letter during the week, to learn that all are well and that you have caught up with things! The doll would seem to be just what we had in mind and we should be pleased if you could purchase and post out to us. Thank you very much indeed.

Here we have been as busy as usual. I have just finished afternoon duty and started on nights last night with rather a bad start! Ten calls - so I didn't feel much like getting up this morning!

We are all well. Peter and Elizabeth are thriving and would seem to be putting on weight - but the scales will tell at the end of this week. They are playing together more and Elizabeth is doing her best to say some words but apart from one or two is quite unintelligible.

Peter occasionally asks when the Pearson boys will be back, or when Andrew Morley will be back but otherwise does not often mention them. Nevertheless I am sure he misses them.

A few days ago we got back the transparencies of our holiday most of which have come out very well. It includes one of all the children taken on our return from Lagos, and last night I showed them to Peter, after his supper and on the wall with the hospital projector. He especially asked for the one of all the children again and went slowly through them.

Last evening we had Mr. and Mrs. Speed in to dinner. He has moved to Ilesha as manager of one of the commercial firms and she is a nurse and is working here as a Sister part time. She is a most extraordinary person with very modern, expensive clothes. As M. remarked she looked like a fashion plate from 'The Lady'. She did her midwifery in the same district of Liverpool as Margaret, but some years later, the winter before the last.

We had quite a pleasant evening on the whole - with a very nice meal. Unfortunately Kay yesterday had a small accident with David Morley's car. No one hurt but the front offside wing is quite badly damaged and will have to go to Ibadan for a replacement I think. She is rather upset about it naturally, as it was her fault she states.

In addition Elsie has gone to Lagos (taking £200) so we shall see what she brings back! I have asked her to get some curtain material for the ante-natal clinic which should be ready very soon, In addition she is going to get a spin dryer for maternity. We have had so much rain recently that the babies clothes are just not getting dry, so we are going to try a dryer.

Our hospital car went down for overhaul and they have found parts broken that they are unable to replace and so are having to send away for it. So at the moment we are rather short of vehicles.

Elsie should be back on Wednesday, the same day as Roy is going up to Ikole and so it all seems to be comings and goings.

Do hope all well with you all. Should be glad to hear from Uncle Twink and Michael about their plans etc. if they have a moment. Love to you all and to Auntie A. from us all, David

PS I asked Peter what he wanted to be when he grew up and he said 'be Uncle Twink'

2.8.59

Sunday again, the week seems to have slipped by. Now afternoon after a rather busy morning, and time to get the letter started before Peter wakes up and compels me to make a seat in an odd box, which is now a boat!

We were very glad to hear how you all were and particularly news of the pond. Does it need topping up? or does it hold water without trouble? Incidentally, when Michael takes some more photos we should like to see one of the new side gate if possible and perhaps one of the front of the house.

We have had busy but not very eventful week. Elsie went to Lagos last week and returned on Wednesday midday. One of the interesting things she brought back was a spin dryer for the Maternity ward. I have never seen one in action before but it certainly gets most of the wet out of material, but what difference there would be after a good squeeze through a wringer and after spin drying I do not know. Anyway as the maternity department does not have a wringer, it works very well. The clothes are then ready for ironing, which in our wet season is a great boon. One has not to overload it - 6lbs of wet washing is damp dry in four minutes. She has also bought the material for the Antenatal Clinic which is almost ready. The material is modern, in bright colours, which will add tone to the department! At the moment the painters are in and the carpenters are finishing off.

In addition we are in the middle of putting in septic tanks for two of the wards and the new sterile supply block and pharmacists office is started, so there is quite a lot to keep an eye on.

Elizabeth has been very well this week and Peter too has been well except for last night when he was very sick after going to bed. I think it must have been something that he had eaten, anyway I hope so. He has been well again today.

Kay has gone to Ibadan, with Margaret Woodland, for the week end, so I have had to do an extra night of duty and keep an eye on the Children's Ward. I hope that they are buying one or two things for the hospital, whilst they are there and take the hospital projector back to UCH to get it repaired.

Now Sunday evening - I have just returned from our hospital service. Peter has been sick over me twice! but once the sickness passed he was as right as a cricket and full of beans but I do hope this episode passes quickly!

Dorothea Taylor and Miss Rance looked in towards the end of the evening, when we were in a bit of a mess, but I think they understood.

Kay and Margaret are safely back from Ibadan. They have had a good time but the car gave a bit of trouble on the way down unfortunately. However they have enjoyed themselves which is the main thing, though they have not got done all the shopping they wished to do.

We are having a visitor at the end of this week for a night or two - Mr. Bamfield from Wesley College. He is coming up to interview candidates for the new year. Later this month the Crossleys are coming for a week or so and the Wainwrights also may come, so we shall be quite busy.

We are wondering if you have seen anything of the Pearsons' who should be at home now - fortunate beings. Love to you all from us all, David

8.8.59

Saturday evening and I am sitting in the children's bedroom! They are both wide awake despite the fact that it is after eight o'clock. As soon as they were put down they began to vie with each other in the amount of noise they could make and would not stop until one of us came in and sat in.

Fortunately the verandah light is so placed that it shines onto the chair and it is possible to get odd jobs done by its light, and I am making the most of it this evening! Elizabeth has now laid down, which is a distinct improvement and Peter has sat down - so it should not be long before they are off. No doubt you have been in much the same sort of situation.

We were very pleased to receive your letter- nice and long in its' two air letters. You seem to have had a most interesting time at Pinewood studios. How interesting that Henry has taken the job of Husky training! What is the film called? You will be going to see it I am sure, perhaps Henry will get tickets for the Premiere.

Glad to hear of Michael's plans and that the dissertationis taking shape. It would be nice to think that it was completed before our return next year. Incidentally we are booked on a boat (Winnebar or Calabar) about the 24th March or 28th or similar, which will get us to Tilbury or Dover about fifteen days later - roll on the day.

One of the nurses has left today and is flying to England on Sept. 6th and is

371

going to St. Lukes Hospital, Guildford. Could you write a letter of welcome to her for her arrival and include the address of the nearest live church which will look after her please? Her name is Miss Christiana Duroza, who is more or less an orphan, and brought up by Frank and Jessie Longley until she started here. I know she would appreciate it. She is a Methodist full member and was one of those who witnessed at our open air meeting.

We are all very well, the children full of beans and in good health. Margaret and I are both very well also, despite much work. Today has been very heavy from the hospital side with Roy at Afon and Kay at Imesi. However hospital is now over, but there is an SCM social to which we must go. Margaret is in fact there now and I hope to get towards the end to close for them. We have had Maurice Bamfield from Wesley College last night and he really is most talkative and doesn't seem to stop!

Eileen has gone to Ibadan for a committee of the Sister Tutors and Elsie has gone up to the Women's Training College for the week end. There cannot be less than 100 unopened letters in her office so she will be rather regretting the acceptance of the invitation made some weeks ago! Applications are coming in for our next Nursing Year and we must have had over a 1000 now for 24 places, so we are going to have rather a job sorting them all out.

The weather is a little warmer the last two days, but we have had some very cool weather indeed with a lot of rain which is rather unpleasant. However it is good growing if not drying weather!

The children are still not asleep, but are lying quietly, so a few minutes more should see them off!

Hope all continues well with you all and your co driver from Spain learns his lesson. Love to you all from us all   David

23.8.59

I am afraid that this letter will be somewhat late as it is now Monday morning. I have had a spot of fever which laid me low yesterday, but is better this morning, however my medical advisor tells me to stay in bed, so I am doing so this morning, then I shall get up later today and be back at work tomorrow. I hope we are going to use the New Ante -natal clinic in the morning and I should be sorry to miss that.

We were very glad indeed to receive your letter last week with its most interesting journey - certainly a long way in two days, but sorry to hear that Auntie Sarah is not too well.

We have had a much as usual sort of week except that we have had a number of visitors of one sort and another and I have been on night duty with very poor nights indeed towards the end. However since then two good nights have helped to make up on sleep.

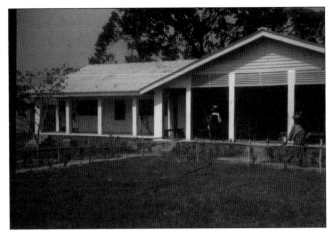

Ante Natal Clinic

The children are very well indeed at the moment. They play together, but not for long because one will take the toy off the other. However during rest time, when they know perfectly well they should be in their own cots, Peter will climb out of his and into Elizabeth's and they will play together with much hilarity and never a tear! Now that Peter can get out of his cot we are putting him in a bed and we hope to get that up today, if all is well.

Saturday we had a number of visitors. David and Mrs. Tew, who are keen Methodists. David is the Radiographer at UCH, brought up the Edmunds who are staying with them for a holiday. The Edmunds we travelled home with last time, she was expecting a baby who is now just over a year, so you can imagine we had quite a luncheon party. In the evening we had Lily and Eileen in to chop and had a quiet evening gossiping

The coming week looks as though it will be busy. There is a Youth Conference being held in Ilesha, starting next weekend. I think there are going to be about 300 delegates. These include a few of our missionaries, so we are expecting the Crossleys, for a week or so. I think John will live in at the conference while it is on, but Margaret stay here and then they are both having a weeks holiday here afterwards. In addition there is Malcolm Wainwright, his wife (of about 8/12 standing), from Badagry who may be coming, but knowing him we don't expect any warning! However we shall be prepared.

Kathleen Owen, our pharmacist will soon be on her way. She sails about two days after the Valedictory service, will you be going? It would be nice if someone could see her before she sails - Andrew will be there also. Her office and laboratory. are now as far as the wall plate and they hope to have it finished by the time she arrives

We have had a spell of dry weather, but it has broken with a vengeance as it has rained almost continuously for 24 hours. Hope all is well at home. Love from us all, David

PS Writing in bed very difficult and untidy - apologies. I hope transparencies arrived safely last week.

30.8.59

We were very thrilled indeed to receive your letter this week including the kodachromes of the house. We have not been able to project them yet but they are rather like photos from Homes and Gardens or 'You too can have a Garden like mine'!

We were most interested in all the activities especially more news of the orchard grass. Glad too, to hear that there is a good crop of fruit. Perhaps there will be some in storage when we return next April - but perhaps they do not last as long as that.

We were glad too to hear from Michael. By now he will be away to Spain but somewhat amazed at future plans for the orchidarium I rather thought it was to be a greenhouse! I imagine it would be rather expensive to run a power line to the green house and it would be quite an expense keeping the place warm, especially during the winter, and one wonders if the expense is justified.

I saw, only yesterday, that two new 850 cars are coming out this year, they should be most interesting. There is a very odd sort of car produced by- I think - Renault which looks very odd indeed, is very crude inside but is cheap and economical to run. I saw one at Swanwick last year, bought to bring out to French West Africa where apparently they are used quite a lot. The Pearsons have bought a 14hp Rover for £65. So far apparently it has run without trouble but you will hear more of it when Andrew comes after the Valedictory.

Here the children and Margaret are very well and I am much better, though have been in bed for the week, which is somewhat unusual. From the fever and allergy of last weekend I developed a very sore mouth, have had a temperature each evening. However it is much better now. I was up in the office yesterday, to check up on things and hope to be back at work shortly. I am afraid it has meant a lot of extra work for Roy and Kay but they seem to be managing quite well. Unfortunately it is the end of the month and the end of the financial year tomorrow, so I simply must get up to the office for some few hours.

The Methodist Youth Conference being held here is well under way. There are over 300 delegates from the whole of the District. John and Margaret Crossley will be staying here from lunchtime today onwards and Malcolm Wainwright and his new wife (who is called Alison) are coming in for High Tea, so Margaret has her hands full at the moment, Elsie also (and probably Kay) will come in after the evening service.

Eileen has gone on local leave. She is going up to Jos with a friend from Shagamu who has a car so she is very fortunate.

At the moment Margaret is getting the children ready for coffee at Elsie's. I shall be content to remain at home! It is a wretched business and I have not had anything but 'slops' for a week and we have a very nice piece of pork this weekend! However a few more days and I should be able to enjoy food and talking again.

We had a letter from the Ashley's this week (she had polio you remember). They sail Sept. 3rd and will stay here whilst Alan gets Afon into shape for living in again. Hope all well at home. Much love from us all David

6.9.59

Sunday afternoon, the children just waking up, so I am trying to get this started whilst there is a little peace! We have had a busy week with one thing and another and fortunately we are all well. The children are in excellent form, Margaret is well though she has been very busy indeed and I am perfectly fit indeed - I have been back at work all this week.

We were very pleased indeed to receive your letter though sorry to hear that cousin Elsie had passed away. We had seen her last furlough when we were staying with Auntie Alice and apart from the Parkinsons disease she seemed quite well.

We had a letter from David Morley about the same day and he told us of his mother's death. She had had angina for some time but had been well until the day before she died.

You seem to have had a very busy week what with one thing and another and before this reaches you, you will have had Andrew to stay for a night and will have been to the Valedictory and perhaps have seen Miss Owen who sails on the 11th I think and should be with us here about the 27th September.

At the moment the roof is just going on the office and the new central sterile supply, so it will be at least a fortnight before it is finished - I hope it will be ready in time. I have just got the carpenters onto making the furniture, there remains one cupboard and have written to all twelve firms from where we buy drugs in Nigeria asking for copies of their price lists so that she can have something to work on when she arrives. I am hoping that she will be able to save me some time along the buying line as soon as she gets settled down and learns which things we buy and use. I hope that when this building is functional we shall have a rest from building for a little while. Peter has now joined me.

During this last week we have had John and Margaret Crossley for a week. They have been very quiet, unobtrusive guests and very good with the children. They went on Friday morning. Then on Friday evening Kay had two guests. A Miss Gibbs who is in charge of Women's Broadcasting for the Nigerian Broadcasting Company who wanted to do a programme about Imesi. She went there and took recordings of Margaret and several other people. This Miss Gibbs brought a friend who is working at WACMR for a short while.

Then yesterday we had Frank and Kay Davey the new Medical Secretary at the Mission House and Fred Hasted to stay for the night (they went this morning).

We are very glad indeed to hear that they are en route for England, sailing on Tuesday. He is speaking to a Medical meeting (with Andrew) in October. Any way if you have the chance of a word with them at the Valedictory I should. He is one of the six world leprosy experts and the most unassuming of people.

Do hope all is well with you all. Michael will soon be back from Spain and Stanley to school! Love from us all David

24.10.59

Saturday evening. Margaret is at a Students Christian Movement meeting, I am sitting in with the children who are fast asleep. Peter and I had a long swim this afternoon and he dropped off almost at once and Elizabeth goes off almost at once as a rule especially if Peter is quiet!

We have not yet received your letter this week, no doubt it will arrive on Monday or so. The week has passed quickly and as usual it has been a busy one. I have been on night duty but it has not been too bad, but Wednesday was quite a busy day.

I left Ilesha at 8.15am and went to Ibadan - taking two patients. I did some shopping, had lunch with the Crossleys and Frank Morton whom you met at the Valedictory service and then went to the UCH for a seminar in the Department of Obstetrics and Gynaecology.

It was most interesting and very pleasant to meet old friends and make new ones. I left just before six and got back just before 8pm in time for a quick bath and meal Fellowship at 8.30 and then I was on night duty. I feel I ought to get down to more of these seminars but on another occasion I should take the hospital driver (it is 74 miles each way) and rest on the way back. We had unexpected guests on Tuesday - the Stringfellows from E Nigeria. He was on his way for a Church Union Committee in Ibadan and brought his wife and daughter (about Peter's age) through also. They ran out of petrol on their way which delayed them, so we provided their lunch at 3pm. They are a very nice family. She went to the same school as Margaret in Chesterfield and he was taught chemistry by Mr. Ingham so they had much in common with Margaret. They said they would look in again on their way back but have not done so.

Margaret had a letter from Thea this week. Ernie has settled in South Africa and his firm have asked him to stay on until May 1960 and do some supervision in two other cities. Thea feels this is rather a long time to have the children without Ernie and wonders if the firm will send her out for a while as apparently it does sometimes. Mr. Ingham is keeping well, not doing so much teaching but *still busy with examination work.*

Here we are jogging along. The Government has given a 10% increase in salaries to all Civil Servants so we have had a request too. It all means extra work in budgeting and finding ways and means.

This week too, office work has been difficult because we have had all the ceilings redone in all the offices - the dirt and mess was indescribable - but the rooms are tidy again .

Elsie and Louie have gone to Lagos together today. Elsie has a Committee next week and she wants to do some shopping for the hospital. I know that they are going to have a good time together! Roy is in Ibadan tonight speaking at a meeting. The rest of us are very well. The children are thriving and Margaret and I are keeping very well.

Love to you all from all of us David

15.11.59

We were very glad indeed to receive your letter on Wednesday this week and to hear that you are all well and to learn of all your activities. Has the fog cleared yet? We have heard that it has caused some serious accidents on the new London to Birmingham Motorway.

Thank you very much for Peter and Elizabeth's Christmas presents which are en route. Peter will be very thrilled with a book - he knows all the present ones off by heart! At the moment he is not sleeping very well. He wakes up about midnight having slept solidly since 7pm, with nightmares - which take a bit of settling and then he is so wide awake he wants a story before he drops off to sleep again.

I note from your letter that the drive is to be widened - is this to allow one car to stand to one side and get the other out of the garage? That would be most useful I think, though perhaps rather too ambitious.

Michael will be preaching on Temperance at Stoneleigh this morning I had to preach on Temperance here a few weeks back - it seems to run in the family!

This week seems to have been very busy again. I have been on night duty so with hospital calls and Peter calls we have had some very broken nights. However we are all very well indeed and the children in fine fettle. Peter thinks things out very well and Elizabeth is as engaging as ever, though unfortunately has got into the habit of taking her pants off - for no obvious reason - I do hope she grows out of it! Last Monday I had to get up at 4.45am to take Mr. Lefebre down to catch a lorry for Benin - we have not heard from him - but presume he did catch it! It was a very early hour.

On Wednesday I went down to UCH to an Obstetric Seminar which was most interesting - Prof. McClure Brown of Hammersmith Hospital was lecturing. I travelled with one of the Doctors from Ife which saved me driving. On Thursday

Kay and Mrs. Lanyian towed David's car to Ibadan to get it repaired and they hope to have it ready for next Saturday. Yesterday Louie came in with a nurse - unfortunately they had a mishap with a lorry en route and so have to get a new wing for the car which will not be very easy. Fortunately no-one was hurt which was a blessing. Bosede came down with them so she and Peter and Elizabeth spent a happy day together.

Last night Marion and Kay came to dinner and we had a lovely meal with chops from cold store and played table croquet afterwards. Unfortunately Peter saw the set this morning at breakfast time so I am going to have to make some hoops and mallets this afternoon for him and there is no chance at all of his forgetting I think.

The next weeks look very busy in prospect with the November Medical Committee on Saturday when we hope all to go down and Margaret doing some Christmas shopping. Then the following Friday I have to go down to the Medical Advisory Board and then we have our HMC ten days later. I shall be very pleased when the minutes of all these committees are on their way! David M arrives Lagos on the 8th and up here about the 10th which will be very nice and we shall not be so hard pressed over Christmas. Andrew arrives about the 14th - then I have Synod for a week or so and then Kay goes home for six weeks.

Much love from us all   David

22.11.59

The weeks slip by, only four and a bit weeks until Christmas and there seems a tremendous amount to be fitted in before then.

We were very pleased to receive your letter and to learn that Michael's sermon went down well and was well received. Elizabeth has just crashed into the front flower bed on Peter's tricycle which she cannot yet ride!

After lunch - it is a very hot afternoon and I have come up to see a patient and Peter has come with me for the moment! I am awaiting a patient who has been bitten by a monkey - the second I have heard of in two days.

We have had a busy week. Wednesday I had to go to Ife to court - High court - to give evidence in a murder case. Fortunately my evidence was straight forward and the Judge was very kindly so it wasn't as bad as it might have been. However it took most of the morning. Wednesday Kay went up to Ikole and that meant I had her work to do on Thursday as Roy was in the theatre all day with a very long operating list.

On Saturday - yesterday, the Medical Committee of Synod met at Wesley College. I am secretary of this in Andrew's absence so perforce had to be there at 8.45am. This meant an early start, up 5.45, breakfast at 6am and Peter was thrilled to be up before light, and he continued to say 'it's all dark, and finally when it became light, that the mosquitoes had put their lights on! We left about 6.30, with Elsie and had a good run through arriving about 8.30 at Wesley College (75 miles). I went over to the committee, Margaret and Peter went out shopping and Elizabeth stayed with the Boshiers. Elizabeth wasn't very happy apparently, but when I got back to the house at 10.30 she seemed happy enough and not overjoyed to see me.

It was very nice seeing Bill Mann again, he was well but Jonah did not seem very fit at all. He had just had a whole week of Committees at three per day and found some of them very heavy I think. Our Medical Committee went very well and we soon completed the business.

Elsie is definitely fixed up for her holiday and flies via Khartoum to Juba on Dec. 7th to stay with her niece and her husband who are CMS missionaries there. She is looking forward to it very much.

Frank Morton was at Wesley Collage, he is coming up around the New Year for a few days. John Crossley is up at Jos for a committee but we had lunch with Margaret Crossley, Jonah and Frank. The children behaved very well the whole day but were very tired when we got back about 4.30pm. I had some patients to see (being on afternoon duty) and then in the evening got out the minutes of the Committee ready for the typist to duplicate them tomorrow.

This morning I have been to chapel and this afternoon hope to get a few letters written. We are all very well and the children (most of the time) perfectly sweet. Elizabeth, yesterday was in really conquering mood!

Next week will be busy - and the week after - committees in both. There is the possibility that I may be going up to Bussa again with another commission but when I do not know. Do hope all well with you. Love from us all   David

6.12.59

Sunday morning and about five minutes before I must set off for the church so I thought I would get this started. We have Dr. and Mrs. (Dr.) Ross here for the week end a very nice young couple who are at UCH for six months but are in fact Quae Ibo missionaries working in Eastern Nigeria, only about 25 miles fro Ituk Mbang. They came Friday evening and spoke to our nurses, helped me yesterday at work and in the theatre and then yesterday afternoon we all went to Imesi for a picnic. The children were very excited and we all enjoyed ourselves very much indeed. They are returning to Ibadan this evening.

It has been a very busy week with one thing and another but we seem to have got through. Tomorrow is a busy day however, we are expecting Jonah and the Manns for our Management Committee in the afternoon. It is quite an ordeal as I have to present our accounts and our budget as well as quite a lot of other business. In addition I have to give evidence in the Senior Magistrates Court in the morning so between them both I shall not get much medical work done. I shall be very glad when the day is over.

The Morleys arrive during the week. I am not sure yet whether they fly on Monday or Tuesday but we expect them here by Thursday in any case- which will mean a considerable help and no doubt some extra work. Elsie flies to Juba tomorrow! she was really quite excited I think at the prospect and no doubt will have a fund of stories to tell on her return.

Your letter and one from Thea arrived yesterday. We were very sorry indeed to hear of Doreen Catterson. As you say they do seem to have had a very rough time during the past ten years or so one way and another.

Most interested to see the diagram of the new cement - it looks very serviceable. Andrew wrote offering us his car at £75. Apparently they are wanting £80 but have only been offered £50, and wondered if we would give the £75 for it without seeing it! I think he is rather hopeful, so I have written back to say we do not want it. In any case there is the problem of the three month gap after they sail and before we arrive and they wondered if it could be housed at No 12 Edenfield Gardens!

Peter and Elizabeth are very well and full of beans but rather demanding in attention. However when Rohan, Andrew and Ruth Morley are here perhaps they will be able to play together more. Margaret is rather tired with entertaining and so forth, but it should ease after tomorrow until Christmas which is less than three weeks away now! and there seems so much to be done before then. Anyway, a day at a time and we shall get through it.

Here we are getting right into the hot season. The grass is drying up and a huge dust hangs over the town when viewed from afar. Hope all is well with you all and that you are not too cold. Love from us all   David

20.12.59

A very Happy Christmas to you all and we shall be thinking of you on Christmas Day, gathered together at No. 12 and wish that we could be with you. I hope that this letter will reach you on Christmas Day, but it may be late with the Christmas rush

We were very glad to receive your letter last week and the cards to Peter and Elizabeth which are delightful and which have been put up in this room! Auntie A and Stanley will have forgathered and no doubt helping with the Christmas preparations.

Here we really seem to be more hectic than ever. Quite without warning Sir Francis Ibiam arrived this afternoon, so I had to take him round. He is now chairman of Ibadan University. He had been to the old compound but had never been to this one and was most interested in all that he saw.

On Friday we had Drs. Collis, Lawson, and Kenstam from UCH through and had a most interesting time. A few weeks ago I got out a report of the Maternity Unit and sent a copy to Mr Lawson, who asked for twelve more and has also asked me to speak to the Obstetrics Seminar in February at UCH - which I shall be pleased to do but must make some preparation for it.

The week has been made busy by having the medical students here- which means that David Morley has had to give quite a bit of time to them.

In addition it was our turn to go up to Ikole - which we did on Wednesday and Thursday. Louie and Bosede were in good form and we started a party for the children at 6.30pm!!! so you can guess what kind of a do it was, having travelled 90 miles, though we arrived at 4.30. The children ate very little and were rather irritable. Peter was put down afterwards and dropped off at once. Elizabeth was put down at the same time and we thought her asleep until a chuckle in the doorway attracted our attention and there was Elizabeth in her nightdress having climbed out from under the mosquito net and from the bed on to the floor!

We had a good trip both ways except that E. was a little sick going up but not coming back but we do not think that had anything to do with the car (we hope not).

Tonight we expect some people (Pritchard) through whom we do not know but one Mr. and Mrs. and child and two students for the night! and then tomorrow our Christmas guests, Joan Ryeland and Pauline Webb arrive. Still we have got our Christmas cards off and have got presents ready if not prepared and no doubt we shall be ready in time. In half an hour it is our Hospital Carol Service - 70 people invited so must be there to welcome them'

We do hope you have a very happy Christmas, with our love from Margaret and David, Peter and Elizabeth

2.1.60

I suddenly decided to type this letter to you. It is a long time since I had my typewriter out and it needs a little work to do.

Your last two letters arrived during the week so we had a lot of home news - but the biggest surprise was the TV set which has been acquired! We look forward to seeing the set and to seeing some of the programmes of which we read and hear so much. Incidentally we now have television in Western Nigeria, but only for 50 miles around Ibadan so far so it has not quite reached us, but Joan Ryeland, at Shagumu has seen it in her compound - the Government has given two sets to each educational institute above the primary schools! I can see that Peter will soon become a devotee of Watch with Mother or the Childrens' Hour programme with the Flowerpot Men. Does it receive Commercial Television?

We are glad to hear that you are all well and have had a good Christmas. Glad you liked our Christmas card - so many folk have asked for a photograph that we thought would serve, we also have some plain enlargements of the photograph which are also quite good and we shall be bringing them home with us if all is well. Incidentally we land at either Tilbury or Dover on April 8th (Friday)

I think it is. The last week has gone very quickly indeed and no doubt the time will very soon slip by especially after the Pearsons are back.

Our guests went back to Ibadan and Shagamu last Monday having had a good time. Pauline sailed last Thursday and as she is on the Aureol she will be back in England in thirteen days and as soon as she settles down again she is going to get in touch with you by phone. The evening after they had gone we had a couple with their son, Roy and Marjorie Dodds, also from Shagumu for the night. They are AOB folk, but very keen Methodists and are working at the Methodist Secondary School in Shagamu They were on their way North for a holiday and stopped for the night en route.

On Tuesday evening the Pritchards turned up unexpectedly. These are the folk from Ghana who were trying to reach Mount Cameroon for Christmas, but unfortunately they had rather a lot of trouble with their car and never got there at all. They have a Morris Oxford Traveller, but it was so overladen that they developed inverted springs and holed their sump. They had to block up the holes with mud etc. refill the oil and try to get back to the nearest agent who could supply the spare part. And this over Christmas - most unfortunate - but we did think they rather underrated the difficulties when they stayed the night on their outward trip. Anyway they stayed the night and are no trouble as they bring all their camping stuff and just set too and do their own cooking - but as they were so tired and worn out they did agree to come into our living room to eat it.

They went on down to Ibadan the next day and that evening Frank Morton arrived, and he is staying with us for a week and taking our Covenant Service in our chapel tomorrow evening. He is an easy guest and gets on well with the children, who are very fond of 'Uncle Frank', He is having a lazy time and is counting it as his holiday tour.

New Years Eve we had a Watch night service in the Chapel led by our senior nurse. She led very well indeed, so it was rather late when I got to bed. Margaret had stayed in with the children and was fast asleep when I returned. New Years Day we spent quietly. Fortunately the hospital was fairly quiet although I had a forceps delivery to do at lunch time, which we had arranged to have as a picnic with the Morleys under the trees on the lawn, and was really very nice indeed.

In the evening we all met together for games at the Morleys house. Frank led them and we all had a most enjoyable evening. Lily Grant wasn't there. She is not very sociable and much prefers to go to bed, and does not go out of her way even on New Years Day to join in with the rest of us with a few party games. This is I feel not a very good sign! Incidentally I don't know whether I mentioned it, that Mabel Rowling has gone home from Ituk Mbang. Apparently her aunt who looked after her was not well and this so preyed on her mind that she felt that she had to go back home to look after her. Also Ituk Mbang has had another disappointment. Dr. Jill Prior had just joined the staff, she came out on the same

382

boat as our Kathleen Owen, felt after a week she was not suited to being a missionary Doctor, and despite intervention by our Chairman of District, she had her passage booked and has retired from the Missionary Society I think.

She had had a year in Kingsmead so we wonder what quite lies behind it. Surely she must have had an inkling of what it was like before she went.

We are all very well indeed, though are having a very severe harmattan indeed, which has given us all colds. Love to you all from us all David

10.1.60

Sunday Morning. Both children are with me in the office - so I fear I shall not get very far with this letter! We have more guests this weekend! Jim and Pamela Parrett who are on the staff of the Nigerian College, Ibadan and who are up for a Scripture Union camp in Ilesha. As she is expecting a baby shortly they are staying with us rather than rough it at the camp. They are a very nice quiet couple but it has meant a great deal of work for Margaret again. They arrived yesterday afternoon and are going back tomorrow.

It has been a busy week. Kay has been examining in Ibadan five days and as she was on night duty I have had to do quite a lot of the work. She arrived back last night and told us that as she was going down to Ibadan she was overtaking a lorry when it swerved out. She braked, the car skidded, slid into a ditch and turned on its' side. Fortunately she was not hurt and before she could get out a crowd of men appeared and lifted the car back onto the road and then she drove on again!

In addition Roy had visitors yesterday and the Morleys too so we have all been a bit busy! Tomorrow the Morleys are having more visitors and again on Wednesday. Next Saturday I am due to go down to Synod and shall be there until the following Thursday I think. The Pearsons arrive on the Wednesday.

Beryl has gone down to Ibadan to await her baby. Unfortunately the ambulance broke down en route and had to be towed back again - but should be back on the road in a day or two - we seem to have much trouble with vehicles!

Marion and Kathleen have gone up to Ikole for the week-end and should be back this evening.

We were very glad to receive your letter during the week and to learn that you are all well. Yes your books for the children arrived safely thank you very much. They arrived before Christmas and were put away to await Christmas Eve. They have given great pleasure to the children.

We are all well, tho M and I are rather tired with broken nights. The children are not sleeping well at all and two nights ago Peter had the most awful croup which has since cleared up but was rather alarming at the time.

Elizabeth is beginning to use more words, still not very clearly - by the time we come home she should be more intelligible.

Now Sunday evening. I have just put E to bed three times! First time as per usual, I was then having a wash etc. when a small naked figure appeared, having taken off nappy and pants, untied the net and climbed out of the cot! Firm words, redressed and put her back. A curious silence so I investigated and she was once again half out of the cot. More firm words and supplemented by mild manual reproof and she is now in bed again! Margaret is attending evening service. I cannot help but feel that she is playing up because daddy is staying in! Peter, Bless him is still under the weather from his cough and still has some fever, so he is watching her antics rather solemnly. No doubt if he was 100% he would be doing likewise. I have just been in again and she has once again extricated the net but appears to be fast asleep.

Our love to you all - only about three months now before we land. David

Lagos, Sat. 16.1.60

Saturday evening and a few quiet moments in which to start this letter. The Synod Committees are past (I did not attend any) and Synod representative sessions start on Monday with the medical business which I am to present on Tuesday morning.

I left Ilesha after lunch, with Eileen, and we had a good journey down, and arrived in Lagos just before dark - about 6.50 Eileen is staying in the GH School at Yaba and I am staying with the Manns at the manse.

I was sorry to leave the family because both children have been out of sorts and irritable, though sleeping quite well. Margaret too has been off colour with cough and sore throat, then as she recovered I got it! but it has just about gone again I am glad to say.

We seem to have had a busy week one way and the other. On Tuesday we were expecting some folk called Postgate - friends of Dr Kendrew who was here two weeks ago. We waited with lunch until 2.30 and as there was still no sign of them had it, and then about five received a telegram saying that they were not able to come. We have not heard from them since - so expect they had some illness with the children or trouble with the car. A pity though because M had been to great trouble with the meals. He is the Director of the NB Corporation

David Morley had to go to Ibadan yesterday, so we were all rather busy and so too, today.

We were very glad indeed to receive your letter and to learn that you are all well and getting out and about! How interesting that Henry has a job with the MRC He has done well. Interested to note too that there is no mention of his wedding day. We had rather gathered from your letters that they were to marry soon after his return to this country. However it appears that all may not yet be settled.

Elsie returns on Monday - we hear that she has had a very good time despite the fact that she was a week in Beirut and a week in Khartoum unexpectedly, but reached her destination in time for Christmas! It will be good to see her when she hoves to.

I have been asked to speak at Handsworth College Missionary Garden Party also! and have arranged to go to Tooting Central Hall May 1st and 2nd. Then we travel to Liverpool on May 3rd and on May 4th I have to go to Cheshire for my first days deputation at Hesby. I thought I would start in the evening but I had a letter today that I am to go to a Grammar School in the morning and WW rally in the afternoon, a JMA rally at six and a discussion group at 7.30. Some day at the start of my Conference Deputation.

Lagos is very sticky, I don't know how they live here! Mr Barnes (ex KS) has not been invited back to the BH School here (Nigerian Principal) on account of his MRA activities! Barnes is a disappointed man I believe! I do hope you are all well despite the cold weather you seem to be having. Love to you all David

WGH, Ilesha, 13.3.60

Sunday morning and Andrew's turn for church so I have a few moments before our coffee morning to start this letter. We were very glad indeed to receive your letter and to hear that you are all well, and that a new garden seat has been purchased. You seem to have established your reputation as a 'speaker to fall back on' at Stoneleigh.

Should you feel inspired to write next Sunday if it was addressed to c/o 22 Marina, P.O.box 161, Lagos it would reach us before sailing and we should be very pleased to hear from you.

We have had a busy week one way and the other. I have been on afternoons and in addition Roy and Beryl have ben unwell and in bed. It seems to have been some sort of virus infection which they have picked up.

It has meant a little extra work for us all and I am on second night call again for the time being.

We had unexpected visitors on Monday who came to tea. Rev. Peter Dagadu of Ghana and Prof King of the Univ Coll. of Accra - Indian and a most interesting couple and they, with Bill Wood will be through again on Wednesday.

On Monday evening we had dinner with Elsie - a quiet evening with a very nice meal and on Tuesday evening we had dinner with Roy and Beryl. Kathleen and Eileen were also there and afterwards we played Bucanna - a very long game which went on til 12.30am! - not our idea of an early night! Roy seems very keen on it so we stuck it out.

Wednesday evening was Fellowship and then Thursday we were to start packing but I had an emergency operation to do in the evening. Friday David Drew came for the night from UCH. He is easy to entertain, and he took our nurses fellowship into the bargain!

Yesterday, Saturday, Margaret had a home perm done by Jean in the morning and in the evening we got started on the packing. We have got a chest filled and ready for crating and another trunk well filled - both of these are to go into the hold. The other things we are using we will pack later on.

We have now got our labels and see that we are landing at Dover, which will make a very pleasant change and we will come up on the boat train. I do not know to which station the train comes but you could ring up Elder Dempster nearer the time and ask. Apparently sometimes Charing Cross, sometimes Waterloo. We shall have a number of trunks so if it should be Waterloo I should try to get them straight down on another train.

Anyway we will take things one step at a time! We have also been asked to bring a trunk home for Roy and Beryl to go to MIH so we shall have that to dispose of. We are all very well indeed - the children getting excited at the prospect of a sixteen day voyage (their parents are not!)

Kay MacD arriving today and Lyn and Louie and chief later in the week! Maternity is as busy as ever - 307 deliveries since January 1st

Looking forward to seeing you all so soon now. Love from us all, David

WGH Ilesha, 21.3.60

It is Saturday morning! and I am starting this letter at Eku, which is 225 miles from Ilesha and down among the creeks, about 30 miles from Sapole. David Morley was invited to speak to a doctors meeting here at the Baptist Hospital and I have come with him as co-driver and Elsie has come also to inspect the nursing school!

We left Ilesha at 10.30am on Thursday morning and had a good run down, picnicking by the roadside, though we had to buy a new tyre in Benin as the red retread on the back tyres was coming through. At Sapele we had to wait an hour for the ferry, then had tea with some friends and then on to Eku, reaching here about 7.15pm. This hospital is run by the American Southern Baptist Church and is much the same size as ours, but does not do nearly as much as we do.

Yesterday we looked around. David M saw some children and I saw the manager (American). We envy them their buildings and the money which has come from the States to go into it but the standard of work is barely up to English standards in some ways.

Do you know that the Baptist Mission grants to Nigeria alone, excluding salaries etc. of missionaries is over ½ million pounds a year?

Last evening David spoke to the nurses and they seemed rather a dim lot to us. Today is the medical meeting which goes on from ten until four and about fifteen doctors from this district are expected - all the doctors for 67 miles radius. David is giving two papers, and I no doubt, will work the projector for my living.

Last evening we went for a swim in a nearby river - the most clear water I have ever seen. The river was fourteen feet deep and quite swift flowing and we could see all the fish swimming about and the sandy bottom of the river.

At home before I left, we had got our packing done to date and we have Monday in which to get all the final packing done. On Tuesday we are going down to Lagos - having lunch at Wesley College, Ibadan en route.

Our labels are ready to stick on. Would you address a packet of stick on and tie on labels, addressed to 12, Edenfield Gardens, to us at the boat at Dover please, then we can use them on trunks etc to redirect them from London.

Kay McWilliams arrived last weekend, looking very well. She is not staying after we get back here, she has been offered a very good job in Uganda.

Miss Ariel, Louie Trott's relief should have arrived by this time. Louie and Bosede fly at the end of this month.

Sunday evening:- Home again after a good journey. Margaret and Elizabeth very well, Peter unfortunately has quite a high fever and has been in bed all day. It is probably an infection which has been going around - I hope it is not measles! otherwise we shall be in the soup!

Tomorrow packing with a farewell party in the evening. Tuesday to Lagos, Wednesday a little shopping and Thursday sail

Will write en route if all is well, love to you all from us all, David

FIFTH TOUR

TSS Calabar, Monday 26th Sept 1960

Monday morning - we have been at sea five days and should pass through the Canaries this afternoon. It is pleasantly warm, the sun is shining brightly, the sea is blue and calm! The children are playing happily with the swing, and Margaret is in the cabin and doing some washing - we are all very well indeed and enjoying ourselves.

It was rather cool when we left the dock at Tilbury and got into the estuary though the first night was quite pleasant. However the following day and Friday as we went down the channel and into the Bay, there was a stiff breeze, rough water and the boat was far from steady. Owing to the delay and tally clerks strike we have virtually no cargo on board and so are riding well up out of the water.

None of us felt well on Thursday or Friday and although we attended each meal it was rather an ordeal and once or twice we left the dining room quite smartly.! One evening less than half turned up for the evening meal! However since then we have all settled down, and the last two days have been quite pleasant. The children have settled down much better - the stewardess is much nicer and wiser in her management of the children - there must be at least 25 of them.

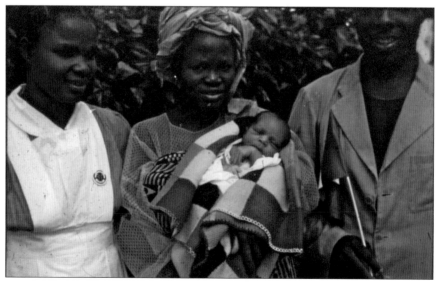

Independence Baby 1960

We are sharing a table with two Sudan Interior Mission missionaries, one of whom is Margaret's distant relative- very distant! The other is Anne Struthers who is a Veterinary Surgeon. Her father is Medical Officer of Health for Westminster, or rather was. They have retired to a small village in Berkshire.

Yesterday I attended the service taken by the Captain in the morning - not very much to write home about, and in the afternoon Margaret and the children attended Sunday school taken by two Assembly of God missionaries who are working in Ghana - which they greatly enjoyed.

There was 'dancing on deck' one evening, but no-one went as it was cold and the boat was moving a great deal.

On Wednesday there is a full day with Childrens' sports, Films, and party in the evening with Carnival night. I shall now tuck this away and finish it just before Freetown.

Thursday evening - Voyage continues well apart from Elizabeth who has a cough and tonight is running a temperature. I have got some penicillin tablets from the ships Doctor and we gave her the first this evening. I hope she will be better in a day or two. The children did not shine in the sports, both being up against older children, but they took part cheerfully! They enjoyed the film yesterday and their party, though Elizabeth was a bit off colour then (yesterday). In the evening we had our Carnival Night and both M and I enjoyed the dancing and games on the deck. In the former we got round very well indeed - so we have gained confidence! We reach Freetown on Saturday at 1pm and will add a further note later.

Saturday morning - Elizabeth much better, but a bout of sickness amongst passengers, which we have fortunately escaped. Freetown in sight but we only dock for three hours so may not see much or anything of Glan and Jean. Weather much hotter and very sticky and shall be glad to reach Ilesha! Hope all well at home - looking forward to having a letter in a few days time.

Love from us all David

TSS Calabar, 3.10.60

Monday morning and tomorrow we reach Takoradi but letters must be ready by this evening as we reach the port at 8am and leave again at 10am.

We arrived in Freetown last Saturday and were very glad indeed to receive your letter and to learn that everything was well at home. You sound to have had a very busy day when the Council men came to enlarge the drive - it must have been a scene of great activity.

Saturday was also Independence Day so the Europeans on board subscribed to a cocktail party given to the Nigerians on board - quite a pleasant event with exciting little biscuits with bits of shrimp and salmon on them to go with our squash.

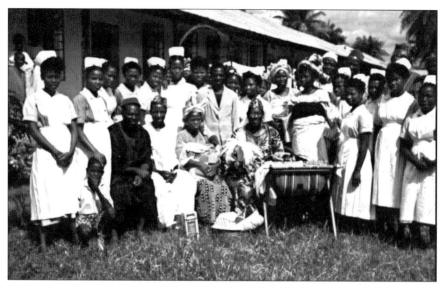

Independence Group

The children had their lunch at mid-day. We docked about 12.30 and saw Glanville and Jean on the quay so they came aboard and then we all went ashore to their home where the rest of us had lunch. It was very nice indeed to get off the boat and the children had a wonderful time playing with Elaine's toys. All three seemed very well indeed and Glanville seems happy in the work he is doing. He is Religious Knowledge tutor at the college and also Protestant chaplain. There are 100 students at the moment, but it is to be increased to 500 in due course. Glanville is permitted to serve in this Government institution and is on a three yearly contract with them.

After lunch we went around Freetown in Glanville's car - there are some lovely views from the hills which surround the town. P and E were very good indeed.

We learned one rather disturbing fact - you may already know - E.J. was sent home last April by the Sierra Leone Government. Apparently there was an argument at the hospital involving the wife of the Minister of Health and E J referred to him in very derogatory terms. She was suspended at once and was home on 'sick leave' within a week. All most unfortunate.

We arrived back just in time and the boat sailed at 4pm. In the evening there was a dinner party for Independence. All the Nigerians sat at the Captains' table. We had a tremendous meal, including trout (whole one each) turkey and all the trimmings. A speech and toast from the Captain and a reply from the Nigerians

Margaret was not feeling very well so we turned in early, but there was a party in the crew's quarters (mainly Nigerian) which went on until 3.00 am - so there was not much sleep that night.

Yesterday was stormy as is today, with a lot of movement on the boat so we *shall be very glad to reach Lagos in two days time. Peter is very well and eating excellently. Elizabeth is still not very well, not sleeping soundly and not eating much at all. I do hope she picks up soon. M and I are quite well and keeping going though it is a bit of an effort sometimes!*

On the whole however we are well and having a good trip. We think and talk of you often and Peter and Elizabeth were very eager to hear what you had to say in the letter!

Love to you all from us all David

5.10.60

Just a line to let you know that we have arrived safely in Lagos. We were very glad to receive your letter at Marina, where Bill and Dorothy welcomed us.

Bill came to the boat and took Margaret and the children off in the car and I stayed to see the loads through customs. I had rather a sticky time and had to pay £4.12.0 duty on the provisions - but even so will be worth while.

At Marina we found 'our' car awaiting us - taxed and insured with roof rack of the same colour! Total cost £536 plus insurance so we feel very pleased about it. Peter was wildly excited so after a drink of squash we packed up tea and motored down to Victoria Beach. By this time Kay McWilliams and Disu in the hospital lorry had arrived, so Kay came with us and we were joined by Bill and Dorothy later.

The children were tired and had a good supper baked beans on toast, the best meal Elizabeth has had for at least a week and she seemed again the Miss Tigger of Edenfield Gardens!

She dropped straight off to sleep and Peter soon after so we went out with Bill in his car to see the illuminations - most impressive. We are very thrilled at the developments made since we went away - it all looks much better.

After we came back I went in to see Jonah who seemed to be in good form and we talked for about an hour.

It is now 10.45 and we are in our bedroom, others having retired for the night. Margaret is writing to Grandpa also, so we can get the letters posted in Lagos to arrive home in good time. Tomorrow we shall do some shopping and then set out mid morning for Ilesha. It will be exciting in the new car.

Will write again at the weekend with a further bulletin. Love to you all from us all, David

Ilesha, 9.10.60

The only air letters we have are one or two from the boat, so I must buy some stamps from the hospital to put on it.

By now you will be settled at home once again after your trip to Sunderland and we look forward to hearing how the journeys and meetings went, and how the front garden is looking.

I wrote last Wednesday evening from Lagos and as you will guess much has happened since then.

The next morning we went out shopping in the Renault and bought in food and a few other things we needed. Meanwhile the lorry was loaded with our luggage, though we were quite pleased to see how much luggage we could get into the boot of our car - the revelation suitcase, the large and small holdalls and my dispatch case. We did not use the roof rack because we did not have any tarpaulin to cover the cases in event of rain.

After we had shopped we spent an hour looking at the Independence Exhibition in Lagos which was most interesting. We left Lagos at 11.40 and jogged safely on as far as Shagamu where we called at the Training College and ate our sandwiches. We bought a picnic because we hadn't time to let folk know we were coming, nor did we know how far we should have got by 1pm. We stayed about three quarters of an hour and set off again. Maximum running in speed is 45 mph but I did not do more than 40 at any time. The children were very good considering it is a six hour journey in the car (160 miles).

We stopped again just outside Ibadan for a picnic tea and then came on to Ilesha arriving about 6.15pm. We were warmly welcomed, had tea with the Pearson's, put the children to bed and then went back for dinner and a talk. We found David Morley not very well so the next morning, I did a clinic from 9.30 - 1.30 in order to give a hand. The rest of the time we unpacked and found that most things had travelled well, only two polythene sandwich boxes had cracked. The bicycle travelled well and is now in going order, apart from the dust caps which must have become lose en route. Elizabeth is very pleased with her tricycle, Ruth has one just like it!

Friday afternoon there was a reunion service in the chapel for 'old nurses' which I attended, and it was addressed by Dr. Hunter. Dr. and Mrs. Hunter arrived last Wednesday and are staying until next Thursday. They have had a royal welcome and seem to be having a wonderful time. They went to Imesi yesterday morning and came here to tea yesterday afternoon. We enjoyed entertaining them. He trained at the London Hospital and two of his children have been there since, so I have carried on the tradition.

Last evening Elsie had a party at her house for us all - a very happy time indeed, though Lily left after the meal and before the games - she is rather odd in this respect.

Unfortunately Peter's cough has got much worse and he and Margaret had a bad night last night, however he has had some medicine and seems a bit better and less feverish this morning. The garden is looking lovely, though not much in our vegetable garden, except beans. The house too, is fresh and looks well. All our cases are unpacked, though the drawers are now a bit of a jumble!

Elizabeth is very well, though she has been a bit clingy since we arrived - it is *an unsettling time, though really they have adapted themselves very well indeed. M and I are very well, though the heat has been a bit much in the afternoons.*

Looking forward to hearing from you in time - hope all is well, love from us all, David

13.10.60

Sunday afternoon again. We have just returned from the trek to Afon having had a pleasant time, more of which anon.

We were very pleased to receive your letter last Thursday and to know that all is well at home. Most interested to hear that you had met Margaret Gregory and heard of Louie Trott. Glad to hear that some of the pictures of the children are good - we look forward to seeing some in due course.

Somehow we seem to have had a very full week again and it has gone past very quickly. Last Monday evening we were invited to the Morleys for dinner and had a very pleasant time. Dr. Sam Katz was there also - he is the measles expert from Boston, USA, and a very nice fellow indeed and very good company. He has five children, the eldest of whom is eight! He is returning to the States on 22nd Nov or so. The measles vaccine has been given and now the children are being observed to see how they react. Wednesday was committee evening which passed off without difficulty. Elsie came in to the wives, who on these evenings have coffee together and sew, as she had attended her last committee a month ago. I was on last Tuesday, Wednesday and Thursday nights with operations and Friday was a very busy morning.

Elsie finally left about 2.30 in our Dauphine. I had hoped that we might take it up to Afon but the loads Margaret Ashley wanted were too great and in addition we took Kathleen Owen, William and a midwife, so the Opel Caravan was pushed to its capacity.

After a busy morning we left about 2.30 and called for stores on the way through. We stopped in Ogbomosho and had a drink of Fanta - a new semi fizzy drink. Unfortunately this proved too much for Elizabeth, who was sick about 100 yards from the house in Afon. However she picked up immediately we got out. We stayed in Kathleen Ormerod's house, a small mud built thatched Yoruba house, very hot and dark and dusty as you can imagine. We all had camp beds in different rooms. There is not a room big enough for two beds. The children shared one bed as we had only got three nets. Peter going off to sleep in Margaret's bed and then, when we went to bed, we lifted him into the same bed but at the opposite end to Elizabeth.

We had our meals with them - but it was all very slow because they have another new house boy, who has only been in the house three months.

On Saturday I saw the patients and in the afternoon we went for a picnic to the Ilorin reservoir and brought back a lot of seedling trees and bushes which we found. A good ride back today and then another week's work. Next week I shall be going to Synod November Medical Committee, but am on duty in the afternoon so shall have to come back in good time. We have heard from Roy and he has got both the Edinburgh and London FRCS. Incredibly good.

We are all very well indeed except Margaret has some backache.

Love to you all, David

23.10.60

Sunday evening and rather later than usual for me to be starting my letter home but we have been up to Ikole and since our return have been to chapel! Thank you for your letter. I hope Father had a good time in Hull.

Here we have had a week of alarms and excursions, and unfortunately there is one at the moment. We missed the phone calls, being in Ikole but Margaret Woodland went down to meet Helen Kohler off the boat yesterday. When she arrived she was welcomed by the crew with the words 'have you come for the patient?' 'No, a nursing sister' but apparently she has been ill ever since they sailed and was so weak she had to be slung off the boat by crane. Even while Margaret Woodland was with her waiting to go ashore she asked her to send for the doctor as she felt she was going to die! A combination of asthma, seasickness and hysteria according to the ship's doctor

This morning there was an urgent phone call from Bill Mann for our big Hospital car to take her out of their house into a hospital as they apparently had an awful night with her. Thus when we got back from Ikole we found that Andrew had set out for Lagos to review the situation. It is all most unfortunate but bears out my impression of her. If the shipping line would have had her I think Andrew would try to get her on the boat back to England, but they will refuse to have her on board until she is better. Olive Osborne who was also on the boat must have had a tottering time. The Sisters here are dreadfully upset about it - their hopes of help vanishing. Margaret has offered and also Aileen, to nurse her if Andrew should feel it necessary. We are hoping Andrew will ring in a few minutes.

We have had a busy week. David Morley and family have been to Tarkua Bay for a holiday, Fred has had a sore throat and not been well, Frank and Kay Davey have been to see the place and interview the staff and then to cap it all trouble has arisen over David M's trial of measles vaccine, so Andrew (in David's absence) had to go to Ibadan last Thursday for the day.

Then Friday we set off for Ikole. We had a good journey up though the Dauphine found the hills hard work with three adults (we took William), two children and a roof rack full of drugs and dressings. However we did about 86 miles in three hours which was quite good going. We are very pleased with the car, especially its road holding properties.

Miss Joan Ariel has made great improvements, painting, furniture, beds for nurses, but is rather critical of Louie's ways. However Joan is in financial difficulties at the moment, no doubt we shall help her out!

We had a very nice time - nice food and the children behaved very well indeed. There were more patients to see but nothing very serious.

Next week looks busy. David Morley has to go to Ibadan tomorrow, Andrew, we hope, will return from Lagos

It is Elsie's last week - at least two parties and two farewell services next Sunday. Tomorrow we are having the Pearson's and Fred in to chop with Elsie we hope. Time now for a drink of Nesquick and then bed! We are all very well indeed and hope you are all also. Love from us all David.

30.10.60

Sunday afternoon and it is very hot indeed and it is certain to rain this evening and will not be cool until it does. We were very glad to receive your letter with all its' news and Stanley is certainly going to try his hardest to get into the University - all strength to his elbow.

Here we have again had a hectic week with another one to come. Andrew and his family went down to Lagos for a weeks holiday on Tarkaru Bay, so once again we are reduced to three Doctors. However Fred Follet our new Doctor who will be feeding with us this week, will pull his weight I feel, so it won't be too bad. However David M will be away two or three days I expect on this measles vaccine trial which starts tomorrow by David Morley going down to fetch the American Doctor who is in charge of the vaccine - and the vaccine as well ! Incidentally he is going in our car which will then receive its 600 mile service whilst in Lagos. We are still very pleased with its performance.

Helena Kohler will be due out of hospital this weekend and Andrew is going to see her tomorrow and see if we can give her a weeks holiday in Ibadan before she comes up to Ilesha. The other sisters are now much more co-operative and willing for her to come to us here to see how she gets on.

We have had three parties this week. On Wednesday Sister Komolafe gave a party for all the senior staff to celebrate the birth of her first child (after waiting six years) which was most enjoyable, though Andrew was very ill afterwards and was in bed until the middle of Thursday afternoon.

On Thursday evening it was our farewell to Elsie. The Sisters, with assistance, put on a lovely meal and afterwards Elsie was presented with an Awka chest (carved wood), a slide projector and a gold broach in the form of Africa. Speeches were made and so forth. Then last night the nurses gave her a farewell party and presented her with a bead cushion and a rig-out of Yoruba dress. It was all very well done.

Yesterday afternoon the male hospital staff staged a football match (we now have a football club) against the police at which Elsie kicked off, and afterwards presented her with a Yoruba costume. Tomorrow the Methodist Church is giving a farewell function for her in the Town Hall and I think on Wednesday the King will give a Garden Party, It is all rather harrowing for Elsie and a little time consuming. Never has the office work been so much behindhand - due largely to Independence Day and to our late arrival back. Andrew has been unable to balance last years accounts yet.

We are all very well. The children get on with their meals! and are in the best of spirits. Margaret keeps well - but the heat at the moment is a bit trying. Hope you are all well. Love from us all   David.

1.11.60

Another Sunday morning is here - cool and very pleasant after a hot and busy week. Andrew is back from his holiday, in good form, and has gone down to church at the moment. Margaret is at home with the children and I am seizing a quiet moment in the office to start this letter.

Our most important piece of news is that we are expecting a brother or sister for Peter and Elizabeth! We are very pleased about it and look forward to the arrival next May or thereabouts. This is, as we hoped before David and Andrew leave and go on furlough respectively next year. Margaret has been a little unwell the last few weeks but is much better the last day or two.

The next piece of news and not yet confirmed is that Roy has got his FRCS We have not heard from him or Beryl but Margaret had a letter from Edith Milner who heard the news when she was in London for committee, in fact you may have heard it too. We feel a little put out that we haven't heard directly, but expect he is waiting until he finishes his London FRCS next week It is the Edinburgh one which we learn he has obtained. We are all naturally very pleased indeed.

David M. has been away several days this week so that Fred and I have had a lot to cope with, In addition there has been a lot to catch up with in the office. Independence Celebrations and visitors seem to have taken up much of the time that we would normally have spent at the desks. However apart from the accounts we are more or less straight though November Medical Committee is a week on Saturday.

Last Saturday Prof. Burn from UCH rang up and said a consultant dermatologist (Dr. Russell) from the London was out, and would like to look round, so we had him from 10.15 to 3.15. He is a very pleasant man indeed and was most interested in all he saw. This was his first contact with a Mission hospital I think. He had come out to look at the possibility of a dermatologist coming out to be based in Ibadan, to do research into skin disorders here. Yesterday was November 5th and the Pearsons' were expected back with fireworks, from Lagos.

We built a very big bonfire, made a guy stuffed with straw and as dusk fell lit *it. It rained slightly but undeterred it blazed away. The Pearsons' just arrived in time with fireworks, simple ones, so a very good, though famous time was had by all and some very tired children dropped off to sleep at once!*

We had the Pearsons' and Fred and David Thompson in to chop afterwards (potatoes baked in the bonfire!) and had a very pleasant evening.

Helena came up from Lagos to Ibadan in the Dauphine - the latter having been serviced - stayed there a few days and has now come on to us. She seems very well but very sorry about the lost time and hopes to fly in future! Anyway we hope and pray all will be well for the next few months.

Dr. Katz, the American measles expert also arrived last night so we are a full compound at the moment. Elsie goes to Lagos finally next Friday. Her farewells are over now. The new Laboratory is in use!

Love to you all from us all   David

27.11.60

We were delighted to receive your letter this week and interested to learn all that had been going on. Especially interested to hear of the visit(s) to Vera and Joe's - we have not done any dancing since we landed, and I hope that the steps come back without trouble else we shall feel to have wasted our time with dancing lessons!

We have had a usual sort of week without anything very dramatic happening. Margaret is feeling better - her backache is less, the children are well but I have developed a sore throat and cough which reduces my activities somewhat. It would not matter much but it is my service in the hospital chapel tonight - I shall be glad when it is over.

Joan Ariel - Louie's successor has had a very near squeak! Last Monday she was returning to Ikole having taken a patient in to Ado when she missed a bridge with her offside wheels and the car rolled off the bridge into the stream. She and the midwife were pulled out by school children, bruised but not seriously injured, fortunately. Later the car was extracted by a contractor and miraculously it still worked though the roof was pushed in, the offside wings and doors pushed in and the wind screen out and back window smashed and the car filled with mud!

Fred went up on trek on Friday and drove it down to Ilesha yesterday which is a stoic effort. Unfortunately from the insurance point of view it is not a complete write-off otherwise we should get several hundred for the car and be able to get a new one. As it is we shall get the repairs only and still be left with rather a decrepit vehicle. The problem of Ikole is still unsolved, with out Louie's parsimony the place is not financially viable, but where the extra £2000 pa is to come from no one is at all sure.

The dry season has come upon us with a vengeance. No rain now for two weeks and none likely until next April. Already the ground is getting dusty and the grass going brown.

The nights are cool and the afternoons are blazing hot. Yesterday, those who felt fit went for a swim in the pool and then we all had a picnic under one of the trees near the pool - very pleasant.

Margaret is having to water the garden assiduously, but last night we had some very nice runner beans for dinner. We had in Mrs. Denia, the new Nigerian assistant sister in the maternity ward, and her husband (PhD Nutrition) and Kathleen and we had a very nice meal - cold store mutton and all went successfully. (I have just taken the nurses and Helena down to church in the lorry. It is the Harvest Festival today - a three hour service at least)

Helena seems to be settling in well with part of the maternity ward and the antenatal clinics to look after, not a great responsibility, but she is doing it very thoroughly. Marion is taking on the Matron's work very well, though finds it a bit of a strain, I think at times and the rest of us jog along.

Peter and Elizabeth are very well indeed and happy!! The other day we had a caravan full of rice parked outside, Peter saw them and would not let them drive off until his little sister had seen them! Very sweet indeed.

Hope you are well, pity we can't swap some of our heat for your rain.

Love from us all David

4.12.60

Sunday morning, and in ten minutes I shall have to go down to church with the nurses, but just time to start this letter. We were very glad indeed to receive your letter, and to learn of the family happenings at No 12. We wonder how Stanley got on at Cambridge - it will be quite an experience for him. You all seem to have been busy, what with the 'tango' to say nothing of addressing meetings.

Here it has been an eventful week unfortunately not all happy ones. On Monday morning Jean Pearson must have blacked out whilst in the garden and fell into a ditch. We think she must have been unconscious at the time because she made no effort to shield her face which was very badly damaged and had to be stitched up, and she had concussion for two days afterwards. She is still in bed but is much brighter now and able to give her mind to her household. Margaret had been managing things for her and until yesterday, has bathed her every day. Aileen has looked after the children and we have had Andrew in to numerous meals.

Whilst Andrew was stitching Jean up in the operating theatre, Marion who was standing by, fainted, knocked her head on the operating table and she had to have stitches in her eyelid, and has also been in bed for a week and is now having a couple of days rest at Ikole! Lily and Helena with Mrs. Dema and Rebecca have been coping with the nursing very well, and Marion should be back again

398

tomorrow. Fortunately Helena is keeping very well and seems very thrilled with all there is to do.

Have been down to chapel - a long hot service - not very inspiring. Tonight it is our Hospital Chapel, the Chaplain is preaching here, which won't be very thrilling either. Last Sunday it was my service and no doubt people made the same remarks about me!

This afternoon is very hot indeed but outside there is the noise of a steamroller, chuffing up and down! We are having our roads laid out and tarred in places and the best day for them to work is Sundays because there are not many folk about. Needless to say the children are fascinated by the 'grader' a machine which levels and cambers the road - a most remarkable piece of machinery.

A few days ago two Roman Catholic nuns came to see me, one had a septic finger and they had been misdirected down to the house. Margaret sat them in the living room and gave them squash whilst she rang up to see where I was. At this point Peter returned to the house, saw them in the living room, and ran to Margaret on the phone in the bedroom 'Mummy, God and Jesus are in our living room'!

Peter and Elizabeth are very well and eating well - we must weigh them again today. Margaret too is keeping well apart from the veins of one leg which are particularly painful. She will be going down to see Mr. Lawson this week again as arranged.

Last Wednesday I received an invitation to the inaugural meeting of the Association of Surgeons of West Africa. I drove down on Friday morning, heard three scientific papers, had a good lunch, saw the medical films, met a number of people and then drove home, this time bringing Larry Longo, the obstetrician from Ife. It made a much more pleasant journey, having someone to talk to. A most interesting day.

Christmas is coming on apace, I am not sure what visitors there will be - probably not many as we shall have a full compound in any case. We are hoping that the new students hostel will be ready in time.

Hope you are all well despite the wet. Love from us all, David

18.12.60

My thoughts were elsewhere, apparently when I started - but this letter brings you all our very best wishes for a Happy Christmas. We can picture you in it so well and wish that we could be with you. Here it does not seem a bit like Christmas - very hot and sticky, no shops with decorations and only a list of events to take place in the next two weeks! However behind the scenes a great deal has been done. Margaret made the cake a month ago. It is sealed up in a tin and we are hoping that it is keeping well. Our fare is ordered and we hope it will arrive on Friday. Our Christmas guest will be Margaret Woodland, but she will not be able to stay very long I fear. The Manns are coming to stay with the Morleys and the Pearsons' are having two guests I believe.

Our Christmas arrangements are much the same as previous years, I will describe them next week. Christmas cards are coming in but are apparently hindering normal mail as we have not had your letter this week, but look forward to receiving it perhaps tomorrow.

We have received three books from Michael which did not contain names of senders, but we are very pleased with the selection, they will be well received by the children.

Peter is very well but Elizabeth has fever today and is most unlike her usual self, heavy eyed, sitting in a chair and looking at a book. She was most unsettled last night and Margaret was up half a dozen times with her.

Margaret is quite well, though her legs are rather troublesome, and she finds the heat a bit trying.

The Dolls house is almost finished, all that remains to be done is a second coat of paint to the surround. The doors are not perfect by any means, but adequate. I have put in some expanding curtain wire over the windows, so that E can make little curtains for them in due course. Anyway we shall be interested to see how it is accepted by the children.

Andrew went up to Ikole last Friday and came back yesterday and tomorrow he and David M are going to Ilorin and then on to Kaiama the next day. The Commission though seems to be disintegrating. Bill M now says he hasn't time to go and Jonah wants to stay longer than the others, anyway we will see what happens. In any case Fred and I are going to have a busy time with the other two away especially as it is the week before Christmas. We shall have to get our presents wrapped one evening this week, and Margaret has the cake to complete, with almond paste, icing and decoration which will take two evenings.

On Wednesday we are to have sacred music instead of Fellowship and next Saturday will be Carol singing.

Last night the Sisters had a party to welcome Helena. Was to have been out of doors but a freak storm as dusk fell , and altered plans. However we had the meal in their lounge by the light of hurricane lamps, had soup in mugs, sausages, bacon, fried bananas and then a potato all with a stick through. it was delicious and would have been very nice indeed outside round a campfire. Afterwards we sang rounds and played charades. Peter has just come in wildly excited 'the Pearsons' are decorating their room', so no doubt we shall be starting ours this afternoon!

A very happy Christmas to you all, Love from us all David

Christmas Day, 1960

A very Happy New Year to you all. It seems rather odd writing this as it is now 10.15 on Christmas morning. The children are playing with their toys at the moment but are due to go to Sunday School any minute. They are very excited, the long awaited day having at last arrived. We were very glad to have received your letters this week. Auntie, thank you very much indeed for your gifts to us we are indeed most grateful.

Thank you very much for the shirt! Mild derision has been pointed at the bathing belles on it! - but it is a lovely shirt. Margaret too is thrilled with her scented cologne and soap.

This week has been a busy one with Andrew and David away from Monday to Wednesday night. However Fred and I managed to get most things done! The sisters have been busy getting all the Christmas things ready for the patients.

On Wednesday evening we had Sacred music (Messiah and Carols) really the beginning of the Christmas festivities. On Friday evening there was a filmstrip service in our chapel for all the staff. I was busy and unable to go but believe it went very well. We had a week of busy evenings, getting things ready, 30 presents to wrap apart from stockings, cake to ice.

The Manns came on Thursday and told me that Mr. Kearsey, Physics master at KS was in Lagos. I rang him and invited him for Christmas, but he was unable to get up, but will come up for the New Year I think! He is acting as a tutor to examiners in the marking of paper I believe, for the West African Examination Council.

Last night was Carol Singing and we went in five cars around the town visiting Methodists and other people, ending up as traditional at the Hon J.O Fadahunsi's house where we had squash, biscuits and nuts. The evening was marred by Helena who fell into a four foot concrete drain and had to be taken home. She is still rather shaken up and bruised.

It was late when we got back, Margaret had stayed in with the children as had Margaret Woodland and Olive who are our guests. However we filled stockings, exchanged them and then put the Dolls House in the room and crept off to bed. Peter woke at 2am but was too sleepy to realise that Father Christmas had been fortunately. This morning I went off to the Communion service in the chapel at 6am. Margaret stayed in to watch for the children and an extra hour's sleep, which she needs.

The children woke at 6.30 and were wildly excited - the Dolls house was an immediate success (as a boat!) and they had some of the furniture in their stockings. They have not yet had their books from Uncles Mick and Twink, nor the motor boat for Peter or the items for Elizabeth from you as they are being kept for the Christmas tree at tea time. They have received numbers of presents, dinky toys, sweets etc. They have just this moment returned from Sunday School.

Peter very pleased because he has learned something. This afternoon there are services in the wards and tonight a carol service in the Chapel. At midday the Doctors and guests and Sisters are having lunch with the nurses, whilst the children have their own lunch. Our Christmas Dinner is tomorrow night followed by a party.

We are all very well indeed, though Margaret's leg is painful unless supported by a bandage which is rather hot Hope you have all had a very Happy Christmas. Love from us all, David

8.1.61

Sunday is here again. I am on duty but am seizing a moment in the office to start this letter. We were very pleased to receive your letter on Thursday and to hear all the news. Auntie A will be back at Brighouse and Stanley back from Oxford. Yes - you are quite right when you state that I am green with envy! A week on the Norfolk Broads! What kind of craft? Are you attempting a yacht and auxiliary engine? Perhaps this will become an annual event! Shall be pleased to hear further details in due course.

We have had a busy week one way and another. Last Sunday an influx of visitors - Mr. Ayres - the senior Chemistry master at the Leys, Cambridge came to see us in the afternoon and stayed overnight. He was most interested in all that he saw and has written us a very nice letter since he returned to Lagos. Monday was a Bank Holiday and most of the compound, including ourselves and Frank Morton who had also come up to us on the Sunday went to Ede (about 27 miles away to a swimming pool in connection with Ede reservoir. We had a lovely time and a picnic and then in the evening we had Dr. Anne Munro who has come to us for two months and Frank and the Morleys in to chop. Turkey which was very nice, though rather small. Afterwards we played Scoop which went down very well.

Dr. Munro is doing the maternity ward and part of the children's work. She will do very well I think, though the danger is that she will start more than we can continue when she has gone.

Yesterday at mid-day I came down to lunch and found a letter waiting from Mr. Kearsey (Physics Master at KS) to say that he would be coming up that afternoon - a double shuffle and we were ready when he arrived about 4pm. He seems much the same as when I last saw him and it must be fifteen years since last we met. He gets on well with the children and seems most interested in all he sees. I don't think he is a very keen churchman though I may well be wrong. He is staying over today and returning to Lagos tomorrow. He knew Margaret's father at Chesterfield Grammar School. Mr. Ingham was the Senior Science master and Mr. Kearsey one of the junior until he came to Kingswood School in 1943.

Yesterday also Prof. Davey (Surgeon at UCH Ibadan) came up to do a couple of operations. He brought his wife and family and the anaesthetist he brought with him, also brought two children. We had the latter to lunch and he returned soon afterwards. Pearsons' entertained the former and they stayed on to swim and a picnic by the pool - eleven children and ten adults altogether! and Mr. Kearsey arrived in time to join in.

Last evening I had to operate on a woman with a ruptured uterus and she seems to be doing well, but fortunately a relatively quiet night.

We are all keeping well. Peter's foot is quite better and he and Elizabeth are irrepressible. They have children to play with and are having a very happy time at the moment. When the Morleys and Pearsons' go they will miss them very much. Margaret is keeping well apart from her leg which is still troublesome.

Next week Andrew will go to Ibadan on Friday for a standing committee and stay down until the Wednesday for Synod. David M will be going for two days, and the following week there is a conference in Lagos to which David M and Andrew will be going so the outlook is 'busy'!

Hope all is well at home, love from us all David

15.1.61

The great piece of news this week is that Peter can ride his bicycle! He has been a bit reluctant to have it out to practice because all the other children could ride it. However yesterday afternoon he was off and although he finds it a bit difficult to start he really manages very well indeed. Now that he is riding it, it will not be long before we require a pair of inner tubes and so should be grateful if you could buy two and send them by sea mail - I will append the size later.

We were very glad to receive your letter earlier this week and to learn that all is well. The boat exhibition must have been most interesting and I look forward to hearing of the Broads arrangements.

We have had a busy week - and Synod starts tomorrow. Andrew will be gong down to Ibadan tomorrow with Marion and Eileen and David will go down on Tuesday for the day. I am going to send, under separate cover, a copy of the report printed of the trip to Borgu - I thought that there might be some material within for talks!

Our 1960 report should be out shortly too, and I have asked the Mission House to send 50 copies to you. Incidentally do you have any copies of the 1958 report left? We have run out completely so would ask you to hang on to any you have left.

Last Monday the Pearsons', Morley and Cannon went out to dinner with some folk who are working in Ilesha. A most interesting meal. The first course was a tepid sort of fruit which was appaling! We did not know what to do! However we managed to eat a little so custom was satisfied. The rest of the meal was very nice indeed.

On Tuesday night we had a party at the Sisters house to welcome Eileen back - a very good party indeed and we played Beetle afterwards. The same day we had a visit from Mr. and Mrs. Wilkinson from Leeds who are retired Post Office workers who bought a Dormobile and left Leeds fourteen months ago and drove through Europe-Asia-Egypt-East Africa-South Africa and West Africa then on to North Africa-Europe and back to Leeds!

An incredible couple, unprepossessing in appearance but must be incredibly hardy. They are hoping to get back to Leeds in May. Mr. Kearsey went on Monday last having enjoyed his stay I think and should be back again in England

We have been rather concerned about our nurses non-attendance at church and prayers and had a meeting on Friday night with all our senior nurses. It was most encouraging and we look forward to better times,

Yesterday we had Prof. Lawson, Mr. Kinston and Dr. Hendricks to inspect the hospital again. They seemed pleased with what they saw.

John Lawson discussed a possible qualification. He had made enquiries about it and feels it would not be worth the effort and cost. It would not make me a 'Consultant' and it would not help in General Practice, so he feels that it would rather be a waste of time.

We are all very well indeed, though Margaret's leg is still painful. Peter and Elizabeth are in very good form and the former attending school for the Spring term! The hens are not laying very well, the garden is dry, but we are still having produce. Marion has just looked in and asks to be remembered to you

Love to you all from all,   David

22.1.61

We were thrilled to hear that Stanley had been offered a place at St. Peters Hall, Oxford and I shall be writing today to him at Kingswood to send our congratulations. We were very pleased to have Michael's letter and to hear details of the Broads trip - I hope the weather is good - and what about a fishing rod or two ?

Any possibility of a visit here during the summer? Always find accommodation for as many as we want - Private Ward beds are excellent.

Here we have had an ordinary sort of week. Andrew and David have been down to Synod, where things went according to plan. They returned on Wednesday evening. There was a suggestion from the Mission House that the tours here should be two years for male Missionaries, except Doctors! This caused some ill feeling at the Missionaries meeting, I believe and also that the first six months of the first tour should be language study.

On Friday I held the first Departmental meeting of the Maternity Unit. It was very well attended indeed and seemed to be appreciated, and this was followed by our nurses fellowship, at 7pm now instead of 8pm. It was a united meeting hymn singing and so on and was very good.

Yesterday we had Jean and Andrew and two teachers from Anglican Girls School in to dinner. We had Yorkshire pudding, followed by roast beef! I imagine that it is the first time in Ilesha that Yorkshire Pudding has started a meal! and it was very nice indeed. Afterwards we played Scoop which seemed to be appreciated by all. Unfortunately there were only five newspapers, so the last twice I had to act as banker and general referee.

Today is my day off and our coffee and as I went down to Otapete last Sunday I shall just drive the nurses down this Sunday.

The tarring of our hospital roads has been started. One day last week I stood and watched for several hours to make sure the right areas were done. I came down when they had finished, for tea and when I went back afterwards I found that they had gone back to the beginning again and done an extra 50 yards, but we hope that they will give us this portion.

The other main item of news is that our new autoclave (£2775) has been installed, but is not functioning quite as we would like It is so automatic that we are powerless to adjust it. It does not attain the correct temperature for a sufficient length of time on one cycle, and on the other it attains the temperature, but again the cycle is too short. So far as working it is concerned it is very simple - just press a button and the cycle is completed automatically. We are going to write to London about it and complain, with one of the temperature charts.

Aileen had a letter from Beryl (in Ceylon) They are also expecting a baby in May, all their three will be younger than Elizabeth. It does not strike us as being a very happy letter. I think she is finding life with Roy's family rather overpowering. She has two ayahs for the children, who dress feed and wash them in their clothes! They would like to remain in Ceylon for Roy's next tour or leave the youngest there. Anyway we will see what we can do by offering to deliver her here.

We are all very fit and well - I have just had to mend a puncture on Peter's bicycle! Love from us all   David

29.1.61

Another Sunday is here and another busy week has passed. We were very pleased to receive your letter and all the news. We can imagine Twink being more Twinkish. I guess he has a most superior air with the small boys at Kingswood now.

We heard from Mr. Ingham the other day too. He is keeping well as are Thea and Ernie and the children. Mr. Kearsey wrote to Mr. Ingham after his visit here and said how much he enjoyed his stay here.

This week has been the Paediatric conference organised by WACMR in Lagos David M went down last Tuesday and is not due back until tomorrow evening.

Andrew, Jean Wingfield and Margaret Woodland went down very early on Wednesday morning and returned very late Thursday night, actually 2.00 am on Friday morning. They had a very busy but interesting time and I think that David M's paper went well. He is hoping to get permission to do more measles inoculations but there is still considerable opposition from Prof. Collard at UCH Ibadan.

Thank you too, for the birthday greetings! As Michael said - he sent greetings and left it at that. There comes a time when birthdays come round too frequently. Margaret gave me a ratchet screw driver, which I had long wanted. Peter had ideas for presents so I drove the family out to the market where a sponge was bought and then on to a shop to buy a tin of salted nuts - both most acceptable gifts - both Peter's own ideas.

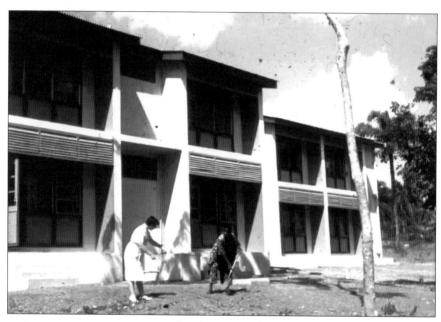

Students hostel

The hospital has been busy and with Andrew away I have had quite a lot of administration to do. We have just had our roads completed and the bill came this morning - just over £1500, which seems a lot when we have already paid £500 for materials. However it is a job well done.

The students hostel is just about complete - I think the builders will be moving out tomorrow. We have all been put in a spot because we have just heard that the Governor of Western Nigeria is coming to look round for an hour on Thursday next. This has meant that we have had to get invitations printed and a plaque made for the Owa to unveil at the hostel as he will open the new building. Glaxo Ltd will be represented and no doubt as this will be one of the Owa's first engagements of this nature there will be pressmen in plenty. The problem is making the plaque, polished wood and paint and to get the lettering satisfactory.

We are all very well. Margaret went down to see Prof. Lawson last Wednesday who found all well. Peter and Elizabeth are in good form - though another two punctures!

One afternoon at rest time there was much merriment from the children. When we went in afterwards Peter had cut off masses of Elizabeth's hair! It does not look as bad as it might but on the crown it is down to one inch in length ! Elizabeth doesn't seem to mind at all!

Peter wrote a very brief note (unaided) in school the other day which we have posted on to you by sea mail! Hens are laying fairly well, garden produce decreasing due to the dry weather. Hope you are all well. Love from us all
David   PS How are the orchids?

12.2.61

Thank you very much for your letter and the card for Elizabeth which arrived on Thursday. We will present the card. The children have made it their chief topic of discussion for the last week and Margaret has instructions to make the birthday cake in the shape of a boat! You seem to have been very busy stripping, wallpaper papering and painting - by the time this letter reaches you will perhaps be nearing the end of it all. So far as we are concerned it is the shape of things to come!

Sorry to hear that Stanley is not yet out of hospital - I should imagine though that it will not be long. We get such patients out on the eighth day. Sorry too, to hear that Mrs. Ranger is unwell. She always did seem on the frail side.

Is the marble topped table going up under the tree? Where did it and the umbrella stand come from?

Here we are all well, busy and happy. It has been an average sort of week, though I managed to get down to the meeting of the Department of Obstetrics and Gynaecology at UCH Ibadan on Wednesday afternoon. It is most refreshing to meet with others engaged in the same work and with the same problems and to learn that their problems are much the same as ours.

Last Sunday I had rather an anxious day with a private patient - a lawyers wife and had to section her in the evening. She has been a most difficult patient and the nurses, both Missionary and Nigerian are heartily tired of her goings on! Anyway she and the baby are well I am glad to say.

This last week we have had in a batch of medical students - the first in the hostel, though as yet the food is prepared in the nurses kitchen However the accommodation seems to be appreciated.

One day last week we were over at the Morleys and I overheard the following conversation between Ruth and Elizabeth. Come and see my new dresses. E New ones? R Yes! Exit both to the bedroom. It is the sort of conversation expected of girls 20 years older!

Peter and Elizabeth are both looking forward to the advent of the new baby. Peter keeps prodding us to get the pram out and carry cot etc. So no doubt we shall have to soon.

Yesterday the Rev John Farley and family arrived to take a weekend at the Hospital Chapel and give a talk on visiting the sick to a number of our clients. He is taking the service in the chapel tonight. Also here this weekend are Ron Morley and Harry Kirk, both Methodists. Mr. Kirk built Queen Elizabeth hospital at Umuahia and Ron Morley is the town and country planning officer. They have drawn up plans for the extension to our Nursing School and are going to design a new nurses home.

Last night we had in Doreen and Ernie Wood - Apostolic missionaries with two young children - one American and one Canadian and we had a pleasant evening. M had ordered a shoulder of local lamb from cold store and got a leg of imported - a vast difference in price and it is almost all bone! However it is a recognised hazard and must be accepted as such.

Next week Andrew is going to Ibadan to do a short course in anaesthetics so I should be having a somewhat busy time. Thank Michael for the rubella booklet and thank you too for the Punches etc. most welcome.

Love to you all from us all, David

WGH, Ilesham, 19.2.61

Another very busy week over. Andrew went on this course in anaesthesia last Monday and is not due back until next Monday (tomorrow) evening. This has meant that I have had all the administration as well as all the palaver to deal with. In a closed community like ours it is very easy for people to get up against each other and it needs a great deal of diplomacy to keep things on an even keel.

We were very pleased to receive your letter on Wednesday this week - a day earlier than usual and to hear all your news. Our greetings to Stanley and we hope his wound heals up in due course.

The last time we had this trouble is when Andrew took the appendix out of Mr. Mackenzie our district officer and it discharged, to our chagrin! It would seem that there was some infection around! We are looking forward to seeing the hall and landing in their new guise - it sounds most attractive.

Last Monday was a day of great excitement. Elizabeth really entered into it. We gave her a baking set, miniature scales, rolling pin, patty tins etc. This was swooped upon by Alison who immediately with Elizabeth's help made some pastry and tarts which were subsequently cooked. Unfortunately the boys spotted them and ate two before they were cooked! The remaining two were very nice indeed. The other families brought in presents, two books so Elizabeth and Peter also were very thrilled.

In the afternoon Elizabeth had a tea party, fancy hats and so forth for the children only. Her birthday cake was sponge in the shape of a ship - looked most realistic. After tea at which they were all presented with whistles they ran off blowing hard!

The last two days have been quiet so I guess they have lost them for the time being! We were to have had some guests last weekend but they are in fact coming next weekend, when we, especially Margaret are likely to be very busy - three adults and a child!

The Pearsons' return tomorrow and then on Tuesday someone will have to go down to meet Margaret Gardener, our new Sister Tutor, who is expected to arrive on Wednesday. We are all looking forward to the arrival.

Anne is still here and doing Maternity. On her return from Ibadan two weeks ago she ran into a bank and damaged her car. She took it into Ibadan and on coming back in Fred's car she was stopped for dangerous driving and they found the car license not in order, so she has to appear in court on Tuesday in Ibadan - all most unfortunate.

We have heard from Beryl, she and Roy and both children will be returning here during the second week in March, it will make a big difference having them back again. Anne sails on March 7th and Fred about the end of March, so once again we shall be down to four Doctors. We hope to hear soon that Dr. David Bowler has agreed to follow David Morley and we hear too that Jonathan Hartfield is to be my successor and will be available in May. Anyway we shall see.

Hope all are well - we are very fit, Love from us all, David

26.2.61

Sunday morning and a few moments in the office to get things sorted out and this letter started. Margaret is taking Sunday School, our guest is going down to the Otapete service. We were very glad to receive your letter and to hear of all your activities. Spring certainly seems to have come early. There is a picture in our Airmail Guardian of crocus in bloom somewhere. I hope it does not bring out fruit blossom prematurely and get it blighted by late frost.

Sorry to hear Stanley is making slow progress. As Dr. Bowen states it is a question of waiting until all the cat gut comes out. We have had two acute appendices here this week and both in young people - but I hope they will be out before the end of this week. Anyway we look forward to seeing a plentiful supply of rugs - perhaps some could go into store for our home!

We were most interested to hear that Michael has obtained application forms for a job near Lagos. If this is a serious application I would suggest that you let me know the address and I could go down and look the place over. *There are one or two snags about applying for jobs such as this, to which one is unable to seek. For example is housing available now, is it furnished (partly or whole)? Is the laboratory ready now? Is it equipped? and so on as establishments tend to apply for personnel whilst building. If it is a serious thought I would be happy to go down and inspect the situation on behalf of one applicant! Women's Work has done very well again hasn't it. The Missionary Society owes a tremendous debt to the women folk for their financial support.*

Incidentally, Joan at Ikole is more than a little chagrined to find that she is not in the prayer manual. Apparently now Women's Work has no interest in Ikole so she does not qualify for prayer! The Broads holiday seems to be coming quite close I trust that all concerned are reading up on nautical terms, the rules of craft sailing. We will expect full details - someone will have to keep the log! and write bulletins at frequent intervals.

We have had a busy week one way and another. The Pearsons' returned on Monday evening, Andrew having had a most enjoyable course in anaesthesia. Unfortunately he heard on Thursday that his Mother died last Monday also. All his family however were at his home and he has a sister living at home who will be able to housekeep for his Father. He is retiring this year and is having a bungalow built not very far away which he will move into in due course.

Last Wednesday Margaret went down to see Prof Lawson again and he found all well. Afterwards she went round to Wesley College where she saw the Principal who is happy for us to have the use of Frank's house, whilst he is away and we shall also be able to have Frank's house boy. This means that I should go down when I start my local leave. It will be quite expensive to have the two households but I think it will be much the best way. Unfortunately there will not be many folk on the Wesley College Compound as the Bookers are leaving for good and the Barfields and Frank all on furlough. I hear that the Principal is hoping to get some replacements who may have arrived by that time. I should get down at week ends except when I am on duty.

Roy and Beryl arrive in Ilesha on March 10th. Miss Gardener the new Sister Tutor arrived on Thursday in good form. We have a visitor with us this week end and two other guests for Friday night. Jean has a sister and Doctor coming today Anne (who leaves in about a week has two visitors also and Frank has one.

Do hope that all is well with you all. We are keeping very fit indeed

Love from us all David

5.3.61

Peter was thrilled with his letter from you all, and took it to bed with him last night. He mentioned then that he was going to write today but whether he will get round to it I don't know.

We were very pleased to receive your letter and to know all is well but commiserate with Stanley over the delayed healing of the wound. It will probably close quite rapidly when the stitches have come out. Meanwhile the rug with roses on it grows apace.

We are all well, Margaret is keeping very fit and the children too. We have had a busy week however, and I shall be glad of a rest this afternoon if all is well.

The Morleys returned last Friday after a good holiday, but David went to Ibadan yesterday and may have to go again so he has not got back to work yet! He has a friend from Newcastle here also Dr. Knox who seems a very nice fellow indeed.

Dr. Mansa ceased work last Tuesday and left on Friday, so we have been a bit pushed to get the work done. However Fred is a great help and a steady stand-by. He leaves in about a fortnight but Roy should be in Lagos on Thursday morning with his family and no doubt at work next week. I have suggested to

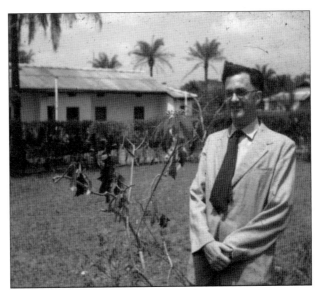

Fred Follet

Andrew that we invite Fred back to do Andrews locum from July to January because we shall again be short. We have not yet heard from Dr. Davy about David M's successor, nor officially about Jonathan Hartfield, my successor though we hear through Marion's mother that he is first going to Ituk Mbang. Incidentally John Baker has resigned from Ituk Mbang, so there is considerable need there I think.

Yesterday the influx of visitors started, John and Nancy Gill from Lagos came with their four children, and we expect Jim Stringfellow and his family this evening - they are on their way to Lagos on leave.

Margaret Woodland had invited us out to tea at Imesi yesterday but as luck would have it a woman came in with a ruptured uterus which I had to repair. This took one and a half hours so we were late getting off and I was played out

411

when we arrived having been up a lot of the previous night! However it was a very pleasant change.

In the evening the sisters gave a party to welcome Margaret Gardener - it was a very good do indeed, but they had taken a number of ideas of ours which we hoped to incorporate in a party we are to give a week on Thursday to welcome the Roys and say farewell to Fred. We have got some thinking to do about that!

Meanwhile it is very hot - we have run out of gas in Nigeria so are cooking on two primus stoves - the water was off for three days. Despite all we are well and enjoying everything. Love to you all, David

12.3.61

It is 12.30am, very early Sunday morning. I am on duty and waiting for the theatre to be prepared for an emergency operation. The patient was admitted to a hospital 50 miles away two days ago, and the Doctor has just decided to send her on here for her operation! I dare not leave it any longer - hence the midnight oil! We were very pleased to receive your letter this week and to learn that all is well - apart from Stanley's slow progress. It cannot be much longer before it heals up.

Very soon it will be time for the Broads - I certainly envy you the trip, especially if the weather holds! for I gather you are enjoying an early spring.

We have had a busy week made the more so by Andrew's sudden decision that I should go down to meet Roy and Beryl. It came as a surprise and I was not mentally prepared for it, if you know what I mean!

I left Ilesha at 2.45 on Wednesday and was in Lagos at 6.55 the swiftest run I have ever done. I went, after some discussion, in the Dauphine, which ran well despite the fact it was over 110F in the sun and 90 in the shade. I spent the night with the Manns (who are coming here on furlough in three weeks time) and the next morning went out to Ileja airport to meet them. They were all rather tired- three days flying, including a day in Rome and two nights in flight, but they all seem very well. Beryl is expecting the baby about the 30th May I think, a little after ours. She has put on quite a lot of weight! Roy seems in very good form and both Rohan and Mithuen are well.

I then did a bit of shopping and in the afternoon Roy and I went to get his trunks out of customs. They had sent them by sea. What a business it was. We spent three hours at it and at the end we could not get them because they had locked the official stamp up for the night!!

The next morning (Friday) Roy asked me if I would bring Beryl and the children up as they were finding the Lagos heat oppressive, which I did. Again we made good time and came straight through apart from a stop for coffee in Ibadan - and arrived here for lunch. The children were very good on the journey.

All was well here. I had the second meeting of the Maternity Department at

6.15 to which I had invited midwives from the town. It was an excellent meeting and afterwards we had our nurses fellowship meeting.

We have done some entertaining also. Last Friday Dr. George Knox and last Wednesday the Gills in to supper though I was in Lagos! Next Tuesday we are giving a party to welcome the Roys and say farewell to Dr. Follett.

We are all well though Peter and Elizabeth have had fleeting colds and Elizabeth is a bit off her food. Margaret is keeping well, though entertaining is tiring and we are reduced to cooking on two primuses as still no gas. How we shall manage a three course meal for 18 on two primuses and a campfire I'm not sure!! I have been busy preparing games.

We have just cut our first stem of bananas and they all ripened yesterday. There are 100 bananas exactly on the stem and there are seven other stems almost ready for cutting and all these from six small banana plants!

The hens are laying quite well but the garden is now so dry that nothing is growing at all. It is very hot indeed in the afternoons and the nights too are very hot - we are longing for some rain.

Hope all goes well with you all. Love from us all, David

19.3.61

Sunday again and the weeks seem to pass and Easter here next week. We were glad indeed to have your letter and to hear of all your activities. The Broads trip is almost here, and no doubt Stanley is reading up the natural history of the fish he hopes to catch. Do you have a map of the area? We eagerly await news of your voyage and of record catches - fish for breakfast, lunch and supper!

Thank you for the inner tubes for Peter's cycle. They look very stout affairs. Another puncture this week! but I repaired the old one as it seems reasonable to get as much out of them as possible.

We are all very well, though on Friday night the children and I had TAB which put us all out of sorts. However today we are all better again, though Elizabeth still seems a bit off her food. Peter can almost swim though a bit reluctant to have lessons! We need two new air rings and hope to get them in Ibadan when Margaret next goes down. Incidentally the Todds are up for a weekend and told us that some new Europeans with children six, three and twins of one are expected in Wesley College in April so that Margaret will have some companionship and the children will have others to play with. We are very pleased indeed to find that this is so. The name is Hobson.

Last Tuesday was the party. Still no gas but plenty of water so William and his helpers had to manage with two primuses and a little gas which had been carefully conserved!

413

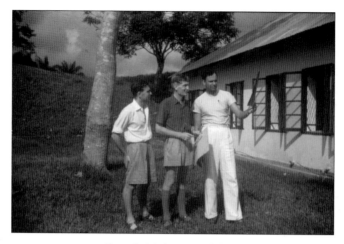

David, Andrew and Roy

We got off to a slow start because Margaret Woodland who had had a very busy day at Imesi, found that the new dresses she expected were not ready and

so had 'nothing to wear'. However she came eventually, but the Morleys too were late. However the meal - tomato soup, curry and rice and grapefruit and ground nuts followed by jellies and whips, then coffee, was greatly appreciated. Afterwards we played games and a treasure hunt, which we played in the dark by the light of torches, went very well. We ended up by the men dressing the ladies in newspapers and one or two were surprisingly good. George apparently does some dressmaking at home and it was obvious from the aplomb with which he tackled the job. Helena's was the best though I think. It requires quite a lot of newspapers for eight couples.

Roy and Beryl are in good form. Roy has taken over the male ward. Fred is having a few days off and will be going to Lagos on Thursday I think. He has agreed to come back and act as locum for Andrew. In effect he will be doing my work so that I can do the administration. However we have no pediatrician and David goes in the middle of May - less than eight weeks now. We shall be in a pickle if we do not not find someone soon and when Andrew goes we shall be very short.

I hope to go to a meeting at UCH on Tuesday evening - it means a late night but worth it I think and Margaret too has to visit Mr. Lawson, the next day.

Easter next weekend - one day a public holiday which will be a respite. Last night very busy. Roy, David and I up until I am and again today. Hope all well at home, love from us all, David

26.3.61

I am afraid this will be a little late for your birthday, nevertheless it brings our love and our best wishes for the anniversary. We shall be thinking of you - I hope you have a happy day. I calculate that Twink should arrive back about that day, and in good form I hope and ready for the Broads.

We were very glad to receive your letter and hear all your news. You seem to be as busy as ever, and to have had quite a lot of entertaining! Interested to hear the cold frame is started - I can see that when we get settled the five will have to come over to continue the good work space permitting! Incidentally I think there is going to be a shortage of Doctors over the next few years, so a job may not be so difficult to find.

We have had a varied sort of week. Margaret had to go down to see Mr. Lawson last Wednesday, so we all went down Tuesday afternoon - stayed over with Frank Morton, the children slept in our camp beds - and then next morning we did some shopping and then went to the hospital and after coffee at the Greensprings Hotel we came back to Ilesha. It was a very happy trip. Margaret saw Mary Boshier and made arrangements about moving in to the house. I heard from Prof. Lawson that he wishes to bring Mr. Gibberd (Guys Hospital) out here for the day on April 15th. This was the day Margaret was going to move into Ibadan, so it will have to be the next day. I shall, of course, take the family down and stay overnight and get them settled in! then get down whenever I can. I shall take my local leave about the time the baby is expected and stay down until we all come back.

We have heard that a new European family (four children) is coming to Wesley College about ten days after Margaret arrives, by name Hobson. They have been engaged by the Principal of Wesley College, so little is known by us about them, and we rather fear that they have little idea of what they are coming to. Anyway they will be company for Margaret and she no doubt will be a great help to them as they settle in.

Today it has been our coffee and my day off so Margaret and I made doughnuts this morning - hot work - smoking hot fat-the chip pan over a primus and the temperature over 80F before starting. We used the doughnut maker which we bought at the food fair, and very well it worked too. We made abut 28 which were much appreciated.

Fred has gone on leave and if all's well will be coming back in July. David Morleys relief is still not forthcoming. Marion goes on furlough in ten days time or so and Helena's six months is running out, so we are going to be short again.

We have had our first rain. A shower two days ago and a real storm last night. The grass is still brown, but if we have regular showers it will soon turn to green. The garden will soon be in production again. One hen died this week but we are still getting about a dozen eggs a week which is very useful.

We are very well. Peter is now swimming without the ring for a few strokes and very pleased with himself. Love to you all and happy Easter, David

9.4.61

By this time the boaters will be home! We have listened to snatches of UK weather forecasts on the shortwave and heard of snow ,rain and winds in the north of England, so we are wondering how all has gone? We look forward with great interest to hearing all about it.

We were very pleased to receive Michael's letter and to learn of his interview. A job such as this is one which greatly widens experience, especially in dealing with people and living and making a home in another country. It would only be a short term appointment as Nigerianisation is the watchword here as you can imagine. Ijeda is just outside Lagos - about ten miles to the Marina for example which is the opposite extreme. The airport is at Ikeja and is on the way up country.

You have had a busy week with seven a side visitors and others, but we find visitors most interesting on the whole. Glad to hear that Auntie is in good form - give her our love. We were imagining you at Easter time with a sudden hush! Easter Monday a quiet day in the garden perhaps or are the bulldozers active at all times? Sorry indeed to hear that Auntie Ruth is not well - I do hope it is not as serious as it seems to be.

We had a happy Easter. Last Sunday morning I went down to Otapete where we had an hour and 50 minute service and the church was packed! sweltering! Anyway in the afternoon David M said he was going to Ire to return a piece of equipment and would we care to go, so we went in two cars and took a picnic - it was about 34 miles each way. David Morley had a new short cut!! It was a magnificent road, tarred, up in the hills but did not lead to Ire! However we had a picnic tea in a spot with a magnificent view found our way to Ire where we had ice creams with the Baptists there and returned home just in time for evening service! This was my one outing over Easter as I was on duty Easter Monday. However Margaret and the children, the Morleys and the Roys went to Ife reservoirs where they built a fire and cooked sausages and beans and eggs and had a picnic lunch. They had a wonderful time! The others went to Oke Imesi and climbed a hill on top of which they had their lunch and then we all had tea together beside the pool in the afternoon. I had had a busy day here with several operations to be done, and sorry not to be able to get out.

On Wednesday Margaret and the children went to Ibadan to see Mr. Lawson who found all well. They returned in the afternoon and I went down to a lecture at UCH returning in time for the hospital committee at 8.30. We both had good trips. Margaret and the children(who were very good) had lunch at the Boshiers.

On Monday evening I forgot to mention that we had a party for Marion who flew last Friday and should be home soon.

Yesterday we had Margaret Gardener in to chop and also Sheila Rivers, a pharmacist from the Nigerian College, Ibadan who has been here for a week of her holiday, helping out in our pharmacy. We all went up to Ikole Friday evening on trek, had tea with Beryl House at Ifaki and then returned yesterday afternoon. We had a very good trip and found all well though I had a lot of work to do.

Last evening Roy and Beryl showed slides of Ceylon - it is a beautiful island and Roy's house quite pretentious. Next Saturday Mr. Gibberd of Guys comes here and then we all go down to Ibadan and I return alone on Monday morning

We are all very well indeed Love to you all, David

16.4.61

Sunday morning. All is bustle as we are packing up for a six week stay in Ibadan! This is complicated by the fact that Margaret has been ill for four days and today is the first day she has been up for breakfast. She developed a fever and had two shivering attacks at night which were rather alarming. However she is much better now though tires easily having had four days in bed. ¯

Peter and Elizabeth are very well and looking forward to going to Ibadan for their holiday. We shall motor down this afternoon. I shall stay overnight and return early tomorrow morning. The Boshiers will be there when we arrive and tomorrow but they leave on Tuesday for England. John hopes that he has a job more or less fixed up in a Technical Institute somewhere in the Midlands. I shall get down each weekend, apart from the one I am on duty. Then in about a month I shall go to stay until the baby comes and we all return again to Ilesha.

We were very pleased to receive two letters this week and to learn that the holiday had been a happy one and all had returned safely. The weather would seem to have been very wet indeed, but perhaps it added to the interest. I am quite determined that we shall have such a holiday in due course!

We were most distressed to hear of Auntie Ruth's ill news. It is a very rare one and unless there is a new treatment which is an improvement the outlook is very poor indeed. Interested to hear Michael's second interview at Nigeria House.

We have had a busy week with Margaret being in bed, but the children have been good and Jean, Aileen and William have been helpful. Yesterday Prof Lawson and Mr. Gibberd of Guys came to look round. They arrived in time for lunch, then we looked round and finally had tea before they left. It seemed to be a most successful visit and I look forward to hearing from John Lawson of his impressions. He said that he would not consider my starting in obstetrics, and trying to scramble up the ladder, so it will be General Practice.

I had a most interesting letter from Frank Davey earlier this week enclosing a letter from a Doctor an ex-CMS missionary in Nigeria, who is looking for a partner and wrote to Frank asking if there was a returning Methodist missionary looking for a job. He wants a Methodist, a missionary, conscientious, but apparently on October 1st not July 1st. and the practice is in Butterknowle about 4 miles from Bishop Aukland , with a live Methodist church. Interestingly the previous partner was David Wright, who is John Wright's brother and is going to join him in his practice near Bristol. I feel this is the sort of man I should like to work with and it is a rural dispensing practice in the Pennines but schooling might be difficult. It is far from London and Liverpool and it is not the time I want.

I have written to John Wright asking him further details about schools. Should be glad to have your comments by return. Almost time for coffee after which I should pack up the car. William is coming down and staying. I have another steward largely untrained who will get my breakfast and tea and I shall have other meals with the Pearsons.

Love to you all from us all, David

30.4.61

Sunday afternoon at Wesley College, the children in the garden talking to some of the college boys - they have just come in and Margaret is reading to them. It is very hot - the hottest day we have had so far since coming to Ibadan but it is at last getting a bit cooler. We are all well. Margaret is much better than when I saw her last week end and feels much more rested. The children are in good form, though at Sunday School this morning they still tended to stay around Margaret.

Last weekend I got back at about 8.30 on the Monday morning and had a cup of coffee and then got on with the weeks work. Work went on much as usual until Thursday when we had our Doctors meeting at the hospital - The students also were there so fifteen of us sat down to a meal in the hostel. They went on talking and so it was quite late before I got to bed. I had an infected toe but it has cleared up satisfactorily now.

Friday was a very busy day. I was on duty and had a string of emergency operations and had a bad night. Saturday I was more or less ready for coming and a patient came in with a ruptured uterus, so I had to cope with this, though I managed to get away at 2.30 and brought back two students. I found the family all well and enjoyed being with them again and a quiet evening.

Afterwards we went for a ride around until it was time for lunch which we had with Dr. and Mrs. Salmon who have three girls and are expecting another baby - they hope a boy! We came back here at about 3.15. Had a rest, it really is terribly warm.

Tomorrow I am going down to Lagos to meet Jonathan and Mrs. Hartfield who are due to arrive at 7.20am on Tuesday morning. I shall spend the night with Jonah if all is well. We shall return to Ilesha on Tuesday afternoon, calling at Wesley College if all goes according to plan.

I have had two letters this week. One from Dr. Davey who asked me to send on the letter from County Durham to another Doctor if I was not interested. This put me in a quandary until I received a letter from John Wright, and reading between the lines he does not recommend it - no schools, scattered practice, no opportunity for study, no expansion of the practice possible and should coal mining fail, as well it might in due course, the people may move away. So I have sent the letter on and told Frank Davey that I will bide my time. John Wright feels that now it is much easier to get into practice and in any case it should only be fixed up when we get home, though of course preliminary discussions could take place. So I am pleased that guidance has come.

We were very pleased to receive your letter this week and to know that all is well at home. We often think and talk of you all and wonder how the building goes on over the fence.

Peter is beginning to write, though at the moment it has little form - it is a beginning. Elizabeth too is fond of scribbling. A little breeze has blown up. I hope a storm comes to clear the air before bed time.

Love to you all from us all, David

7.5.61

Saturday evening and I am once again in Ibadan after a busy week! However very pleased to receive your letter and one from Michael too. I wrote a note to him for his birthday. Congratulations on being elected President of the Luncheon Club - I know you will do it very well and I don't suppose they will mind you visiting West Africa! Yes the children have the Flower Fairy books. Actually they are still in Margaret's present drawer, but we have them ready to give.

Glad you had a good time at the May Meetings - quite an Ilesha gathering!

Last Monday I travelled down to Lagos and spent the night with Jonah - he was in good form though he had plenty of grouses! I was up at 6.00 am and got to the airport at Ileja at 7.10. The plane was late so I went to the cafe and had breakfast, Fruit juice, cornflakes, two eggs, three rashers of bacon, two slices of toast - pot of coffee - six shillings, I guess the best value in Lagos.

Unfortunately the plane arrived before the scheduled time so I had to leave half the toast but I was in time to see Jonathan and Meg Hartfield come down from the plane. They are a nice couple and will be a real asset to the compound. Their child Sheila is fifteen-months-old. After some shopping in the morning, we motored to Ibadan and had tea with Margaret and then on to Ilesha for 6.45. They are living in the downstairs flat in the new hostel and it is just about right for them and will do until one of the houses is available.

Wednesday evening was the Committee and fortunately a pleasant one though long. Thursday I was out to chop with the Morleys, they had an American family staying with them. Yesterday was my day on duty this week, busy but not too heavy and this afternoon I came here.

Elizabeth has been rather unwell with diarrhoea but sulphonamides have put her right, though she is still a bit fretful

Margaret has been well till today when she has had a tummy upset but seems better this evening. They have had a good week. The Morleys came down to see them on Wednesday and again on Thursday they went out to lunch and tea.

The latter part of this week has been preparing for the new teacher at Wesley College here, the Hobsons, who have four children, six, four and twins of two, so they will make good companions for Peter and Elizabeth. We have just been up to salute them and to get their loads off the lorry. One very heavy box containing an electric cooker and a washing machine!

They are coming in here for lunch tomorrow, so we shall get to know them a little, they seem nice however, and they are Methodists.

I shall return very early Monday morning but am on duty next week -end so shall not be down again until the baby is about due and we shall both be pleased when it is all over.,and I shall be pleased to be able to get down and stay down with Margaret.

Next Saturday is a farewell party for the Morleys. They still have not got their sailing date but it will be about two weeks off now. Our love to you all, David

PS Why not come here September/October and spend a week in Rome on the way home?

at Wesley College, 14th May 1961

By the time this reaches you, you will have had my cable if all is well with the good news. At the moment it is 11.30am on Sunday morning- I have been around to the post office and there is no chance to get the cable off till 8.00 am tomorrow morning so am feeling rather disappointed. Richard David Cannon arrived after alarms and excursions!

I was at Ilesha last night - 11pm and we were having a farewell party for the Morleys. I was on duty and as you know expecting to come down next Tuesday, prior to Thursday when the baby was due.

I had had several phone calls about patients and when this one came I thought it was another patient! It was Margaret to say would I come down as there were indications that labour might be commencing. Everyone was helpful - flask of coffee, eggs packed up, loan of suitcase, medicines and by 11.50 I was on the way. It was a bad journey - 75 miles, pitch black, bumpy anxious expectant father!

I was at Wesley College by 1.45am, 14.5.61 and was met by Margaret who said she thought she ought to go in straight away. We were there at 2.50am. Prof. Lawson was there by 3.30 and Richard was born with a little assistance from John Lawson. I saw both Margaret and Richard afterwards - both very well and saw Richard weighed - 6lbs 3oz.

Every one was very kind and John Lawson and I had tea together afterwards. I was home by 4.30. William had been dozing in a chair listening for the children

- who had not stirred. Peter woke at 5.30am and wondered where Margaret was and I told him and he was very thrilled - and any chance of sleep disappeared - and I shall be ready for my rest this afternoon!

After breakfast I tried to ring Ilesha without success and then went to the post office again without success.

Richard Hughes has just looked in. The children are very good - Elizabeth is doing a jigsaw and Peter is cutting out paper and sticking it onto other paper. I shall go to University College Hospital at 4pm which is visiting time and I will let you know how I find Margaret and Richard.

Congratulations to Michael on being offered his lectureship in Physics. We shall be most interested to hear of decisions taken - very difficult indeed I think.

You all seem to have had a busy week - sorry Garth still seems so unsettled. His prospects hardly look fair enough to get employed I think.

At Ilesha we had a busy week. On Thursday night there was a farewell party for David Morley at the History Hotel to which I went with the Morleys. We had such a nice meal but conversation flagged a bit - but quite enjoyable on the whole. We have given the Morleys an elephant tusk carved into elephants as a parting gift which they seem to appreciate greatly - they are going to be sadly missed.

It is 7.30pm Peter and Elizabeth in bed and asleep. Margaret and Richard were very well today. Richard looks very much as Peter did as a baby with the reddish hair. What a 24 hours!

Love from the five! of us to you all, David

21.5.61

It is 8pm and there is considerable noise as Elizabeth is irrepressible and Richard is thirsty. There is no water and the fridge is still not functioning!

Margaret and Richard came home yesterday - both very well, but the weather is so hot that both are somewhat exhausted! However it is grand to be all together again.

We were very pleased to receive your letter on Friday, brought down by Jean Wingfield who is en route for furlough and is having six days in Rome. Glad to know all is well with you all.

Here we have had a happy week. I have been in each evening to see Margaret and quite a number of other folk too have visited, including four of our ex-nurses who are now staff nurses here and doing quite well I think

Margaret has had a restful week, eating well and making good progress and Richard on discharge was 6lbs 8oz - 5oz over his birth weight which is quite remarkable.

Most days I have been out to the shops in the morning, often taking Mrs. Hobson and her eldest two, so we had quite a car full.

Then some school with Peter, and in the afternoon to the zoological gardens,

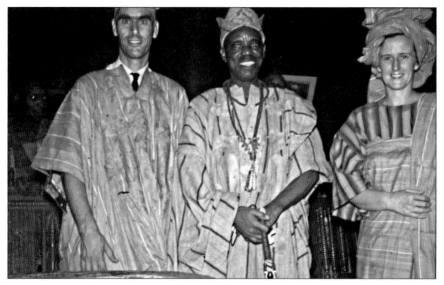

Morleys farewell

and another day up a local memorial tower and so forth, and then back in the evening after seeing Margaret to bath them and put them to bed. William has not been very co-operative. He feels he is not getting enough money - at the moment he is getting about £10-£11 per month, which is a reasonable wage here but is quite a slice of our income and we feel we cannot afford any more. We are hoping however that William will take over the laundry and we will employ a girl to help with the children when we get back to Ilesha. Anyway we shall see how it works out. In addition we shall be moving into the Morleys House, which is considerably larger than ours, so we shall have to see what transpires.

There has been no water in the taps today - terribly difficult with a baby/nappies and two energetic children who require pints of squash to replace their fluid loss.

I fear that the washing up is not done. I got tea William is off but we literally haven't a drop apart from some water which has been filtered which we keep for drinking. The toilet has not been flushed all day - very trying in this heat!

We shall spend next week here, but probably travel back to Ilesha next Saturday so that we have Sunday to settle down before I begin work again, though I shall have to have a day or two off to move house.

On Monday we expect the Morleys in for morning coffee, on their way to Lagos - they sail on Thursday. They are in the midst of their 'good byes' - a very gruelling time! Should think they will be very pleased when it is all over. I think they will settle down near London. David is hoping to get a job at the School of Tropical Medicine and they are situated near Euston station.

Peter and Elizabeth are asleep and Richard still vocal - now about time for his feed I think. Hope all well with you, Love from us all, David

28.5.61

Richard is two weeks old today, and is doing very well. At the moment he is having his bath and morning feed and we hope to get him weighed in a while. Likewise Peter and Elizabeth are at the moment in Sunday School and so I am seizing the moment to begin this letter.

As you will see we are back again in our little house in Ilesha and how nice it is to be home again. The compound is looking at its best with the flowering shrubs and trees in full bloom and the grass is deep green.

We were very pleased to receive your letter whilst we were at Wesley College and one by the same post from Grandpa Ingham, and we have also heard from Auntie Alice. I wrote to her when Richard arrived. We were most interested to hear of all your activities.

As you know Jane Sutton is in Ilesha now and in fact visited the hospital when I was there. She said her home letter was full of the Flower Show and her father's display (Sutton of Sutton Seeds).

We have had a lively week at Ibadan. Margaret came out a week ago yesterday and the next two or three days we spent quietly at home. Peter and Elizabeth have accepted Richard very well, though Elizabeth is acting in rather a babyish way at times in order to attract attention. Peter seems little affected psychologically. I have been out shopping with them each morning, but on Wednesday we had to make a special expedition because Thursday and Friday were Public Holidays and no shops open at all! The main Muslim festival.

On Tuesday the Morleys came in for coffee. They seemed in good form and got off to time. Unfortunately instead of sailing on the Thursday they sail today (a cargo boat) but they should be away by now if all is well. They have most luxurious accommodation I believe. They are not yet fixed up but hope to settle near London- I will let you have their address when I know it.

Wednesday we went to the plantation, about five miles from Ibadan to order some fruit trees and after much trying we found the right department . Thursday and Friday we spent at home - though Wednesday afternoon we went to the Friendship Hotel for a swim which we all enjoyed. Peter and Elizabeth and I went in - though a bit expensive - eight shillings per dip.

Friday was a lovely day - the Longleys had invited us to go to see them in their new station for the day, so we set off after Richard had been bathed and fed and went the 60 miles to their home which is between Ibadan and the Dahomey border. It is not well wooded, rocky and very sparsely inhabited. The road was tarred and we made good time. We had a lovely lunch, soup, chicken in sauce, coffee and then a rest. Then Frank and the children and I went to look at the site where Dr. Stephens first began work in Nigeria, and I spoke to one old man

423

who remembered him going there in 1912! Most interesting. We set off home after tea and returned through the game reserve and in the twilight saw two large snakes on the road and three mysterious birds which we could not identify on the roadside. A lovely day.

Yesterday I collected 18 fruit trees - grapefruit, lime, lemon and orange (cost 22/- the lot) and they have been put in and are awaiting watering tomorrow. All well here though Beryl not yet delivered. In a week or two we shall begin to move over to the Morley House in easy stages - a drawer at a time so to speak.

Tomorrow I start work again. Love to you all from us all   David
PS Richard now 7lbs 3oz

29.5.61

Dear Michael,
Just a line to say that I hope to dispatch a film to you by 2nd class airmail by the same post. It is NOT developed. It contains mostly exposures of the family including Richard at two weeks of age! Frank and Jessie Longley also appear on some, taken on our visit to Igbora. I put a filter on the last 20 and hope the exposure was OK. Could you have it developed please and then examine and have enlarged those you feel to be satisfactory and let me have prints of six good ones. The developing and printing is so poor here I do not want to risk any of the film being spoilt.

Most interested to hear of your two interviews at Borough. I should have thought that if you were offered the job, that is the one to take. I have made enquiries and no PhDs are supervised yet at Ibadan.

Love to you all from us all   David

5.6.61

Saturday evening and about time for our evening meal. Margaret is just finishing her bath and all the children are asleep. Richard is a model child and sleeps very well when he should do but is a bit lazy over his feeds. He seems to be thriving well and we shall weigh him again tomorrow to see how he has got on.

Margaret is keeping well and we are once again settled down. We looked round the Morley house today with an eye to cupboards and drawers and find it is barely as well supplied as this house and certainly the fabric is not so good However we feel it right to move so shall do so slowly. Peter is well and lively but Elizabeth has fever this evening. She has been out of sorts for a day or two and this evening she has just slept. They are both excited at the thought of moving and have already taken over some books. I hope to go through some drawers this weekend and sort the rubbish.

We were glad to receive your letter- you have all been very busy indeed- but we are most distressed to hear of Stanley's disorder and shall be glad to hear more details - such as why he went to the Doctor in the first place and any further news. I seem to remember listening to his heart some years ago and finding it normal. It may not be serious of course and we shall see what has to be said.

Our main items of news is the safe arrival of Beryl's baby yesterday, It is another boy! She is very disappointed, Roy is very pleased - Asians prefer boys. Anyway both Beryl and the baby are well and every one is pleased the event is safely over.

We have had a busy week, but the children have all been very good indeed and kept well except for Elizabeth the last two days.

On Thursday Jonathan and I motored over to Ogbomosho to the Doctors meeting that was held there. It was a very good talk given by a Doctor from UCH, Ibadan, with an excellent meal

Returning about 11.30pm we got into a bad skid due to loose gravel on the road (I was driving) but apart from being a bit shaken there was no trouble and the car is none the worse for it - it behaved very well indeed.

We have had a number of callers to salute Margaret and Richard and all the compound seemed pleased to have us back again.

Again we have had a number of letters which must have been inspired by the notice which we put in the Methodist Recorder and which must have been inserted on the 25th.

Richard's birth certificate arrived today and so at the first opportunity we must get him added to Margaret's passport.

I hope that by now the film I dispatched to Michael has arrived and I hope that there are some reasonably good photos of the children. Should they not be very good, if Michael could let me know what was wrong with them I will run off some more. We look forward to seeing some in due course.

Incidentally we had a letter from Gladys this week as I wrote to her from Ibadan also and she seems to be thinking of summer holidays.

How goes the building at the lower end of the garden? Is the cold frame in use and successful? Perhaps there isn't room in the greenhouse for producing seedlings. We have been very short of rain and the farmers are worried. The new yams which should be ready are not and we have seen several children with malnutrition. Very little is growing in our vegetable garden, though the grass is a good green. The hens are picking up and the Morleys left us two so we now have seven hens and a cock but one is broody.

Hope all is well with you all. Love from us all, David

11.6.61

It is Sunday morning, and my weekend on duty. I have been round the wards and just cleared the administration of emergency patients - it took one and a half *hours!*

Now a few minutes before time to go down to coffee and then at 11.30 I have an operation to do so the rest of the time will be filled in. We are all very well. Elizabeth is quite better, though she has spells of wanting to be picked up and carried - a delayed reaction to Richard and being not very well last weekend. Richard seems to be flourishing. Last Sunday he weighed 7lbs 14oz. - we have not weighed him today.

I have not been very fit, with fever, pains in the back and so forth, but am better again today I am glad to say. Jonathan has had two days off with Dengue fever, but is better now. This made last Friday a very busy morning.

We were very glad to receive two letters this week. Michael's arrived on Wednesday - very quick - and we were interested to hear of his visit to the West Country and Kingswood School and so on, and also his decision to stay at college as lecturer in Physics. I feel sure the PhD job not being available, it is the right thing to do at the moment. The job here might have been very interesting and useful but might have been very frustrating if they hadn't the equipment you needed and so on.

Mother seems to have had an incredibly busy week - difficult to know how you have fitted everything in and it contained the activities of several people. We are sorry to hear of Stanley's aortic stenosis and wonder what it was that sent him to cardiologist? I should think that when he returns for the holiday it would be worth getting a letter from our own Doctor to see a Cardiologist in London and go under his wing so to speak. Stanley won't be going back to Bath after this term. Any of the large London Hospitals or the National Heart Hospital would do, so long as he sees a cardiologist. Dr. Brigden at the London Hospital I know and is very good.

The week here has slipped by, we have sorted out drawers and taken some things over to the Morleys house. We have had a bathroom cupboard made and I hope to get it fixed today if I get a few minutes with the tool chest. Margaret succumbed to Peter's entreaties to make a rainbow cake for her birthday and he brought out all the food colourings from the store, so you can imagine the result, which however tasted very nice. They also insisted that we wore hats, so we must have looked decidedly odd when Mr. Ogarijobi, vice principal of the Ilesha Grammar School walked in at tea time! He graciously accepted a cup of tea.

This morning coffee was at the sisters. They have had their room done out in yellow and grey with reflected lighting and it looks very nice indeed. In a lull in the conversation a small voice attracted attention by saying 19, 20, my plate's empty! Richard was weighed again this morning and is now 8 lbs 9 oz, gained another 11oz this week. We must start the inoculations as he is a month old today.

Next week or rather this week Andrew and I are going up to Kaiama. As you know we are hoping to open up a welfare centre there (It is in Borgu 200 miles from here). Building has started on the foundations of the dispensary and we wish to inspect those before the building starts. We should go on Friday afternoon and return on Saturday evening.

Hope you have got some good photos of Richard! and that you are all well. Love from us all, David

18.6.61

Sunday morning and a very wet one too - Margaret is feeding Richard and Peter and Elizabeth are playing with Alison and Bryan in their bedroom and in a few minutes folk will be arriving for our coffee and one of my tasks, that of putting cream into brandy snaps is delayed as the cream is frozen.!

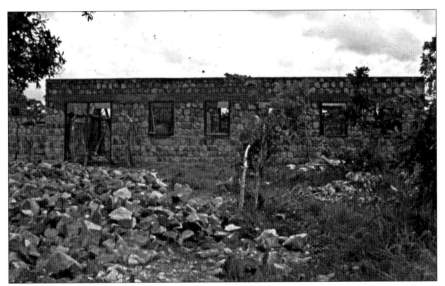

Kaiama being built

We are all well apart from Margaret who is feeling a bit under the weather, but she should be better in a day or two. On Wednesday she is due for a post natal examination in Ibadan so will be travelling down in the morning and back for lunch if all is well. Peter has had a cold but is now improving and he seems well in himself. We were very glad to receive your letter during the week including a photograph which we thought very good and a letter from Michael.

We were very interested to note that Michael is considering coming for a holiday. The fare of £180 would be the only cost of course, and the question of justification for spending so much on a fare needs to be thought out. A month's holiday at least - perhaps some investigation into local food factories - canning, fruit bottling in Ibadan and there is a firm producing pounded yam and of course

427

many bakeries - would the National College of food Technology be interested? A paper in a food technology journal ? A scholarship from the College or a journal?

We should be delighted to have you and if it would help make up your mind be prepared to meet part of the air fare Have you enquired about student flights?

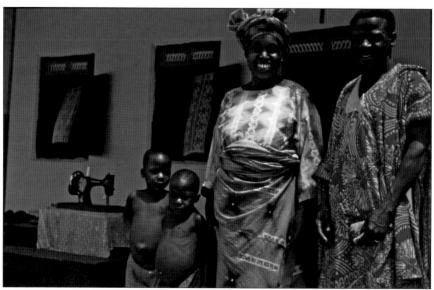

Kaiama catechist / family

though on second thoughts they would probably not apply! Anyway we shall be interested to hear your conclusions! Pity you are not secretary of a Methodist Department.

We were glad to have Mothers letter with news of the invalids and to hear that Auntie Ruth has less pain. and is home again. Glad also to hear that Stanley is in better spirits. We must certainly get him on the books of a London cardiologist as I mentioned last week.

The garden sounds lovely. Here we are in the midst of the wet season and everything is very green. Vegetables are just beginning in the gardens ours and ours to be (the Morleys). Corn is about ready - on the cob - and we had some for our evening meal (cost Id a cob), one done for five minutes in the pressure cooker and the other done over the open fire and roasted both delicious with salt and butter and very filling! (almost worth the £180!)

We have had a usual sort of week. Our Wedding Anniversary last Monday was acknowledged by ourselves! but unremembered by others! the main item of news was my visit to Kaiama last Friday/Saturday. Andrew, Eileen and I set off, Jean and Margaret having prepared our food and water(no small job) about 2.30pm and arrived at Afon about 5pm. We got tea and made up beds (the house is empty now) We went to see the village head and then returned. I lit the

428

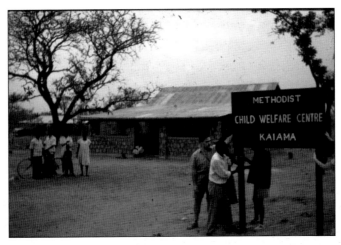

Kaiama sign

lamps and cooked the supper. Onion soup, sausages, peas and potatoes, followed by an instant whip and coffee. An early night and then off at 6am. I cooked breakfast, porridge, bacon and fried eggs, coffee. Then 118 miles to Kaiama where we met the Minister Rev. Osinuga, Stephen the catechist and the contractor. We examined the foundations of the new welfare centre and then had lunch on the verandah with Stephen and Louie. We set out for Ilesha. On the way we saw two families of monkeys crossing the road and a large snake. We got back about 7.45pm on Saturday night, having travelled about 300 miles in the day, at 20 miles an hour for every hour of daylight we were away.

In two months I shall have to go up again to check the building and give a certificate of completion - a longish way. This week we shall have to move into the Morley house as Fred Follet will be coming in a fortnights time. We shall then be well doctored. Hope you are all well and fit Love from us all   David

PS Urgent. Could your send me my birth certificate - needed for Richard's passport. If not with you at Mission House.

2.7.61

Sunday afternoon and we have just had a very heavy rain storm and every where outside is very soggy. The children have got on swimming things! and are playing with the Pearsons'. It is very pleasant and cool though damp! Richard is sleeping - he weighs 10lbs. today and for the last four nights he has slept through from 10 until 6am which is much more restful for Margaret.

Peter's birthday was greatly enjoyed yesterday. Unfortunately I had to go on trek to Ikole - Roy should have gone but he had to go to University College Hospital for a small operation. Jonathan was in Lagos waiting for his loads (which still have not come) and Andrew was on duty. Margaret and I gave him a signal

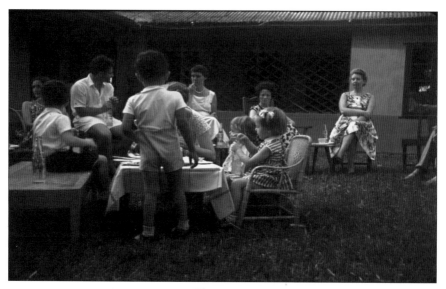

Tea party

for his railway and the other children in the compound gave him gifts. At tea time (by which time I had returned) they had a lovely party - hats, sausages on sticks and a cake in the shape of an aeroplane were Peters requests and were all fulfiled. He looked and behaved in a very grown up sort of way. It seems hardly possible that Margaret and I have a son of five! If we were at home, he would be in uniform with cap and satchel and going of to school.

We all got weighed this morning and all of us apart from Margaret are either satisfactory or gaining but Margaret is only 6 stone 10lbs. which does not seem much. Feeding Richard of course is quite a drain on protein which is not in great supply here, though we are taking extra protein on our porridge.

Jonathan went down last Wednesday to Lagos to collect his loads but as we forecast has had a most frustrating time. The ship has not yet berthed, however he waited for Kathleen Owen who landed yesterday and they travelled up this morning. Kathleen looks very well indeed, very sunburned compared with the rest of us who are very pale! Fred Follett arrives tomorrow morning on the early plane and Disu is there to bring him up so we shall be well staffed. Andrew however is not doing any more duty and is going to have a shot at his second language exam, so probably won't be much in evidence.

I had a good run up to Ikole in the Dauphine, all the other cars or rather the other cars were in Lagos with Jonathan. Helena wasn't very well, though it is very difficult looking after Ikole for someone else! There were not a great number of patients so I was back home by 4.15 in good time for Peters party,

We were glad to have your letter and hear all your news though sorry to hear about Doreen Catterson - it is very sad indeed.

Michael seems to be having an interesting interlude at College at the moment! How about coming out here to visit his odd Nigerian student.

With Fred Follett here I shall be giving him quite a lot of my medical work as I take up the administration as I have also to be acting Medical Secretary of the Christian Council of Nigeria which will involve me in a number of committees and boards, so I shall not be seeing many patients I fear.

Incidentally David Morleys relief, a Dr. and Mrs. Dr. Clapp of the USA will be coming in due course so we shall be well off for doctors.

Hope you are all well, David

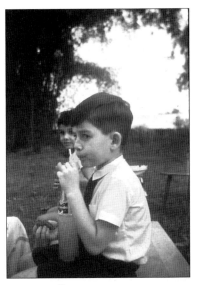

Peter at party

16.7.61

Another week over, a few moments in which to start this letter in a rather busy day! Richard is to be Christened this evening and we are getting preparations made. Margaret made six dozen sausage rolls yesterday, iced two cakes as we expect about 60 down at the house after the service. We have sent out printed invitations largely to hospital staff.

We are having lamps (hurricane) on poles outside on the lawn with benches and offering a plate to each person with a sausage roll, sandwiches and biscuits and a bit of Christening cake, with coffee or a soft drink. We only hope it keeps fine! We are in the middle of a very wet wet-season. and in fact we have only had the sun for one afternoon for the last week and very little of our washing has dried and even when ironed won't air - we have no stove in the kitchen! The font from Otapete has been stolen so we are using a locally made brass bowl and putting a small pyrex dish inside.

Beryl, Jean and Meg are all assisting with the sandwich cutting this afternoon.

This week has been under a cloud rather, for on Thursday Fred Follett had a telegram from his mother to say his father had died suddenly. His only brother is in South America. He rang up and apparently his cousin a widow had moved in and his mother said she did not want him to come home, though we of course said it was perfectly in order for him to do so. He has picked up very well and has just been in talking about the future.

The Pearsons' are preparing to go. They are leaving first thing on Thursday morning ready for the plane on Thursday evening. They are staying two days in

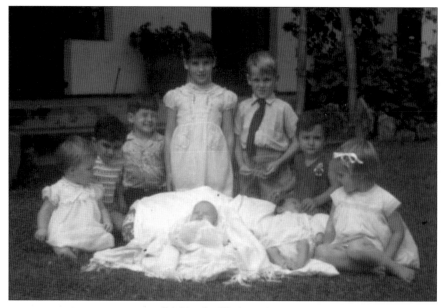

Richards Christening

Rome on the way and arrive in London on Sunday or Monday I think. They have taken a house in Bury St. Edmunds so that they can be near their boys.

Next weekend therefore, I shall be the Acting Medical Superintendent for the fifth and last time, and shall be glad when it is over no doubt. In addition I have to be acting secretary Medical Board of the Christian Council in Nigeria.

We are all keeping well. Richard had his second triple vaccine injection overnight and gave us a bad night but was better the next day. Two nights ago we gave Peter and Elizabeth their measles vaccination (this is very new and not available in the UK yet). It meant two injections each, Jonathan and I gave them and although they both woke up they neither of them had any recollection of them. We expect them to be fretful in a week or so and then be immune to measles which can be a very severe disease here in Nigeria as there is no herd immunity.

We were very glad to receive your letter from Fort William. We remember

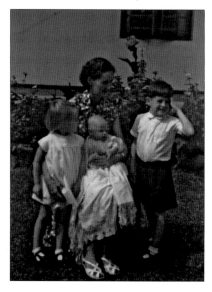

M,P,E at R's chr

432

your route part of the way from our honeymoon, but your weather seems to be much as ours was! I hope it improves later on.

We heard from David and Aileen Morley yesterday. They have got a house in St. Albans and David will travel up to the School of Tropical Medicine daily by train. It would be nice if we got a practice in the same sort of area. John Wright says I should be able to pick and choose jobs if I do not want to be near London, so we shall see what transpires.

Next Thursday I hope to go to Shaki and then on to Kaiama to see about the building there. Tomorrow Frank and Jessie Longley come to stay for two or three days. The new laundry equipment has come and is being installed - I hope it works! Love to you all, and Auntie A, from us all David

21.7.61

Dear Michael,

We were thrilled to have your letter this morning, the children are wildly excited It is perfectly convenient to us and if all is well I shall be at the airport to meet you, or if I cannot be there our Hospital driver Disu will be there.

With regard to clothes - shorts and shirts, sandals, socks two shirts for evening not sports. If you want to wear a tie (optional though customary!) One light weight suit, Sundays jackets are necessary, few ties/cravats. One pair shoes.

We have all the linen of course. Evenings I wear grey bags (terylene usually). We can get washing done daily so a vast supply underwear and pyjamas not necessary - a change would do. Swimming trunks if you want to swim. Camera for photos!

This morning's post was certainly the most exciting we have ever had. David had only just time to begin this reply before setting off on two day trip to Shaki and Kaiama, so he asked me to get it off by this afternoon. It gives me an opportunity to say how delighted I am that you can come. The future looked gloomy this morning as we have just said farewell to the Pearsons' and Peter and Elizabeth are going to miss their playmates, but now we have all cheered up.

The children are very fond of dressing up and I wonder if something in the way of Cowboy and Nurse outfits (two cowboys if there is one small enough for Elizabeth) are available and not too bulky. Dinky toys are always acceptable. Peter is now reduced to two vans, but these can be obtained here so are not so highly prized. Inflatable rubber toys for the pool would be welcome and easy to pack.

David will be writing again on his return at the weekend. Sorry this is in such haste. We look forward very much to your visit. With love from us all, Margaret

9th Sept. 1961

It is Saturday evening and Margaret is cutting out on the table, the wireless has

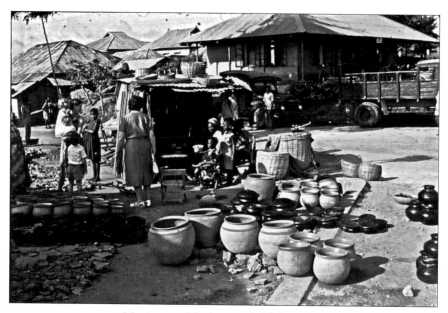

Mother at Market with M, P and E

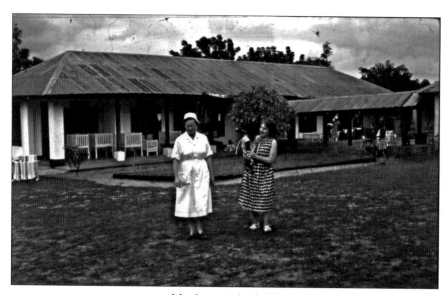

Mother with child

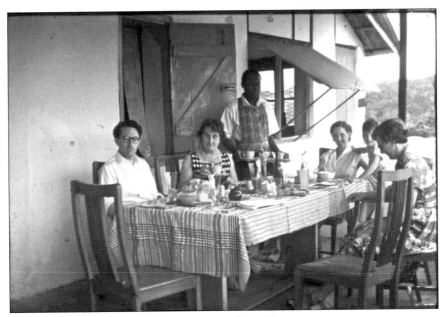

Mother and M at Imesi

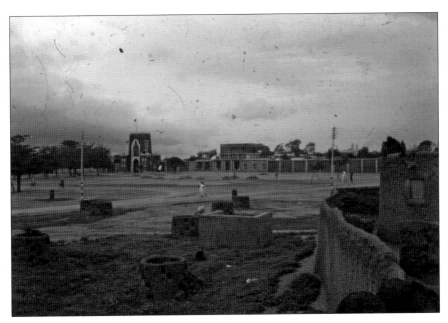

Kano

been playing soft music, the children are asleep - so you can picture the scene. I have had a leisurely afternoon at home, done one or two odd jobs, read and annotated one of the journals, so am feeling better for the change.

We were very pleased to receive your letter on Tuesday and your letter from last weekend, today. You seem to have been very fortunate in Kano with the assistant manager of the food factory. You did not comment on the city of Kano itself though - how does it compare with Southern Nigeria? Also rather curious to know approximately the cost of the Central Hotel though we gather you had most of your meals out.!

Did you get the orchid and seeds through without much trouble. No doubt the orchid was identical with the one over the door in the greenhouse or was it a new variety. Although I have kept my eyes open I have not seen another yet! Strange it should be just outside the house!

Here we have had a normal sort of week. I was on duty last weekend and had quite a bit of surgery. Any odd moments that I have had, I have spent on the accounts. We are still unable to trace £64-6-10 which we appear to have been spent in excess of our income!

I have begun writing the hospital report for this year and must get it completed in a week or two and ready for the Medical Committee of synod which comes in November.

In addition there are reports of Kaiama and Afon to make. Incidentally I had a letter from Kaiama the other day to say that the welfare centre is completed so if you see Mr. McNeil you might mention it to him.

I have had a notice of a meeting of the midwives Board in Lagos on Monday so I have rung Jonah and intend to travel down tomorrow afternoon and arrive in time for service there, and the hymn singing afterwards. Jonah was not in but I left a message with a guest who happened to be staying there so I hope it is acceptable. It seems a long way to drive for a two hour meeting.

Peter, Elizabeth and Richard are well and full of beans and the kitten is as playful and co-operative as ever. They play quite a lot with Rohan now and took their tea over to his house today which gave us a very quiet tea time.

Roy is not very well and is going into University College Hospital for a check up on Thursday and may be in over the weekend. Joan is still in, but I expect she will be coming out during this coming week and will be staying with us for a week or two. Marion is going to be two weeks late coming back we hear. If all is well we are going to have a party for Lily and Margaret Woodland's farewell three weeks today and probably another for Marion's arrival.

Last Monday, John, the Ikole driver had a smash in the Ikole car at Effan Aloha on the way to Ikole and apparently the car was a complete wreck. Fortunately John was not hurt but was in court on Friday and we have not yet heard of the outcome of the case I had to get a breakdown van from Ibadan to tow it in, and *it will have cost £30 just to get it towed in. Jean is therefore up at Ikole and without a car, so feels rather cut off I expect.*

By the time this reaches you, you will have been home a fortnight and already Nigeria will be slipping into the past. We were so very pleased that you could come here and anything we did to make your stay happy is but a fraction of the love and care we receive when we come on furlough.

Do hope all continues to be well with you all - we look forward so much to your weekly letters. Love from us all, David.

16.9.61

Saturday evening, Margaret is sewing, the children all fast asleep and I am writing this sitting on the settee with the help of the ginger kitten.

We were very pleased to receive your letter on Thursday and have sent Mrs. Oluyie's letter on to her. We were most interested to hear the cost of the Central Hotel! I am sure two nights were sufficient!

I was very sorry to hear of Doreen's death, it must be very sad for David as you say. Hope the Valedictory Service went well and Andrew was in good form - I believe he was returning to Birmingham the same night. We feel very sorry for them in that they have been unable to find anywhere to live near Bury St Edmunds and the Missionary Guest flats seem to have deteriorated appreciably.

Incidentally, whilst I remember, Peter has mentioned several times the kindness of Auntie Pop in getting a cactus garden for him and Elizabeth wonders if she will have one too! So if you could make two from one for them I know they would be very pleased.

We are all very well. The children are in excellent fettle and Richard is as good as ever. Peter has managed to fix the push chair to his bike and last week-end could be seen struggling to pull Elizabeth and Rohan on this contraption, plus their loads, which included a picnic. They went right up to the lower gate and back and finally had the picnic on the netball pitch!

Amos has settled down again and seems happy in his rooms. He is getting the laboratory in order and is getting some good work done. I heard yesterday that the London University examiners will be coming on 19 October and they will be staying a night.

Last Sunday I went down to Lagos and stayed the night with Jonah and then went to the Midwives Board Meeting at the Federal Ministry of Health. It was quite an interesting meeting but went on for over three hours. I had lunch with Jonah and travelled back in the afternoon, to find all well at home. On the way back I looked at the Ikole car - it is a complete write off. Unfortunately too Joan Ariel, who was due to come to us yesterday, is far from well again and not fit to leave hospital. I am rather concerned about this as she has now been in five weeks and should be about ready for coming out. I believe she is in very low spirits again and will perhaps be unwilling to continue her tour. If she does not go back to Ikole I do not know what we shall do. Marion will not be back until 24th October, so Eileen and Margaret Gardener will be alone for a time as Lily is due home on October 4th.

Roy has not been very well and was in UCH last night as a patient but is back again today. On Thursday night the Todds stayed with us - from Immanuel College Ibadan - and then the next day we had 18 visitors including children. A Dutch doctor and his family rolled up, the Ashleys came unexpectedly - they seem well but not pleased at going to Ikole , then Olive Osborne and Margaret Woodland. Mr. and Mrs. Reeves the new teacher is at Olives school also came. In addition we had Sheila for the day as Meg went out for the day to Ibadan. However today has been a much more settled sort of day and I have spent the afternoon and evening with the children. Elizabeth is very quick at dominoes! Almost time for bed. I am not on first or second call so it should be a quiet night. Next week would appear straight forward! but you can never tell. The autoclave is not working again!

Hope all is well with you all, any Nigerian seeds coming up? The Uzuakoli ones have been planted out! Love from us all, David

24.9.61

Sunday morning and I am in the office having just been round the maternity ward, and hope to complete this letter before it is time to go down to Otapete. We were very pleased to receive your long letter on Thursday. Glad to hear the orchid is hanging. Although we have kept our eyes open we have not seem another!

Glad the Valedictory was well attended. I think Andrew must have slipped out to catch a train back to Birmingham from what he said in a letter a while ago.

We have had an ordinary sort of week! The children are in great form and even more irrepressible than ever - at least Elizabeth is. Peter at times can appear quite school boyish, and he is beginning to frown on Elizabeth's misbehaviour at times to keep her on the straight and narrow.

Last Sunday we went for lunch at the GTTC with Nan Dalton. The children behaved quite well considering that there were no toys of any description and we all had a very good meal.

Monday Alan Ashley rang up to ask if he could stay the night as he was down in Ibadan buying furniture for the new house. He did not arrive until 10.30 pm without having had any meal for hours so we set to and produced a meal for him we had expected him about 8pm. Also on Monday a policeman arrived and said that Fred and I were to be in the court in Ibadan to give evidence on the Tuesday morning at 9am so I had a short night. We drove down as soon as it was light - 6.30 and arrived at the court at 9am. We gave the evidence and then did some shopping finally going to see Joan Ariel. She is better again and hope will be coming out next Tuesday. We had a letter from her yesterday and she seems much more cheerful.

On Thursday we had Miss Jadesimi in for the day, also Friday. She is a medical student at St. Andrews, has two years to go, and the daughter of the archdeacon who was in Ilesha until a year or so ago. She is interested in the work of a Mission Hospital when she qualifies - so we were very pleased that she was able to come.

Friday we had the Todds from Immanuel College, Ibadan, in to lunch. They were on their way back to Ibadan and have taken the white mice with them. They were a little nonplussed at the number but no doubt they will be returning here when the Pearsons' return.

On Friday Fred went up to Ikole on trek. Jean Wingfield is managing but she still has the Ashleys with her! All most unsatisfactory. The Ashleys house at the school is still not finished and it does not seem likely to be finished for a few weeks yet. I hope most sincerely that they are out before Joan is ready to go up or there will be fireworks.

There is a standing committee of Synod on Tuesday in Lagos but I have told Jonah that I am not going down for it. It is a long way when there is nothing relating to medical matters.

Joan will be coming up on Thursday, we shall have to make the arrangements to put her up, so I hope she is feeling more cheerful it will be a lot of trouble for Margaret. She has been rather difficult in the Hospital I believe.

Next Thursday is the Doctors meeting here. Mr. Hanson of UCH is coming up to talk to us. Next Saturday is a party to welcome Amos and say goodbye to Lily and Margaret Woodland who both go the following week. Tonight I am preaching in the hospital chapel, and I am struggling to get the Maternity report completed. When does Stanley go up?

We shall be thinking of him, Love from us all to you all, David

WGH, 8.10.61

Sunday morning and I am on duty and have just done a caesarean section and cleared the Admission room of patients, done my rounds and there are a few minutes until coffee time.

We were pleased to receive your letter with all its news. You must have had a very worrying journey to Doncaster and Brighouse and we are wondering how Auntie Sarah got on last Monday - it would be a serious undertaking. We are glad to hear of the flowers in the garden - ours are just the same in this season less place!

Here we are all very well. The children are in good form and irrepressible. Richard is as good as ever and taking to his mixed feeding very well. He is getting used to a number of new 'swallows' and seems to enjoy them. Joan Ariel is still

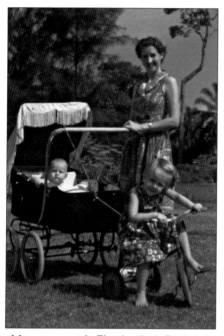

Margaret with Elizabeth & Richard

with us but we think she will be going up to Ikole on Wednesday next. The Ashleys are out of the Ikole house at last, and are living in the school compound, in their own house. Alan came down on Monday, wanting to go to Ibadan. I lent him our car which he used, coming back on the Tuesday and going on up to Ikole in it on the same day. They used it I think for carrying their loads from Ikole to the school anyway they seem most grateful for it. Jean came down in it on Friday. She seems in good form and will be going to Imesi early tomorrow morning.

Lily and Margaret Woodland got off at last after a rather unpleasant scene, one wanted to go in the lorry, the other in the Morris car and they went in the car and it broke down just as they turned off the main road to go to the airport! Apparently Margaret Woodland was in a real stew. However they got a lift to the airport and Margaret caught her plane and Lily stayed at the Marina one night and then off to the boat on Thursday morning which she caught without trouble!

Roy went up to Kaiama on Tuesday but unfortunately did not stay long enough to meet the Minister or Contractor. However Mr. Lanija is going up on Tuesday in the lorry to take up the plumbing fittings and to get the various pipes laid to carry rain water from the roof to the tank and so forth.

When Miss Stennet comes we intend to take her up, and Marion, Jean Wingfield and I spending two nights at Afon as we have done on previous occasions I only hope all are on speaking terms!

We had some excitement yesterday. Peter was on the front verandah when a snake fell out of the palm trees on the lawn. He called out and as they watched it, it went back up again. Margaret phoned me and we all stood trying to see it and I got my gun. Anyway I went to see some patients and mentioned it to Hezekiah who happened to be there. He went home and got his gun and after about five minutes looking he saw its head and shot it and it fell out - between five and six feet long a black tree snake! We are going to give it to James Sutton!

Last Monday we went there for coffee in the morning and in the afternoon we went for a bush walk after which the children had tea at Rohan's birthday party.

440

On Friday Rebecca's girl Olivia, gave a first year Birthday party in our house - at lunch time - liver and rice with about twelve guests - complete with photographer in the living room! We are all well and hope you are too.

Love from us all, David

15.10.61

Your letter with the sad news of Auntie's passing arrived this week - and we were very grieved to receive it. We have been thinking often of you and Auntie Alice, and Mary and remembering you all in our prayers. It is good to know that Auntie Alice is with you at Worcester Park and we send our love to her.

You have all had a busy week last week and I hope that this week which has just passed has been an easier one for you all.

Stanley should be about ready for Oxford I guess and is probably there now, and Michael's new term with his new duties and responsibilities will have started and we hope all is going well.

Here we are all keeping well, though as it happens we were up with Elizabeth in the night- she had some diarrhoea but this morning she seems much better. She is growing fast and catching Peter up in stature. I expect he will have a spurt in due course.

Richard, who is just five months old doesn't time fly! is as good as ever and appreciates his mixed feeding. He is gaining weight steadily, though not spectacularly. Peter's swimming is improving and he can now swim across the pool with ease, about fifteen feet.

We have had a usual sort of week. Roy went down last Friday to meet Beryl's friend but she wasn't on the plane, but he didn't know that until the plane came ,so he was very late back on Monday. He has gone down again, as they had a wire to say she would be in today. I do hope she is.

Last Monday we went out to chop with Dorothea Taylor and Jill at St. Margarets School. After dinner - a Chinese meal - they permed Margaret's hair which looks very well indeed now. There was a tremendous storm and all the lights went out so it had to be completed by candle light and by torch light!

On Friday, Roy organised films in the chapel- but the machine broke and it took us a long time to get it going. After that however all was well.

Yesterday we had a pool picnic and Mary Allen from St. Margaret's came and we all had a swim and the a picnic by the pool. In the evening we went to the Hartfields for chop and afterwards listened to records. They have at last got their new record player - a Pye Black Box- and it is first class. I think we shall get one when we get settled down.

We had some Bach played by Schweitzer on the organ in the Parish Church in his village - does Michael know it? Also a record with Kathleen Ferrier and Isobel Bailey singing a duet? The recording of the first is not perfect but has great *historic interest I think.*

This morning I have been to Otapete - Sunday School Anniversary and a long do - but out eventually!

Next Thursday is the visitation by the L. University examiners and we are all getting on to our toes about it. The dates of Miss Strudwick's visit to Ilesha have been changed so I have had to remake arrangements! Heigh Ho!

Last Tuesday I went down to University College Hospital to hear Mr. Flew (Obstetrician from UCH London) lecturer. He is a very nice man and a Methodist! He is coming next Thursday.

Hope all is well. Our love to you all, David

22.10.61

We were very pleased to receive your letter this week and to know that you are all well but very busy. Sorry to hear that Twink's room was not up to much at Oxford - but no doubt he will be able to make something of it. We should be able to visit him next year if all is well - perhaps we shall not be far away from him. Incidentally I wrote to the BMA Practice Advisory Bureau and I had a good letter from them stating that there was nothing I could do about a job until I got home and then he suggested that I went along and saw them after I arrived in England. The secretary does not think that I shall have difficulty getting a job if I don't mind urban or industrial practice! In any case I can get locums without difficulty which would keep the wolf from the door, 30gns week, but not provide a settled home.

We have had a busy week with the visitation of the London University Examiners. They arrived about 10.45 and we settled Mr. and Mrs. Nicholls surgeon from St Georges also Dean of St Georges Medical School, in our guest room and Prof. Kelswick (Middlesex Hospital) in the Pearsons" guest room, and Mr. Flew, the obstetrician used our bathroom as he was not staying the night. They were all very pleasant but very shrewd. The Nicholls had lunch with the Roys and we had Prof Kelswick and Mr. Flew and the Mountfields so we were a pleasant party. They had looked all round the hospital and seemed interested in all they saw. After lunch they retired for a while and afterwards the doctors all had tea together. Meanwhile I had produced some details which they required.

After tea and a very heavy shower we went for a stroll on the lawns and suddenly got covered with ants down by the fruit trees, so our walk ended in farce!

In the evening we all had dinner together in the hostel - soup, ground nut stew, trifle and coffee - eighteen of us all together. It meant a great deal of work - but a very pleasant evening and it gave everyone a chance to meet everyone else.

Next morning they had breakfast with us and then went on to Elsie's. They had rather a wait for transport but Prof. Kelswick played with the children, he has four of his own! It was pleasant having them, though a bit of a strain really. We are now awaiting their report, but this will no doubt be a while coming as they have to report to the General Medical Council.

Next week is going to be busy too, I think. Marion and Fred are coming in for chop tomorrow evening and on Tuesday I have to go to Oyo for a medical committee. Roy goes on holiday on Monday - tomorrow - for a fortnight so Fred and I are dividing up his work, but it means I shall have an outpatient clinic each day.

The Hobsons, they arrived at Wesley College whilst Margaret was awaiting Richard, are coming up on Friday morning for the weekend, two and a half days! They have four children so we really are going to be busy - or rather Margaret will be, though I expect Mrs. H will lend a hand.

The following week is our entrance exam which is going to be a very busy time for us all and the week after, Miss Stennet comes. Incidentally I had a letter from Elizabeth Johnson (now in N Nigeria) - wants to come the same week as Miss S

We are all very well indeed and send our love to you all,   David

5.11.61

Sunday morning and a few moments in the office, having done my rounds and before going to church in the lorry! We were very glad to hear that all was well with you all. You certainly seem to be up to your eyes with speaking at meetings but no doubt the winter spate of meetings is in full bore so to speak. Glad to hear of your outing with Auntie to Bedford and that they are all well.

We too were surprised to hear of David Cattersons engagement It certainly does seem to be somewhat swift!

We should be pleased to welcome Miss McKnight if things work out that way and we would of course look after her at this end.

Here we have had a busy week with one thing and another, rather overshadowed by the fact that all the children have had very bad coughs and colds and Richard, bless him, is still not very well. He is much more cheerful today but even he has been grizzly and fretful which is most unlike his usual self. However his smile and gurgle are in evidence this morning so he is on the mend I think. He has had a temperature for four or five days. Peter and Elizabeth are better but Elizabeth is still rather difficult, off her food and wants attention, though they are all sleeping well.

Margaret and I are keeping well, but both getting tired. The work is very heavy at the moment, Roy is on holiday till tomorrow. I shall have been on either first or second call for twelve nights out of the last fourteen.

Next week is to be a busy one, with the Synod Medical Committee on Friday, which day is the beginning of Miss Stennet's visit to us here! I am secretary of the committee so have had to complete the agenda and so forth and prepare for the meeting, which is likely to be long. After the meeting we bring Miss S. back with us.

Joan Ariel is also a problem! She does not want to come down and now says she does not know whether she wants to leave or not, so I don't really know what to say at the committee. In addition she will require fetching from Ikole!

Next Saturday I shall be going to Afon with Miss Stennet and Gwen Davies who will be accompanying her I understand. I am not looking forward to this trip very much. I really must get up to Kaiama also if I can in the near future to see what is happening to the house. The week after that I have to go down to Lagos for a meeting of the Midwives Board.

This last week we had two medical students from Bristol University staying in the hostel for three days. We had them to a meal on Monday - they were a pleasant couple. Then on Tuesday we had a party in the Sisters' house to welcome Marion and Jean Wingfield. Wednesday night was our staff committee at which we discussed our Christmas arrangements - not long now!

On Thursday Roy and Beryl came back. Their children had not been well, but they are picking up now. It will be good to have Roy back at work again - I have had his outpatients to do!

Last night we had a quiet evening and I did some work in the office and a long uninterrupted night so feel more rested this morning.

Elizabeth Johnson is not coming next weekend, instead I have sent her all our publications. Incidentally she is only a Rural Medical Officer - the lowest form of Government Medical Officer. However we have an American, his wife and child from Friday to Sunday instead!

On Thursday last we were to have been visited by the Minister of Health. He had to cancel his visit but suddenly the Owa turned up! Apparently it had been put about that he was dead - so he came around to show people that he was well. Hope you are all well. Love to Auntie A and you all from us all, David

H. O. Awodiya, WGH, 6.11.61

Dear Mrs. Cannon,
Your letter of 6.10.61 was received with many thanks and I am indeed grateful for it. Nothing will be too great to give on behalf of your dear son - David. We really appreciate his services to we Africans especially Ijeyshas among whom he has been working since these days. His leaving at the end of this tour is a very heavy blow on us which I hope will take some years to recover.

David has done quite a lot for me as an individual, he contributed largely to raise me to my present position as the Hospital Manager and it was he, who helped me through thick and thin and I am very grateful to him and I should like you also to thank him wholeheartedly on my behalf. Thanks

Hope the family is all well and greetings to all.

How is Michael? Hope his work is going on well - warm wishes.

It is becoming too hot here now, but we still expect some heavy storms more before the real hot season sets in.

You must have been getting ready for the Birth of our Lord and I wish you and the family a merry Christmas and Happy New Year in advance. Thank you very much,

Yours sincerely, H O Awodiya

13.11.61

This is a very rushed note to let you know that all is well with us all.

We were very pleased to receive letters both from Mother and Michael this week and should love to have heard 'Glory Hallelujah'! I wonder if you did play choruses for the collection? I am pleased to say that all our family is well. The children's colds have all cleared up and we are very fit. Margaret is bearing up with all the visitors, who incidentally have all been very pleasant and at the moment we haven't any, though our next lot are coming on Friday - Rev. Peter Paris and wife with the Student Christian Movement he is a travelling Secretary. I think they are French Canadians.

The week has been very busy. We have had Keith Smith for the whole time but he was very interesting to entertain and very good with the children.

Then Bob Mitchell, wife and child arrived on the Friday to Sunday. They were Americans, but a very nice couple and Stuart who is nine months old interested the children, who are now very keen for Richard to walk.

Thursday we sent the car up for Joan Ariel who seemed in good form. Friday was very busy. We, Marion Joan and myself left at 6.45am and arrived at Wesley College before nine. I was secretary of the committee and Miss Stennet was there. There was some plain speaking on both sides! and I am having much difficulty preparing the minutes, in fact I have asked Miss S. to run through my first draft!

Joan was upset on the way back and I pointed out quite plainly to her that she was a Missionary in spirit but locally engaged. She said she wanted either full missionary status, which she cannot have as she is a Pentecostalist on government salary. Incidentally she told us she was receiving £2400 pa with the World Health Organisation in India so no doubt she feels £360 pa somewhat lower. Miss Stennet and Gwen Davies came back with us but in their own car. I was unable to get out to shop as there is a Standing Committee I had to attend.

Yesterday, or rather, Saturday we set out for Afon. Marion, Gwen, Miss Stennet and I. Between Ilesha and Oshogbo they decided that they wanted to go to Kaiama! Despite the fact that we had barely enough food, we set off. We stopped for coffee en route and Marion left the back of the Opel open so after 100 yards the chop box fell out. Bang went the staple part of our lunch! However we had a good trip and the house is going on well and we hope Joan W might well move in in January

Coming back last night I got a headache and so went to bed early and had a very good night - for which I was ready and am very fit again today.

This afternoon I go down to Lagos for the Midwives Board and hope to get back tomorrow. Hope all well at home, Love from us all, David

19.11.61

We were very glad to have your letter this week, to learn that all was well with you all. We were very pleased to learn that Stanley has been chosen to run for Oxford Freshmen and look forward to hearing how he got on.

Yes the Morlings were in Ibadan and have been to Ilesha many times. It was he who redid our site plans for us. She was a deaconess before marriage. Her first name is May. I should get in touch if you can, they are very nice people indeed and have two children now I think.

Here we have had a very busy time. I wrote last weeks letter on the Monday morning feeling quite unwell! However I drove down to Lagos in the afternoon and felt much better on arrival. I stayed with Bill and Dorothy Mann. The next morning I did a bit of shopping and then the Midwives Board at 9am. This went on until 1.30! I then had lunch and returned to Ilesha in the evening.

Miss Stennet had been to Ikole and spent the night with Joan! They both survived but they were both uncommunicative about it!

On Wednesday Miss Stennet looked round the hospital with Marion - again she made few remarks, and then in the evening, we had Roy, Beryl, Jonathan, Meg, Jean W and Miss S in for dinner! We had quite a happy and hilarious time! After dinner was Fellowship, led by Marion, which did not seem to catch fire.

Miss Stennet left on Thursday - again uncommunicative. In her fifteen years as secretary of MMS I feel she has learned to keep her mouth shut!

On Friday our weekend visitors arrived Rev Peter Paris and wife. They are both Canadian, she is white, he is coloured and are a very nice couple. They have not been married very long and are Travelling Secretaries for the SCM.

I went up to Ikole on Friday evening and found Joan in quite good form. I had a lot of work to do, but had a long nights sleep. I brought a patient in labour back with me - but she had a normal delivery later I am glad to say. Last night we had Jill and Dorothea in for chop from St. Margaret's with the Paris family.

After chop we put on a film (sound) 'Song of Ceylon' for the senior staff. it was good but made in 1935! so it was a bit dated. However it made a very good evening entertainment. Roy was very pleased indeed to see it and hopes to show it round one or two places.

Today I hope to have a quieter day. Roy has gone to service at Otapete and I am writing in the office. Jonathan is on duty. Next Thursday I have to go to Ibadan for a meeting of the Medical Advisory Board and hope to be able to do some shopping at that time. Christmas is coming so soon that it will be here before we know about it.

Incidentally Bill and Dorothy gave me some fairy lights for the Christmas tree and the children are very pleased.

We are all very well. The children have quite recovered and are full of beans. Richard is now in a big cot in the children's bedroom - they do look a family!

The Ashleys are due through here today on their way back to Ikole - they have been shopping in Ibadan. Hope you are all well, Love from us all,   David

2.12.61

December is here - time is certainly slipping past and no doubt soon you will have Stanley home and perhaps Auntie Alice coming. Here the children are becoming increasingly excited about Christmas, and each have one of these cards on which you open a window each day until the Day, so there is quite a ritual!

It is Saturday night and we are enjoying an evening on our own! No visitors - though we had Prof. and Mrs. Jolly from Ibadan, Thursday/Friday and then on Monday we have Rev. Solovin and Bill Mann for the night plus Prof. Lawson, Harold Garling for lunch as well. It is our Hospital Management Committee on Monday afternoon - I shall be glad when it is over.

Your letter arrived on Friday and we were as usual pleased to receive it and hear all your news, though we were sorry to hear of Ruby's depression and hope it soon improves with therapy. The bungalows opposite seem also to feature prominently!

No! We do not wish to continue our membership of the National Geographic Society! It was a gift to us originally from Uncle Fred Craddock, which we greatly appreciated but we did not feel it sufficiently worthwhile to continue. Perhaps if I get into a pleasant practice I might get it for the waiting room!

Here we are all in good form though Roy is really quite sick with chicken pox. He noticed the spots on Monday and has had quite a high fever- 104 most days. He has been really quite ill with it and it is likely to be a couple of weeks before he is back again. This means that we are all having to do extra work and with the medical students here for 20 days it is really very hard at the moment. He was to examine in Ibadan next week so I have had to cancel this- rather short notice, I am afraid, to find someone else.

The vehicles, too, have been in the wars. Jean W had a smash in the Imesi car on Thursday and had the front and rear wings dented, a door and wheel hubs damaged. However we have got it straightened locally. Then yesterday the Sisters went to Ife for a meeting and a stone was thrown up by a passing vehicle and the windscreen shattered, so the Opel is having to go into Ibadan on Monday for a new windscreen!

Today the Hartfields have been to Ibadan to do their Christmas shopping but seem rather disappointed with their visit , they do not seem to have got what they wanted. Apparently, being Saturday, the shops were full and Sheila was rather a weight to carry round.

We enjoyed having Prof. and Mrs. Jolly here. They were easy to entertain and asked many questions of many things, and I think were quite impressed. They have three children aged eighteen, sixteen and fourteen, all at boarding school at the moment, but coming out for Christmas. They may well bring them out here for a day.

Richard has cut his first tooth! We are all thrilled, especially Peter and Elizabeth who take an extraordinary interest in their young brother. He is as good as ever and is taking a whole selection of foods very well. Tomorrow is weighing day again - we shall wait and see how the children have done, with their coughs and colds last month both Peter and Elizabeth lost, but have been eating better this month.

Apart from the Management Committee the coming week would seem easier - apart from Roy being in bed!

Hope you all keep well, Love from us all, David

10.12.61

The weeks are rushing past, and we seem to be almost at Christmas again - it will be our tenth in a row here in Ilesha. I shall have to get down to thinking of Christmas gifts for the clerks. There are so many now it is a real problem.

The gifts from Michael for the children arrived yesterday, thank you very much indeed! Thank you too for the address of the Pattersons.

Twink will be home now and we wonder how he got on the second visit to Cambridge, running. We note your reaction to Stewardship Campaign - is it really April '63? a year and a half hence?

Thank you for the offer of the desk in Twink's room. I am sure Peter would love it, it might help him to do some work! Though at the moment Margaret says he is trying much more consistently at school. He is good at numbers but seems to make little headway at reading, though no doubt it will suddenly 'come' one day.

Here we have had a very busy week again. Roy is still not at work, though he is much better, but yesterday both their children went down with chicken pox! one feels that we can hardly escape!

Last Monday was our management Committee. The Rev. A. S. Slamin came and stayed with us over night and in addition we had Bill Mann, Harold Garling and Prof. Lawson for lunch.

The committee was at 3pm and was attended by the above, plus Mr. Fadahunsi, the Chairman of Nigerian Airways, Dr. Sasingbu, the chief Medical Officer Western Nigeria and others. It went well and afterwards we had tea together, organised by Margaret, but in the Hostel.

At 7.30 we had a valedictory service for our outgoing nurses plus the presentation of badges, some prizes - quite an interesting service, though not well *attended except for hospital staff.*

On Wednesday Mr. Laniyan went off to Kaiama with a bath! to put in the house there. I have not seen him since his return, but if all is well the house should be complete apart from furnishing, but the plumbing and painting should be complete.

Wednesday evening it was Margaret's Fellowship. On Tuesday a consultant anaesthetist turned up and gave a talk and showed a film on artificial respiration to the nurses - excellent. He stayed with us for lunch.

Then on Wednesday Prof. David Allbrook arrived, he rang up first. He is Professor of Anatomy at Makereri - Uganda and would you believe it - I knew him in the IVF when we were students in London, so we had a very pleasant time together and he seemed most interested in all he saw.

On Thursday Bill and Mrs. Wood came for the night, they are travelling through to the East and may well be here on Monday night also.

Yesterday (Saturday) Joan Ariel had called her Committee so we were up at 6am and on the way at 6.30 I called for coffee at Ifaki at 8.00 and arrived in time for the committee. I called also on the Ashleys and had more coffee! I then saw some patients, had lunch and returned to Ilesha

In the evening St Margaret's were doing a Nativity play so I took Peter and Elizabeth. It should have started at 6.30 but didn't until 6.50 so we were late home - quite dark. The children were thrilled and enjoyed it and Peter followed it mostly, some of it was beyond him. Jane Sutton had produced it.

Richard has not been well. He was vaccinated 2/52 ago, and it is very inflamed. He has been feverish, not willing to feed and most unlike himself. However he is much better this morning. Margaret has had a bad cold but now better. I am in the midst of one. However if Roy is back next week it should be easier. Hope you are all well, love from us all here, David

16.12.61

It is Saturday evening and we have just finished our meal - roast corn, followed by a grill and coffee, so I am feeling at peace with the world. Margaret is preparing for 'school' next week and then get off some more of our local Christmas cards. Marion is coming in this evening to use the sewing machine for making curtains and decorations for the wards.

Thank you all very much for the cards which arrived for each member of the family this week. They have been attached to the pelmet of the window overlooking the sandpit, so you can picture them there.

We were glad to receive your letter - you seem to have been as busy as ever , though it would appear that the garden (and bungalow) is in a poor state! Our garden is as dry as a bone. The grass is getting quite brown and the road is very dusty so the children can become clean/dirty in a surprisingly short time!

Here we seem to be as busy as ever. We had the Ado Doctor on Tuesday and Wednesday and also on Wednesday we had a Dutch Sociologist who was seeking information, not that we were able to help him very much.

The children are getting excited about Christmas. I have just realised that this is the last letter before Christmas day - A very Happy Christmas to you all! We went out shopping for the stockings the other day leaving the children with Meg. We had a good run round and walked through the market where we bought a number of gifts including some for Williams progeny! We are giving William a torch like our new one as he showed great interest in it so we hope he will be pleased. We have had two miniature tool boxes made for Peter and Elizabeth into which we have put a real hammer, pincers, screwdriver and small bradawl-feeling it is better they get used to the feel of real tools from the beginning our poor furniture!

Joan Ariel's new car has come and is already up at Ikole, as is her new gas stove so she should be well set up for Christmas. She sent down a long list of provisions she wanted, which we have sent up with Roy, who went up on trek yesterday - and came back today. He is improving and is back at work, though because of his scabs he is not willing to scrub up in the theatre as yet. Rohan and Mithra have been most unwell, with chicken pox, but Mithra 'came to' today, so Beryl is feeling more cheerful. If our two get it, it will be just before Christmas - most unfortunate.

We have just started wrapping presents and will do a few each day as a ploy for the children - they do enjoy it.

There seems a bit of doubt at the moment about the Clapps. It is possible they may not be here until April, which would be rather disappointing. Also they appear to have doubts as to working with British Methodism! Anyway we shall see.

Our Christmas guests, Kathleen Moore from University College Hospital, Ibadan - we had lunch there the first day you were here and Monica Humble from Shagamu, are coming on the Friday before Christmas and staying until the following Thursday so we shall have our hands full. In addition Mr. Esan has asked us to arrange accommodation for the 22 Missionaries who will be attending Synod in January! No small task.

Well time and space have fled... We do hope you all have a lovely time this Christmas and perhaps next year we shall all be together some of the time!

Much love to you all from us all, David

23.12.61

We were very pleased to receive your letter this week with your Christmas wishes, and with this, we send you our best wishes for the New Year - it will not be long now before we are home again.

Thank you very much Auntie A for your Christmas presents to us all, we appreciate your kindness very much indeed. I will get a mid-week letter in if all is well, and let you know how we are getting on.

It is now Saturday night, and most folk are at Carol Singing. I am on duty, Roy, Jonathan and Fred have gone with Marion and Margaret Grant our visitors and 35 nurses, so it is a large party. They have gone up to the leprosy patients village at the moment and will be going down to the Owa afterwards.

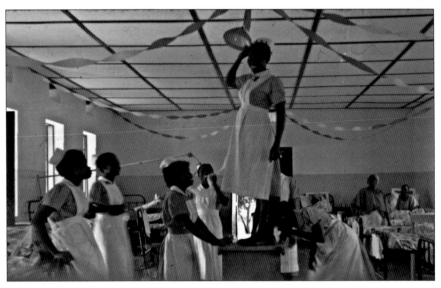

Decorating the ward

At home the children are getting very excited. We have decorated the living room and Peter and Elizabeth have 'decorated' their room too! Our visitors came yesterday - Kathleen Moore and Monica Humble - you will recall both of them. We have got some Cassia tree in the corner of the room by the settee and have on it the fairy lights which blink on and off. Needless to say Peter and Elizabeth are very pleased with it.

We have done very well for local presents so far - two turkeys, and a complete Yoruba rig out for me and for Margaret and Peter, and Margaret has just run one up for Elizabeth so we are all set for Christmas Day.

Today has been busy with the decoration of the wards, nurses dining room and so on and last minute rehearsal of the Nativity Play which is tomorrow afternoon and to which we shall all go. Tomorrow evening is our Carol Service, in which I am reading and afterwards we are going down to Hon. J. Fadahunsi's to sing carols - he is returning specially for it from Lagos, and then that brings us to Christmas Eve. Somehow this year we seem to be a day in advance of our usual timetable.

Thinking for the moment of our furlough, we wonder if you could enquire about the possibility of Peter and possibly Elizabeth going to school for the summer term at either the school opposite the hairdresser or the school on the Avenue? Would Pop see the Principals and ask about the possibility please, costs and dates of terms. We feel that it would be a good thing for Peter to get into a school for a term until we get settled down somewhere for the new school year. The school on the Avenue is nearer, but probably rather expensive and we might have to buy special uniform, which we should not want to do for a short while.

If it was possible for Peter to go for the term then we shall probably go up to Liverpool to see Grandpa soon after arriving and be back in Worcester Park for the start of the term. My only engagement is in Plymouth by the way at a midweek meeting, at Charles Day's church, about 16 May. I must not get involved with deputation until I have a job in view.

Incidentally Frank Davey rang on Thursday - the Clapps are coming in March, and Andrew has been in touch with a Methodist couple, both Doctors, no children, who are in practice in Castle Bromwich, east of Birmingham, who might well come out later in the year. They have a Christian practice and I wondered if there might be an opening there. A suburb of Birmingham 107 miles from London on the M1 and 90 miles from Liverpool - quite conveniently situated   But it is only a pipe dream! However I will let Andrew know what I have in mind.

Time is slipping past and it will soon be time for my night round. I was up last night and no rest today! I hope it is a quiet one. We shall be thinking of you often and can picture you all at home.

Love from us all, to you all, and every good wish for the New Year! David

PS I fear this will be late as Monday and Tuesday are public holidays.

30.12.61

Thank you very much indeed for your Christmas presents to us all! Margaret was very pleased with her blouse and I with the cravat. The drawing frame for Peter is just what he needs at the moment and to encourage him to draw. Elizabeth is very pleased with her xylophone! We have all had a most enjoyable Christmas and hope you have had a pleasant one too.

Your letter has not arrived this week and it is more than likely that ours has not reached you as I understand that there is postal confusion in England at the moment. I wrote to Auntie Alice last night but unfortunately the letter has not gone so it will be Tuesday before they go I expect.. After doing rounds, we all set off between 10.45 and 11.30 in the cars to go to Imesi where we had elevenses with Jean Wingfield in the Imesi house. It was very pleasant indeed and we all ate a great feast to the point where lunch held no interest! However it was surprising how our appetites returned when we went to the Imesi High School, to Roy Bowcocks for lunch. There we had cold turkey, ham rolls and cheese -

absolutely wonderful! Just my favourite swallow.

The children played on some massive rocks outside and had a lovely time. Only Fred and Marion stayed behind.

We returned for tea about 4pm and in the evening we had the nurses party. Our guests organised the games, and Doctors and Sisters did a 'sort of play' with a few lyrics written by Marion. It seemed to be appreciated but was hard and tiring work!

Wednesday we were back in the normal routine again, with a heavy outpatients as we had not had outpatients for three and a half days. In the evening we had a Staff Committee followed by listening to the tape recording of our carol service - not very good with much extraneous noise! I have just been out to put some chestnuts to roast in the fire! I tried some last night and most of them charred, so I have put them in a tin in the ashes tonight!

Monica left on Wednesday and on Thursday Kathleen left - Gwen Davies and Jennifer came to eat their sandwiches and at the same time Harold Garling, his wife, and two daughters came for the same thing so eleven of us were here for lunch - twelve including Richard who now sits in his chair at meal times and eats most enthusiastically more than either Peter or Elizabeth at the moment.

Friday was again a busy day - four folk dropped in at tea time to look round, one being Margery Rushworth from Ituk Mbang.. Last evening was a quiet one with an eight hour night for the first time for some time.

Today has been the staff children's party - about 70 of them turned up for games Krola and biscuits - then a film strip.

Margaret Woodland arrived today in very good form and will be going out to Imesi tomorrow I think and picking up from there. Margaret Gardener has flown to Zaria. She is to examine next week and to have a little local leave at the same time. Margaret Woodland brought the news that the Pearsons' may be here earlier than expected - in time for Synod, so I may have much less to do than I expected, though hospitality will be more difficult than we had imagined as we had planned to have Jonah in their house.

Our hospitality plans for Synod are about ready - just a question of when and where to put folk. On Wednesday 17th we are having an 'open day' when they can all visit the hospital.

Tomorrow night is Watch night and the beginning of a new year which is likely to be a most eventful one certainly for us. Do hope you are all well, with love from all of us here, David

PS Have written the AA for help in clearing the car on April 6th!

7.1.62

Sunday morning and there are a few minutes before I need to set out for church, in which to start this letter. We were very pleased to receive two letters this week, one written on Christmas Eve with the story of your preparations and the other written a week later in which you describe the snow in the garden. From all accounts it has been very cold indeed! Fred was saying that he has never before known snow in his home which is very close to the Thames Estuary in Kent. Here we have had it as hot as usual, though there is a bit of a harmattan again at the moment. Elizabeth has got a cold which may well run round the family, as has William, but the children are in fine fettle really.

Last Sunday our Watchnight was somewhat marred by the burning of one of our wires in the gatehouse and our inability to start our own generator - however it was repaired on New Years Day so all was well.

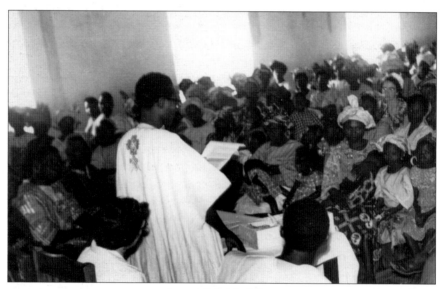

Imesi 5th birthday

We had hymn singing in the Sisters house and then we returned to our house for roast potatoes, done in the fire, and then went to the chapel at 11pm for the service taken by Pastor Osinguna and the nurses.

New Years Day was spent quietly at home. We half expected some visitors who however never came, though some unexpected ones came in for tea. Work then was much as usual for the week. Mr. and Mrs. Deeks and two children came to stay en-route for Lagos on Wednesday night and then Frank Morton arrived yesterday. He will be with us for almost three weeks!

Yesterday however was the Imesi Scheme 5th Birthday.

There was great preparation and I left at nine with a very full car (Meg H and Mrs. Jolly plus her three children (17, 14 and 11)There was a service in the Imesi Methodist church 10-11, followed by speeches. The Minister of Health spoke first, Judge Oguntoge followed and I spoke third. The church was full of women and children and a truly amazing sight. After this we all went up to the

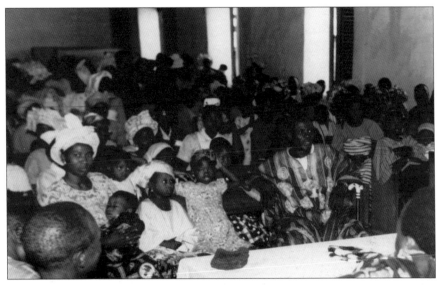

Imesi 5th birthday

house for squash and biscuits and then Prof. Jolly, Jonathan and I went to the local Rural Health Centre, which is built but not staffed yet and after this we all went to the Boys High School for a sit down lunch of curry and rice, one dish of curry being very much hotter for our Nigerian brethren! A very happy occasion. Then we went to Roy Bowcock's house for coffee and then Margaret's house again for tea after which we went down to see the traditional dancing which would be

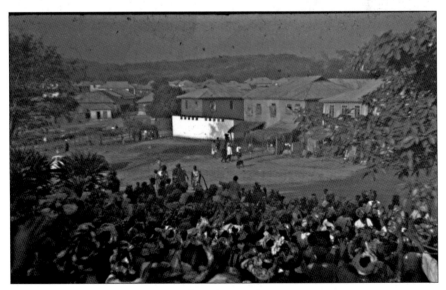

Imesi crowd

followed by a candlelight procession and a cinema show. Most of us from Ilesha returned before that however.

This coming week marks the start of Synod and by this time next week Ilesha will be full of Methodists. Committees start on Wednesday and Synod proper a week tomorrow

The Pearsons' fly 18th and land 19th and come up 20th, just before the pastoral session and after all the work is done! Frank and Jessie Longley will stay with us and we shall feed Jonah and Frank as well so we shall have a great deal to do - especially Margaret, bless her. We do hope you are all well at home - Auntie as well. and the weather is not too cold I hope there will be an improvement before April!   Love from us all,   David

14.1.62

Your letter of the 7th arrived in good time this week, so it seems as though the postal hold up is at the distribution end rather than the sending. I hope our letters are not too delayed. You seem to have been having quite a gay time what with the Chinese Restaurant and plays. Thank you for the assurance that Pop will enquire at the schools - we look forward to hearing details in due course.

Here we are in far from arctic conditions and we are in the midst of entertaining in a big way! We have Jonah and Mrs. Jonah, Mr. and Mrs. Longley and Frank Morton as permanent guests, so you can imagine how busy Margaret is! We were very surprised on ringing Lagos last Friday night to hear that Mrs. Jones had come back with Jonah - apparently a last minute decision. However she seems quite well and cheerful, though is taking things very quietly. They are in the Pearsons' bedroom with the use of their living room, so are quite a way from the children and come over for meals. Frank and Jessie Longley are in our guest room and Frank Morton is in the private ward. All the other houses have their quota, but none with so many or with such incapacities! However we are jogging along quite well and have got a few days over! The Synod Committees have been meeting so far, plus the opening and dedication of another church in Ilesha yesterday.

I went down for the beginning at 4.30pm and left at 6.30 - just before the end - quite a marathon task but an interesting event. Then last night we had a barbecue on our lawn for 36 folk. We had three fires, two for cooking and one for sitting round- the latter vast - one could not get near to it. Meg Hartfield had made six chef hats and aprons for the men and we cooked soup and sausages fried, baked beans and potatoes followed by bananas and biscuits and coffee. I think everyone enjoyed it and our men guests did the cooking. Margaret was organiser in chief!

Afterwards we sat round the fire and sang rounds and songs with one or two solos by Roy and Rebecca! A most enjoyable evening.

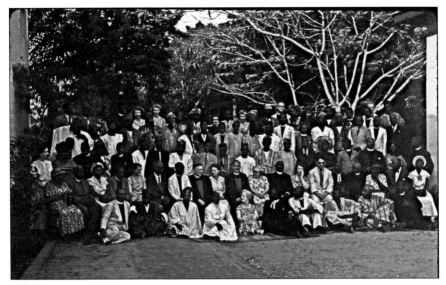

Synod

Today I am staying in this morning to prepare for the ward service this afternoon and also to prepare for the medical business which I have to present to Synod on Tuesday and I shall be very glad when this is over. On the following day, Wednesday we are having an Open Day at the hospital and inviting the whole Synod to come and look round (about 150). This will be quite a special occasion. After this, apart from hospitality which will go on until Thursday week, I shall have no more responsibility and Andrew will be back next week end. They fly on Thursday, arrive Lagos on Friday and intend to come to Ilesha on Saturday. We shall be pleased to see them but in some ways I shall be sorry to relinquish the post of Acting Superintendent - which though it has been heavy, is rewarding in other ways.

We have had three book boxes made and a box for the sewing machine so we feel to have made a start with our packing. In addition we have been through some drawers. I have approached the AA to clear and cope with the Dauphine on arrival in the UK and also have it serviced and two wing mirrors fitted.

We are all very well, though having so many guests for so long is tiring.

Love from us all to you all, David

21.1.62

Sunday morning, a few minutes between an operation and coffee in which to write this letter. The Pearsons' are back! They arrived last evening and seem in good form despite the rapid change from cold to hot. They came in for supper last night with the Jonahs - we had a pleasant evening and then in came John Mellanby, entirely unexpected, so we really do have a full house still!

We are very well apart from Richard who is not well at all. He has had fever and has developed severe diarrhoea. We all feel he will soon be better, but he is a very pathetic little scrap at the moment and both Margaret and I feel rather anxious.

Synod began last Monday and I spent most of the time there, as on Tuesday we had the Medical business. This went quite well and Jonah said a few words of appreciation, after which the Synod rose as a token of respect for your truly- all rather embarrassing.

Tuesday evening was the Missionary Meeting in Otapete at which Frank Longley spoke. The music was accompanied by 'talking drums' which really sounded most attractive.

In the evening we had the Missionaries meeting at which all the Missionaries were present - this went on until almost midnight. Wednesday, Roy went to Synod and in the evening the Hon. J. O. Fadahunsi gave a dinner for all Synod which was very nice - a buffet serving - as it were - of a proper meal. I had a very satisfying meal.

On Thursday most of the lay folk returned so we were left with our Ministerial brethren. The Pastoral session starts tomorrow and they hope to finish by Wednesday at 2pm so we shall be back to our normal sort of number by next weekend, though we hope to have a party on Saturday, to welcome the Pearsons' and Margaret Woodland and to say farewell to Fred.

We have had another letter from Elizabeth Johnson who wishes to come from Feb 12 -19th, so we shall be busy right to the end it would seem. We may well have the Crossleys too for a week or so whilst he is doing some work in Ilesha.

We have got three book boxes made - I don't think we have enough books to fill them all- but we can always use one to pack toys and so forth in. They are similar too, but smaller than my tool box and as solidly constructed.

Peter and Elizabeth are very excited at Alison and Bryan's return and went out to play with them very early this morning.

The Pearsons' will spend a day or two unpacking I expect and then Andrew will get back into work again. It will certainly be pleasant to hand over the responsibility - but I have enjoyed acting as Superintendent the last few months.

We were very glad to receive your letter earlier this week - you will feel somewhat depleted without Stanley and Auntie Alice but your deputation seems on the increase!

I have heard from Arthur Miller and agreed to speak to Young Peoples Fellowship on April 29 provisionally- our movements won't be definite till we hear about the schools, the results of Pop's investigations. I wish we could send you some of our warmth - but we are looking forward to getting home whatever the weather. Love from us all David

PS Monday, Richard is much better this morning, M.

28.1.62

Another Sunday, and a few moments in the office to write this letter. I am pleased to say that Richard is completely recovered and is his own cheerful self again. He had a severe dysentery, which made him rather more ill than the diarrhoea would account for. Anyway we are all in good health and good spirits now.

Thank you for you letter and Michael's too and also for the photographs which came yesterday. I fear that I left the film in the camera too long - hence the spots etc. Since then I have had a colour film in - just over Christmas and got it away quickly and it is perfectly OK so I am sure it was just delay in getting it off.

I have written to Dorothy (of Boston) saying I should be very happy to go, but asking if they could swap weekends, as the one they chose is very close to my promised visit to Plymouth, and I don't think I could fit it in, but have offered two further weekends. I have told Harold Johnson that I cannot manage July- I hope to have a job by then or at least be house hunting in the area.

We were thrilled to hear that Stanley wished to go 'on note' I hope he keeps it up. I think that Jean Pearson is rather concerned about her brother David who seems to be making money rather too easily in television and have rather a broad outlook on life!

Michael seems busy at College with lectures, and no doubt finds many extra curricular activities to fill his odd moments!

Here we are resting after Synod! Our last guest went on Wednesday and our house seemed empty without them. Jonah said it was the best synod they had had for years, in a quiet relatively cool phase without much travelling to be done so Mr. Esan is pleased, as are we all.

Andrew has been gradually taking over this week so I am feeling rather a displaced person. I now have no desk in the office! However it is very pleasant not to have the responsibility.

Last night Margaret and I gave a party - there were 20 all told. Tomato soup, cold turkey and stuffing of two varieties, peas potatoes and apple sauce, in lieu of jelly, trifle and coffee. The turkey is magnificent and cooked to a turn and there are still some lovely bits left! Then we played games, had two charades and to bed about 11.30. I think everyone enjoyed it very much.

We have got our first crate packed but there will be many more still to do but it is good to get started in time I think.

The arrangements about the car are taking shape and insurance on landing. I am arranging all through the AA and the Motor Insurance Co. for marine insurance and after landing.

We have been considering the sleeping of the children on our arrival and feel that the following scheme has much to commend it :- Both Peter and Elizabeth sleep well on our camp beds, and the beds themselves are easy to dispose of by pushing under another bed. It would seem satisfactory then for the cot, if it could be borrowed again, to be beside our bed on Margaret's side, then at night Elizabeth in a bed across the bottom of ours, (tucked under the bed during the day) and Peter on a camp bed in Michael's room if Michael would be agreeable and the bed pushed under his bed during the day, on the understanding that Peter only goes into the room for sleeping and all his clothes are kept in our room. This means that all the regular inhabitants need not be disturbed from their beds, unless Auntie Alice arrives, when the loft could be used - but normally all could sleep on the same floor.

The children would be thrilled, and we should feel happier if there was as little disturbance as possible to others. I realise what an influx it is going to be and what a lot of extra work. Would a furnished flat be available do you think? Somewhere nearby? or can we manage for the weeks until I get a job.

Next week Prof. Lawson and Mr. Gwillim (the chap from St Georges) are coming on Tuesday and then Dr. Pearson senior is expected next Saturday and Mr. Holgate, the architect. The same day we are expecting John and Margaret Crossley (and Jonah) for a week or so! Thus we are still going to be busy!

Do hope you are all well, and the weather is warming up. Ten weeks and we shall be home! Looking forward to it. Love to you all, David

5.2.62

Saturday evening and the Crossleys, Margaret and I are sitting quietly after dinner having been out to Ede pool in the afternoon for a swim and a picnic which we all enjoyed very much indeed.

We were delighted to receive your two letters and to hear that Peter is fixed up in a school. We are very pleased and grateful and Peter is thrilled. I do hope we can locate a Nursery School for Elizabeth or there will be tears! We note that term begins on April 30th so we must fix our visit to Liverpool before this date. I have promised May 6th and 7th to Dorothy in Boston, I think this is mutually satisfactory. They have had rather a shock at Grandpa's. The couple upstairs - the husband Ken had pneumonia but was recovering but went to the toilet, collapsed and died before the Doctor could arrive. Thea and Ernie rallied round and took Lesley and the child home and coped - but they had the police round and an inquest and so forth - he must have had an embolism I think. Anyway they are straight again but it must have been a shock for them all. I gather the flat will be empty till after we have been there so we shall have room to spare for our visit.

Last week I did not mention my birthday, which was a very pleasant day - gifts from all the members of the family - a little pointed, towel, soap, sponge and powder! We had a birthday tea and cake (three candles) and in the evening lamb chops - a special treat.

We were very sorry to hear that the Shears are moving I do hope we get some pleasant neighbours again. We have had a busy week with one thing and another.

On Tuesday Prof Lawson and Mr. Gwillim (the senior obstetrician for St. Georges Hospital, London, came about 11.30 and before lunch we looked round, then had lunch. Afterwards Andrew came in and talked. Mr. Gwillim said he would help Jonathan to get a job, he is going to sit the MRCOG and will require two years posts in the UK prior to sitting.

Both Prof. Lawson and Mr. Gwillim said they thought it was a pity that I was not continuing in obstetrics on my return to the UK and suggested I took the MRCOG. This would mean two years in hospital appointments to qualify for the exams (though I have written to the Royal College to confirm this) and would mean quite a lot of study and in addition a residential appointment for part of this period 6/12 or a year. Very few hospitals provide married accommodation so it would mean having a flat or renting a house nearby for the family. This would be expensive as I should have to pay for my residence, but not impossible to manage. I should be home at the weekends and perhaps one day a week off duty but should not see much of the family for a year. The second year during the gynaecology appointment I might well be able to live at home if it was not too far away. Again it is possible that I might have to do several jobs - though more likely - as the appointment is for one year, renewable, I should be in the same place.

If I got the MRCOG - what then? I could either go into General Practice or continue in hospital service, which ever door opened. Prof. Lawson seems to think I could pass the examination but it would mean a lot of preparation - 40 cases to write up in detail and two dissertations which have to be accepted before it is permitted to sit the papers and have clinical examinations. I think it would take two years from June or July if I got a job then (the exam is in Jan and June) but one has to apply six months in advance and have the casebooks in three months before the exams so it might well be January 1965 before I was able to sit. Afterwards and probably before, I should be living at home and doing a more or less 9 to 5 job with spells of being on call. In General Practice I should be better off more quickly and probably settled more quickly, though an assistantship might not go on to a partnership and a move or two be entailed. Anyway we shall see! What do you think?

Here we are all well. The Crossleys arrived yesterday and stay till Wednesday. Roy goes into UCH for an operation, not serious, on Thursday, and Andrew does the Umuahia trip Wednesday, Thursday and Friday. His father has not arrived yet! Our new chaplain has arrived - the Rev A. O. Idiston from Immanuel College - a young man who will fit in well we think

Do hope you are all well   Love from us all,   David

Again it is Saturday evening - the weeks are passing very quickly now and all is quiet. I am not on call, Margaret is at Beryl's and John Crossley is reading. It is getting very cool again and we are having a very severe harmattan and the nights are positively cold, for here. We have two blankets again! Incidentally the third box is almost completed and I managed to get some wood straw today so that I can make a nest of some sort for the glassware. I have got most of the Pyrex ware packed.

We were very pleased to receive your letter this week - you seem to be very busy with spring cleaning, and Mr. Painter the painter. Michael's suggestion for fitting us all in would seem to be a good one, though it is putting him out a bit I fear. Sorry to hear that the birds have had some of the buds from the fruit trees, perhaps there will be more fruit than expected. Glad to hear that Stanley is preaching and long may it continue. Have got Boston fixed up I think- though I have not heard again from Dorothy but I think I told you that last week.

Here we have had a 'much as usual' week, though it has been busy with Andrew off to Umuahia for three days. Roy is in Ibadan Thursday onwards and Jonathan off to Ikole Friday and Saturday. However we are now three again and as it happens my week end off. Margaret and John Crossley set off for Ibadan on Wednesday, had car trouble and had to come back. Then John came back yesterday for a meeting last night and will stay until Thursday. Elizabeth Johnson arrives on Monday for the best part of a week, but will be staying with the Pearsons.

We are all very well though both Peter and Elizabeth have colds and sore noses. It is Sheila's second birthday today, Mithra's second tomorrow and Elizabeth's fourth on Thursday. We are compromising and having a party on Monday and regarding this as Elizabeth's birthday. We are having all the children and all the grownups and a combined effort, Beryl, Meg and Margaret. In school Peter and Elizabeth have been busy making birthday cards for the other children and they are quite interesting arrangements of colour.

We have had two severe fires this week - the first accidental, the second controlled. It has been very dry indeed and the bush caught fire round the back of Roy and Beryl's house - flames 20-30 feet high. Chains of buckets, to the fire organised by Hezekiah and nurses, and in half an hour all was well. We decided therefore that we had better burn it all for if it had caught when we were asleep and no men on hand it could have been very serious. So Friday afternoon Hezekiah stationed his men and burnt it - quite a frightening sight - but no more damage done.

Our time here is running out and we keep wondering what the future has for us. I have rather swung back to General Practice again in view of the family and home - it would not be very satisfactory living in hospital with two or three moves, though probably less trouble than two or three moves in *General Practice.* However if I get locum or two in June/July it would give time to settle down and get re-orientated. I have no wish I think on reflection to be a consultant gynaecologist - MRCOG. Virtually every one qualified in the past ten years has taken the D. Obstetrics, I think. Anyway we shall see what comes forth. Eight weeks today we shall be home not long is it?

Margaret is busy with Elizabeth's cake which has to be a boat cake!

Do hope all is well with you all. Love from us all here, David

18.2.62

As you say in your letter, which we were pleased to receive this week, not many more letters to Ilesha, and similarly not many letters from Ilesha. Four weeks today will be our last Sunday. We have got a further two boxes packed during the week - one of glass ware and one of books, to date a total of five, but this is only a start! I am not sure where they will go when we arrive home. Ten at least we shall not require until we have our own home and I wonder if there is anywhere they could be stored? Stoneleigh Chapel? - probably not.

Here we are well apart from Richard who has got the children's cold, added to which he has cut one of his upper incisor teeth, but he is better today and has his appetite back. He has slept well, fortunately at nights. Peter has learned to swim underwater, can jump in from the side and almost but not quite dive! He"s very pleased with himself over this and both he and Elizabeth are trying much harder at school now they have Alison and Bryan with them.

We had an excellent birthday party last Monday at Beryl's for the three children with birthdays, Elizabeth, Sheila and Mithra. All the staff were there as well as some Auntie's from St. Margarets. The children had sausages on sticks and egg sandwiches, which are their favourite, fancy hats, crackers, and Fanta - so were well pleased. There were three Birthday cakes. Margaret made one in the shape of a boat and the other two were Teddy cakes, all very nice The grown-ups had sausage rolls. After tea the children had a treasure hunt followed by games. In the midst of this Elizabeth Johnson arrived. She was in very good form and has enjoyed her stay I think. We had John Crossley until Wednesday, so she stayed with the Pearsons' but came to us for chop on Tuesday. She went to University College Hospital on Thursday and stayed two nights and again had a very interesting time returning to Ilesha yesterday. She and the Hartfields came in to chop last night and we had a very pleasant evening, and could have gone on talking a long time. She has certainly been impressed with the work and standard of the hospital and no doubt will give it a boost in the right circles.

We are still turning over the future and have come to no decisions yet. Either course it all depends on the sort of job and ease of accommodation and so on. For example there was a job advertised at the Walter Hospital, Liverpool. Not a job I should choose but the flat at 76, Oxford Rd would have been at our disposal. Some jobs, too, have married quarters provided but with room for children? Anyway we shall see. I have written off for certain certificates to send to the RCOG to see what they have to say.

I must now break off to go to a village about 8 miles away to take the chaplain to an appointment which Andrew should be taking but cannot because he is on duty!

Have now returned - a good service in a small village chapel - about 30 adults and 30 children. This afternoon I have to take a ward service and then give an anaesthetic for one of the patients.

Still later! Margaret now in our chapel for evening service, the children are in bed and I can hear Peter and Elizabeth talking in their room. A busy week lies ahead and next weekend will be my last weekend on duty

A letter at last from the Clapps but it seems unlikely they will be here before mid April so the three Doctors here are going to have rather a busy time for a month or so.

Hope all well with you all at home - and the weather warming up a bit - it is very hot here just now, though we had a few spots of rain on Friday.

Love from us all to you all,   David

10.3.62

Saturday night and we are all at Ikole, it is rather hot and late, but we are shortly going to have chop. We were very pleased indeed to hear of Michael's engagement to Audrey, and send him our congratulations here, but I hope to get a letter to him inn the same post. The Pearsons' too, send their best wishes to him and Audrey.

We were glad to have news of Uncle Kingsley and Auntie Ruth, though sorry to hear that the former is rather under the weather. We look forward to seeing them, and of course Uncle Stanley and Auntie Theda, in the summer, as you say it will be quite a family re-union.

We will try to get a letter to Mrs. Weir re blankets when Lily arrives. The boat should have arrived today and if they got off in good time, Lily and Eileen, who went down to meet her, were hoping to get up to Ilesha this evening. We are so short of drivers that Jean Pearson has had to drive down to meet her, though she was not looking forward to driving to Lagos.

We are up to the eyes in packing and these two nights at Ikole has rather set us back a bit. It is odd to think that four weeks tonight we should be in Worcester Park, having left Nigeria for the last time.

Already folk are looking in to say goodbye and to our surprise, last night here at Ikole, the nurses gave a party, and this morning before outpatients, the welfare mothers gave a 'send off' and gave us about three dozen eggs and a duck. As we have already been given a small turkey we shall live well for the last week.

Our diary next week is very full, farewell meals and events each afternoon and evening. The most difficult day will be next Thursday, when we have the Hospital farewell in the afternoon chaired by the Owa, and the farewell from the staff in the evening. Quite what I shall say at these events I do not know.

We have heard by the way, that our boat is docking at Dover again. This would seem to be O.K apart from the car - I don't know where this is off loaded, nor when. I picture the cars stay on board whilst the boat goes to Rotterdam, and then is off loaded at Tilbury later, so it may be a while before we can get hold of it. Anyway the AA is coping with its clearance, but I shall have to go to some port to bring it back home.

Last week Phyllis Garden of Ado turned up for a chat and to say farewell and in the evening it was my Fellowship.

On Thursday we went to a party at Marion's to welcome our new Chaplain the Rev. Idowu. We had a nice meal and then showed transparencies.

Yesterday (Friday) was busy as Jonathan has been on local leave for a week.

However I shall be stopping work on Wednesday I think and give time to the packing and listing and so forth. So far we have 11 boxes packed and labelled black and white paint put on by a hospital carpenter!

I hope to pick up travellers cheques this week, and I hope too, to have disposed of my gun. We have also sold our camp beds, complete with nets and we shall get two more, without nets and attachments when we come home if we require them. We are hoping too to sell our wireless which is a shortwave set and unsuitable for home. I have also sold my typewriter and I shall get a more suitable model when we get home and settled.

Thank you for the note in your letter referring to the acknowledgement from the R.C.O.G. I wait to hear their views with interest.

I should think there will be one more letter from Ilesha and perhaps a note from the boat! Our love to you all, David

WGH, 18.3.62

Sunday morning and no round to do - it feels very strange. In a short while Margaret and I are going down to Otapete at which there will be a farewell - we hope most sincerely that this will be the last. They are rather harrowing, to put it mildly. It has been an eventful week, none the less so by receiving McKay- Hart's letter, after Father's cable. I have replied that I am most regretful that I cannot accept his offer. I shall not be home until 6th April, a rest and I have deputation commitments. I have already written him on this line , though saying what I would like to do - I and Prof. Lawson are sure that he will help me as much as he can. I went into Ibadan last Friday to see John Lawson and to thank him for his kindness and he feels sure I shall find a job, but recommends that I apply for a

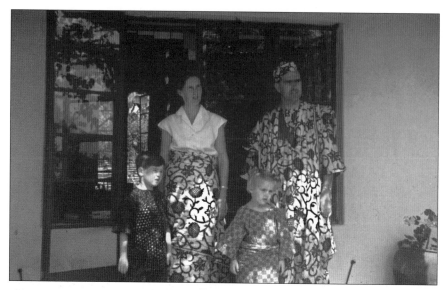

Farewell

Registrar post, rather than as a House Officer. However, if I had coped with it, it could have led to other things.

Glad that you had a nice time at the Celebration - it sounds to have been a very good occasion.

To return again to the RCOG - as you gather I am awaiting their decision on what I have to do, so would appreciate it, if the letter comes you could send the gist of it in an air letter en route and I can mull it over on my bunk! Takoradi 23rd, Freetown 28th, Madeira possibly April 1st, the latter not very good airmail service! You could check dates with Elder.

We had an excellent ride down last Sunday from Ikole and I went to service in the evening here. Monday, Tuesday and Wednesday I worked in the hospital in addition to other things.

Monday we drove down to see the Reeves for tea. She has been a staff nurse with us for some months. In the evening we had dinner with Vernon and Doreen Woods and had a very pleasant time.

Unfortunately the first part of the week was slightly marred by my not having the car insured due to the inefficiency of the Motor Centre Insurance Company in Lagos.

On Tuesday in the afternoon we drove over to Ede where they had prepared a tea party for us with seventeen children under seven years of age, including ours most of which I have cared for at some time or another. They presented us with six poufs - two large and four small. In the evening we went out to Roy and Beryl's and had a very nice meal.

Wednesday I operated in the morning and then had a ruptured uterus to cope

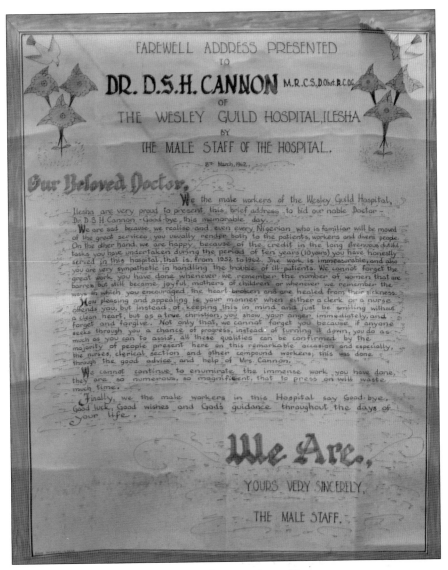

FAREWELL ADDRESS PRESENTED
TO
DR. D.S.H. CANNON M.R.C.S.,D.Obst.R.C.O.G.
OF
THE WESLEY GUILD HOSPITAL, ILESHA
BY
THE MALE STAFF OF THE HOSPITAL.

8th March, 1962.

Our Beloved Doctor,

We the male workers of the Wesley Guild Hospital, Ilesha are very proud to present this brief address to bid our noble Doctor - Dr. D.S.H Cannon - Good-bye, this memorable day.

We are sad because we realise and even every Nigerian who is familiar will be moved of the great services you usually render both to the patients, workers and divers people. On the other hand, we are happy because of the credit in the long strenuous dutiful tasks you have undertaken during the period of ten years (10years) you have honestly served in this hospital, that is, from 1952 to 1962. The work is immeasurable, and also you are very sympathetic in handling the trouble of ill-patients. We cannot forget the great work you have done whenever we remember the number of women that are barren but still became joyful mothers of children or whenever we remember the ways in which you encouraged the heart-broken and are healed from their sickness.

How pleasing and appealing is your manner when either a clerk or a nurse offends you, but instead of keeping this in mind and just be smiling without a clean heart, but as a true christian, you show your anger immediately, and forget and forgive. Not only that, we cannot forget you because if anyone seeks through you a chance of progress, instead of turning it down, you do as much as you can to assist, all these qualities can be confirmed by the majority of people present here on this remarkable occasion and especially, the nurses, clerical section and other compound workers, this was done through the good advice and help of Mrs Cannon.

We cannot continue to enumirate the immense work you have done, they are so numerous, so magnificent, that to press on will waste much time.

Finally, we the male workers in this Hospital say Good-bye, Good luck, Good wishes and God's guidance throughout the days of your life.

We Are,

YOURS VERY SINCERELY,

THE MALE STAFF.

Citation from male staff

with in the afternoon. However I got down to the bank and collected travellers cheques etc. and got the car insured at last £5 odd for a week. In the evening we went to the Sisters for chop and afterwards we had Fellowship here as the Hartfields were unwell. Jonathan has had fever for a week and Meg had some rather alarming lower abdominal pain - she is only 32 weeks (out of 40). However they both picked up.

On Thursday afternoon the male staff gave us a farewell - speeches- a set of Yoruba dress each and a large illuminated address we have had a frightful job to pack. I forgot to say that Wednesday afternoon we had a farewell in the town given by a Committee of women who were all my patients. This was a very good occasion - we each got a set of Yoruba dress and a Bible!

At all these functions and at odd times we have had 'group' photo - fourteen so far! but only four have been given to us to date, this makes final packing very difficult. The male staff farewell was rather marred by lack of organisation and a very heavy storm.

Thursday evening, the missionaries gave us a farewell party and presented us with a gold Ilesha necklace and bangle for Margaret. I was given a small projector for looking at transparencies and a painting done by Meg of our old house which I think is most talented. A very pleasant evening in which Andrew and I made speeches,

Friday I took a patient into Ibadan, saw Mr. Lawson, visited Frank Morton who is in a Nursing Home, though now recovered from his fever, called to see Larry Longo in Ife and then returned home

Yesterday Richard was not very well, so I took the children to Imesi, where we found Margaret Woodland not very well either. However it was a pleasant visit. In the evening the nurses gave us a hilarious farewell party and dance and presented us with a lovely Bible and a pair of double sheets and a pair of single sheets and two of the group photos. A very pleasant evening, though it was exhausting. This morning we go down to Otapete. Richard seems better and has eaten his breakfast. Meg is going to look after him.

Now back from service. They gave us a beautiful beaded pouf and £10.10.0 - very generous indeed. Hope all well, Love from us all David

21, Marina, Lagos, 6.4.62

Here we are Wednesday afternoon and very hot indeed in Lagos. The loads, apart from hand luggage are already on the wharf and the car has been left there also.

We are all in good form, but shall be glad now when we are actually away!

Last Sunday we had a Communion Service, followed by hymn singing and then Monday was full of folk coming to say good-bye so we did not actually get much done until 10.30pm and got to bed around 1am.

Tuesday we were up betimes and had breakfast with the Pearsons', loaded up and were off by 9.15. We had elevenses with the Hobsons at Wesley College, then had lunch at Shagamu with Joyce Proctor, Gwen was in Badagry and the folk there came to salute us good-bye.

We called at the airport to get some vaccine from customs to send back with the lorry and then had tea with the Garlings in Yaba, arriving at the Marina about 6.30pm. We are staying with the Jonahs who seem in good form.

This morning I went to Apapa to leave the car and the heavy loads, went to the bank for some English currency and Margaret did some last minute shopping with the three children!

The Longleys have arrived and seem in reasonably good form! In a few minutes tea, then we hope to get down to the beach by hook or by crook - no car!

We have to be on board tomorrow by 8am so it means an early start, so I will finish this letter then if all is well.

Tuesday morning:- Safely on board, with all our loads we hope. They are just about to cast off. Thank you for your letter to the boat - just arrived.

Love to you all, David

DESTINIES

I became a General Practitioner in Watford. For seventeen years I did two sessions per week in the Antenatal Clinic of Watford General Hospital.

Margaret very sadly died suddenly from a brain haemorrhage on June 20th 1975.

Michael, my brother, became a Methodist Minister, now retired.

Peter, reached middle management in Sanyo UK, Watford. He died 2005 from a brain tumour.

Elizabeth became a nurse, and is now an endoscopist to two hospitals.

Richard is Professor of Micro-genetics in the University of Otago, New Zealand

Stanley 'Twink' is the son of my cousin and came into our family on the death of his mother. He is now Professor of Inorganic Chemistry (Retired), Dalhousie University, Canada.

Henry is the son of friends of my parents, who came to stay with us for a week to seek digs, stayed five years! He is now an ophthalmic surgeon in remote parts of Canada, flying his own plane.

The Wesley Guild Hospital was taken over by the Nigerian Government in 1975 and became part of Ife University Teaching Hospital Complex.

A sad note. Helena Kohler who was so unwell on the boat coming out to Nigeria, worked at Ilesha for some months before being posted to Ikole. Some weeks later a message came through to Ilesha that she was ill, and she was brought to Ilesha immediately. She was obviously very ill but neither Roy nor I could determine the cause, and she was transferred to UCH Ibadan. I kept in touch daily with the hospital and also London. She died a few days later and was laid to rest in the Cemetery in Ilesha. It transpired that she was taking cortisone and had not informed anyone. I did not put this in my letters home - I did not wish to add to the concern of my family. When I was settled in Watford I was appointed to the Medical Board of the Methodist Missionary Society and was able to ensure that this set of circumstances did not occur again.

Andrew Pearson, OBE continued working in Nigeria and became Chief Medical Officer for the University of Ibadan's Community Health Programme. He died in 1997 from a brain tumour identical to the tumour that caused my son's death.

Dr David Morley CBE became Professor of Tropical Child Health, in London University. He also set up the Charity TALC, (Teaching aids at low cost) which *supplies books and filmstrips for medical fieldworkers in developing countries. He died in 2009.*

Jonathan Hartfield became a Consultant Obstetrician and Gynaecologist in New Zealand. He also took Holy Orders and was ordained into the Anglican Church.

Medical note. My predecessors performed Classical Caesarean Sections that were prone to rupture. I introduced the Lower segment Caesarean section, which avoids this hazard.

Cannon DSH, Hartfield VJ. Obstetrics in a developing country. *J Obs Gyn Cwlth,* 1964; 71: 940-950

Editoral. Obstetrics in developing countries. *Lancet,* 1965 (i): 791.